Oxford Specialist Handbooks published and forthcoming

Hand Surgery

OXFORD MEDICAL PUBLICATIONS

Oxford Specialist Handbooks in Surgery
Hand Surgery

EDITED AND AUTHORED BY

David Warwick MD FRCS FRCS (Orth) EDHS

Consultant Hand Surgeon
Southampton University Hospitals
Reader in Orthopaedic Surgery, University of
Southampton, UK

ALSO AUTHORED BY

Roderick Dunn MB BS DMCC FRCS(Plast)

Consultant Plastic, Reconstructive and Hand Surgeon
Odstock Centre for Burns, Plastic and Maxillofacial Surgery
Salisbury Hospital and Honorary Visiting Senior Lecturer
University of Southampton, UK

Erman Melikyan, MD, Dip (Orth Engineering), European Diploma of Hand Surgery FRCS

Associate Specialist Hand Surgeon
Honorary Clinical Lecturer
Southampton University Hospitals, UK

Jane Vadher Dip COT SROT Dip Hand Therapy BAHT

Clinical Specialist Occupational Therapist
Southampton University Hospitals, UK

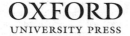

OXFORD
UNIVERSITY PRESS

OXFORD
UNIVERSITY PRESS

Great Clarendon Street, Oxford OX2 6DP

Oxford University Press is a department of the University of Oxford.
It furthers the University's objective of excellence in research, scholarship,
and education by publishing worldwide in

Oxford New York

Auckland Cape Town Dar es Salaam Hong Kong Karachi
Kuala Lumpur Madrid Melbourne Mexico City Nairobi
New Delhi Shanghai Taipei Toronto

With offices in

Argentina Austria Brazil Chile Czech Republic France Greece
Guatemala Hungary Italy Japan Poland Portugal Singapore
South Korea Switzerland Thailand Turkey Ukraine Vietnam

Oxford is a registered trade mark of Oxford University Press
in the UK and in certain other countries

Published in the United States
by Oxford University Press Inc., New York

British Library Cataloguing in Publication Data
Data available

Library of Congress Cataloging-in-Publication-Data
Data available

Typeset by Cepha Imaging Private Ltd., Bangalore, India
Printed in Italy
on acid-free paper by
L.E.G.O S.p.A.—Lavis TN

ISBN 978–0–19–922723–5

10 9 8 7 6 5 4 3 2 1

Foreword

It is a privilege for me, as a hand therapist, to be invited to write the foreword for this book.

In the United Kingdom we are very fortunate to have so many excellent teams of surgeons and hand therapists in our hospital units. This teamwork is a tradition that began in the early days of hand rehabilitation. It was started by enthusiastic skilled therapists such as Nathalie Barr and Maureen Salter who gained the respect of eminent clinicians and surgeons with whom they worked—Guy Pulvertaft, Paul Brand, Kit Wynn-Parry, and it continues to this day.

This book is a manual which will be welcomed by surgeons and therapists alike, an excellent teaching tool in postgraduate education and an aide memoire to the more experienced practitioners. The British Association of Hand Therapists has established guidelines for postgraduate courses in many aspects of hand therapy. These courses, which run in numerous centres across the United Kingdom, benefit from the generous willingness of hand surgeons to lecture to the delegates, enhancing their understanding of hand management. This is a demonstration of the close cooperation that exists in so many centres today.

The authors, David Warwick, Roderick Dunn, Erman Melikyan, and Jane Vadher, are an excellent example of this teamwork. They are front runners in surgery and rehabilitation of the hand and also in the provision of continuing education to both surgeons and therapists who have an interest and expertise in management of hand conditions.

This is a book that will sit very comfortably on a bookshelf, desk or in a pocket, easily handled and likely to have well thumbed pages. Thank you team!

Annette Leveridge
Past Chair
British Association of Hand Therapists
Past President
International Federation of Societies for Hand Therapy
Current Chair
Education Committee IFSHT

Foreword

Hand Surgery is a significant achievement for its four authors. It is a daunting task to cover all hand surgery topics in a single book. This publication includes definitions, diagnoses, mechanisms of injury, pathology, principles, indications, treatments, outcomes, and complications. By necessity it is written in point form and with few illustrations. The intent is not to explain or discuss extensively. However, the degree of detail is admirable and is a consequence of a thoughtful and precise format and pithy writing.

The sections on assessment, anaesthesia and rehabilitation are invaluable. They highlight the symbiosis between patient, therapist, surgeon, and anaesthetist, and also complement the chapters concentrating on surgical conditions.

In reading this book, one is reminded of the extensive and varied nature of hand surgery: it involves the management of the skin and its contents, and demands orthopaedic, plastic, vascular and neurosurgical expertise, as well as an understanding of the principles and practice of hand therapy, splinting and rehabilitation. The content of current orthopaedic and plastic surgery training programmes is less than adequate for the purpose of training a hand surgeon.

It is a privilege to teach. It is gratifying to see those one has taught teaching others. This book will be a rewarding companion for all involved in the management of hand injury and disease, be they therapist or surgeon, trainee or consultant.

Michael Tonkin
Professor of Hand Surgery
University of Sydney

Preface

Hand surgery is perhaps the most intricate and diverse surgical sub-speciality, which connects orthopaedic surgery and plastic surgery, occupational therapy and physiotherapy seamlessly. For this reason, this book has been written by an orthopaedic hand surgeon, a plastic hand surgeon as well as a hand therapist

Without the hand, wrist and nerves of the arm, we cannot work, play or gesticulate. So many things can happen—birth defects, injury, arthritis, nerve compression, tumours, work-related pain. Over 20% of A&E attendees have a hand injury; 1:500 babies are born with a hand defect, 1:30 of us get a nerve compression syndrome. Anyone of us, from goal-keeper to violinist, can have our work or hobbies curtailed by a hand problem; hand surgeons and hand therapists do their best to give people their lives back.

Most hand surgery problems are fairly routine and within the practice of a fairly generalized orthopaedic or plastic surgeon. Some problems are rather more sophisticated and are dealt with in local or regional centres. Occasionally problems are so rare or complex that only a few people in the country deal with them.

Even the most routine hand problem may require specific hand therapy to achieve the best outcome.

In this book, we have tried to cover most of hand surgery, from common to rare, from easy to complex. The layout should give a simple overview and the text should give the fine detail. We hope this book will become a well-worn pocket companion for hand surgeons, for trainees on hand surgery firms and for hand therapists. It should serve as a concise, comprehensive revision aid for surgical trainees and therapists sitting professional exams. Perhaps the more general orthopaedic surgeon or plastic surgeon, physiotherapist, occupational therapist and general practitioner will find it a useful reference on their bookshelf.

We would really appreciate comments from the reader: please send any suggestions or criticisms to davidwarwick@handsurgery.co.uk so we can improve the book next time.

Acknowledgements

Richard van der Star MRCP, Consultant Neurophysiologist, Southampton University Hospitals for the section on Neurophysiology in the Nerves chapter.
Chris Edwards MD MRCP, Consultant Rheumatologist, Southampton University Hospitals for the medical information in the Rheumatoid chapter.
Alex Crick MD FRCS(Plast), Consultant Plastic, Reconstructive and Hand Surgeon, Odstock Centre for Burns, Plastic and Maxillofacial Surgery, for her contribution on sarcoma.

We all acknowledge our trainers, colleagues and above all, our patients.

Dedications

David Warwick

To my parents, my wife and especially my kids James, Louisa, and Alicia who make life and work so worthwhile.

Roderick Dunn

For Pete, Kuki, Finn, Sam, Bede and Ailsa—thanks for making me one of the family.

Erman Melikyan

In loving memory of my father Azad Melikyan, MD, a man of kindness, wisdom and humour; to my mother Sona Melikyan, a woman of infallible judgement, remarkable character and enduring principles; for their selfless dedication to my upbringing.

To my dear wife Neslin, who has stuck with me against all odds; to my children Arev and Lusin, without whom this life would not be worth living.

Jane Vadher

To my family: my parents, husband and children, Josh, Mollie, and Daniel—without their love and support this would never have come to fruition.

Contents

Detailed contents

Symbols and abbreviations

📖	Cross reference
↑	Increased
↓	Decreased
❶	Warning
⚠	Caution
2PD	Two-point discrimination
ABC	Aneurysmal bone cyst
ADL	Activities of daily living
ADM	Abductor digiti minimi
AdP	Adductor pollicis
AEDs	Anti-epilepsy drugs
AER	Apical ectodermal ridge
AIMS	Arthritis Impact Measure Scales
AIN	Anteria interosseous nerve
AJCC	American Joint Committee on Cancer
AK	Actinic keratosis
AMC	Arthrogryposis multiplex congenital
ANA	Antinuclear antibodies
AP	Anteroposterior
APB	Abductor pollicis brevis
APL	Abductor pollicis longus
APS	Anti-phospholipid syndrome
ARDS	Acute respiratory distress syndrome
AROM	Active range of motion
ASD	Atrial septal defect
ASSH	American Society for Surgery of the Hand
ATLS	Advanced trauma life support
ATT	Automated tactile tester
AVM	Arteriovenous malformations
BCC	Basal cell carcinoma
BMP	Bone morphogenetic proteins
BR	Brachioradialis
BSA	Body surface area
CCT	Congenital clasped thumb
CHA	Circumflex numeral artery
CID	Carpal instability dissociative
CIND	Carpal instability non-dissociative

CK	Creatine kinase
CM	Capillary malformations
CMC	Carpo-metacarpal joint
CMAP	Compound motor action potential
CMMS	Casting motion to mobilize stiffness
CNS	Central nervous system
CPM	Continuous passive motion (device)
CPS	Cycles per second
CREST	Calcinosis, Reynaud's syndrome, oesophageal stricture, scleroderma and telangectasia
CRP	C-reactive protein
CRPS	Complex Regional Pain Syndrome
CT	Computerized tomography
CTD	Cumulative trauma disorder
CVA	Cerebro-vascular accident
CVLM	Capillary–venous–lymphatic malformations
CVP	Central venous pressure
DASH	Disability of the Arm, Shoulder and Hand
DBS	Dorsal blocking splint
DD	Dupuytren's disease
DES	Dynamic extension splint
DI	Dorsal interosseous
DIPJ	Distal interphalangeal joint
DISI	Dorsal intercalated segment instability
DREZ	Dorsal root entry zone
DRUJ	Distal radio-ulnar joint
ECRB	Extensor carpi radialis brevis
ECRL	Extensor carpi radialis longus
ECU	Extensor carpi ulnaris
EDC	Extensor digitorum communis
EDM	Extensor digit minimi
EDQ	Extensor digiti quinti
EEC	Ectrodactyly. ectodermal dysplasia, cleft lip and palate
EI	Extensor indicis
EIP	Extensor inclicis propnus
EMG	Electromyography
EMLA	Eutectic mixture local anaesthetic
EPB	Extensor pollicis brevis
EPL	Extensor pollicis longus
ESR	Erythrocyte sedimentation rate
FBC	Full blood count
FCR	Flexor carpi radialis

FCU	Flexor carpi ulnaris
FDM	Flexor digiti minimi
FDP	Flexor digitorum profundus
FDS	Flexor digitorum superficialis
FGF	Fibroblast growth factors
FNAC	Fine-needle aspiration cytology
FPB	Flexor pollicis brevis
FPL	Flexor pollicis longus
FSS	Functional Status Scale
FTSG	Full thickness skin graft
GA	General anaesthetic
GCT	Giant cell tumour
GM	Germinal matrix (of nailbed)
G & S	Group & save
GSW	Gunshot wound
HAQ	Health Assessment Questionnaire
HAVS	Hand–arm vibration syndrome
Hb	Haemoglobin
HF	Hydrofluoric acid
HIV	Human immunodeficiency virus
HLA	Human leukocyte antigen
HME	Hereditary multiple exostosis
HPV	Human papilloma virus
ICSA	Intercompartmental supraretinacular artery
IFSSH	International Federation of Societies for Surgery of the Hand
II	Image intensification
IOM	Interosseous membrane
IPJ	Interphalangeal joint
ITU	Intensive care unit
IV	Intravenous
IVRA	Intravenous regional anaesthesia
KA	Keratoacanthoma
LA	Local anaesthetic
LM	Lymphatic malformations
LMM	Lentigo maligna melanoma
LTIL	Luno-triquetral interosseous ligament
LVM	Lymphatic–venous malformations
MC	Metacarpal
MCPJ	Metacarpophalangeal joint
MCV	Motor conduction velocity
MFH	Malignant fibrous histiocytoma

MM	Malignant melanoma
MMP	Matrix metalloproteinase inhibitors
MMT	Manual muscle testing
MN	Median nerve
MRA	Magnetic resonance angiography
MRC	Medical research council
MRI	Magnetic resonance imaging
MRSA	Methicillin-resistant *staphylococcus aureus*
MSTS	Musculoskeletal Tumor Society
MUA	Manipulation under anaesthetic
MULE	Microprocessor upper limb exerciser
MUP	Motor unit potential
NA	Noradrenaline
NCS	Nerve conduction studies
NE	Norepinephrine
NSAIDs	Non-steroidal anti-inflammatory drugs
NVB	Neurovascular bundle
NVI	Neurovascular island
ODM	Opponens digiti minimi
OO	Osteoid osteoma
ORIF	Open reduction and internal fixation
P1	Proximal phalanx
P2	Middle phalanx
P3	Distal phalanx
PA	Posteroanterior
PABA	Para-aminobenzoic acid
PEM	Patient Evaluation Measure
PIA	Posterior interosseous artery
PIPJ	Proximal interphalangeal joint
PIN	Posterior interosseous nerve
PL	Palmaris longus
POSI	Position of safe immobilization
PRC	Proximal row carpectomy
PROM	Passive range of motion
PRUJ	Proximal radioulnar joint
PSLS	Posterior superior liac spine
PT	Pronator teres
PTSD	Post-traumatic stress disorder
PVNS	Pigmented villonodular synovilis
PZ	Progress zone
QST	Quantitative Sensory Testing

RFF	Radial forearm flap
RCL	Radial collateral ligament
RCT	Randomized controlled trial
RDA	Radial digital artery
RF	Rheumatoid factor
RFA	Radio-frequency ablation
RFF	Radial forearm flap
RMC	Radial mid-carpal
ROM	Range of motion
ROS	Reactive oxygen species
RSD	Reflex sympathetic dystrophy
RSI	Repetitive strain injury
SBRN	Superficial branch of radial nerve
SCC	Squamous cell cancer
SCIA	Superficial circumflex iliac artery
SCS	Splint Classification System
SCV	Sensory conduction velocity
SFCF	Scaphoidectomy with four-corner fusion
S-H	Salter–Harris
SLAC	Scapho-lunate advanced collapse
SLIL	Scapho-lunate interosseous ligament
SMP	Sympathetically maintained pain
SNAC	Scaphoid non-union advanced collapse
SNAP	Sensory nerve action potential
SNB	Sentinel node biopsy
SODA	Serial Occupational Dexterity Assessment
SSG	Split skin graft
SSS	Symptom Severity Scale
ST	Scaphotrapezial
STI	Shape–texture identification
STS	Soft tissue sarcoma
STT	Scaphoid–trapezium–trapezoid
SWMT	Semmes–Weinstein monofilaments test
TAG	Tactile Acuity Grids
TAM	Total active motion
TAP	Thoracodorsal artery perforator
TAR	Thrombocytopenia—absent radius (syndrome)
TAROM	Total active range of motion
TCAs	Tryciclic antidepressants
TENS	Trans-ultaneous electrical nerve stimulation
TFCC	Triangular fibrocartilage complex

TICAS	Trauma-induced cold-associated symptoms
TM	Trapezio Metacarpal
TNFα	Tumour necrosis factor α
TNM	Thickness, nodal, metastasis
TOS	Thoracic outlet syndrome
TPM	Total passive motion
TPROM	Total passive range of motion
TROM	Torque range of motion
U&E	Urea and electrolytes
UCL	Ulnar collateral ligament
UDA	Ulnar digital artery
UMC	Ulnar mid-carpal
USS	Ultrasound scan
VACTERL	Vertebral anomalies, anal atresia, cardiovascular anomalies, tracheo–esophalgeal fistula, renal anomalies, limb defects, Fanconi
VAS	Visual analogue scale
VBG	Vascularized bone graft
VM	Venous malformations
VWF	Vibration white finger
WCC	White cell count
WEST	Weinstein Enhanced Sensory Test
WRULD	Work-related upper limb disorders
XFF	Cross-finger flap
ZPA	Zone of polarizing activity

Assessment

Assessment

Why do we assess?

Patient's perspective
- Identifying the underlying cause of their problems
- Prioritizing their problems
- Monitoring their progress

Clinician's perspective
- Identifying underlying cause of the patient's problems
- Establishing an appropriate treatment programme
- Baseline for treatment
- Justification for treatment
- Monitoring effectiveness of treatment
- Provide patient feedback
- Identifying patients suitability for surgery
- Medico-legal reports
- Information for other clinicians

Types of assessment

History
- History:
  - When the injury/condition occurred
  - Mechanism of injury
  - Pattern of symptoms
  - Handedness
  - Patient's attitude towards injury/condition
  - Level of discomfort
- Social information:
  - Work status
  - Home status
  - Hobbies
  - Mental state
- Past medical history:
  - Drug history
  - Diabetes, rheumatoid etc.
  - Surgery

Subjective observation
- Body language/posture
- Skin colour/circulation
- Wound status
- Oedema
- Scars
- Deformity
- Muscle wasting

Tactile assessment
- Joint/soft tissue tightness
- Sweating/drying of skin
- Temperature

- Sensitivity
- Scar tethering
- Nodules/thickenings
- Swelling
- Tenderness

Investigations
- X-rays
- Ultrasound
- Magnetic resonance imaging (MRI)
- Computerized tomography (CT)
- Bone scan
- Blood tests

Objective assessment
This is part of the assessment that can be measured with specific assessment tools. Certain principles or guidelines optimize assessment.

Guidelines for assessment
General guidelines
- The same therapist should assess the patient on each occasion
- The repeat assessment should ideally be performed at the same time of day and at the same point in the patient's therapy session
- Therapists in a department should assess in the same way and should develop local assessment protocols/assessment forms
- Consider other factors that may affect the assessment (open wounds, oedema, scars)
- Previous activity levels should be considered
- Alterations in weather conditions should be considered
- Consider location of assessment, ideally choose a quiet area free from distraction that maintains confidentiality
- Be prepared! Ensure you have all the relevant tools and paperwork
- Record carefully and accurately
- Does the patient need glasses?
- Does the patient have a cognitive impairment?

Equipment guidelines
Ideally standardized tools should be used that meet basic criteria:
- Tools must be *reliable* and *valid*
- Tools should have administration, scoring and interpretation standards
- Normative data should be available
- Ideally a statement of purpose and a bibliography should be available
- All tools should be regularly calibrated to ensure accuracy and handled and stored with care

Range of motion

The *available arc of movement* within a joint which can be classified into:
- Active range of motion (AROM)
- Passive range of motion (PROM)
- Total active range of motion (TAROM), also known as total active motion (TAM)
- Total passive range of motion (TPROM), also known as total passive motion (TPM)
- Torque range of motion (TROM)

AROM

Defined as the range of motion (ROM) that is achieved when an individual utilizes their own muscle power to initiate movement at a specific joint. This is typically measured first and can reflect the presence of joint irritability and an individual's willingness/ability to move a joint.

PROM

Refers to the ROM that is achieved when an external force is used to move the joint, i.e. the clinician's hand.

TAROM or TAM

Defined as the total ROM achieved when all three joints—metacarpophalangeal (MCP), proximal interphalangeal (PIP) and distal interphalangeal (DIP) of a digit are actively flexed or extended simultaneously, minus any extension deficit at any of the three joints (🕮 see Fig. 1.1).

TPROM or TPM

Analogous to TAROM, however this measurement is achieved through passively moving the joint.

TROM

Refers to a joint being moved passively through its full available ROM with a known constant force applied. Brand advocates the use of a Haldex gauge, a calibrated spring gauge that can either pull or push and is measured in grams.

Standard position for measuring

- For finger and wrist measurements, position the elbow on a table at 90° and wrist in neutral
- For elbow pronation and supination, tuck arm into trunk with the forearm in mid-position

Instruments

- Goniometer
- Ruler/tape measure
- Solder wire
- Fluid goniometer
- MULE (microprocessor upper limb exerciser)—used as an assessment and rehabilitation tool.

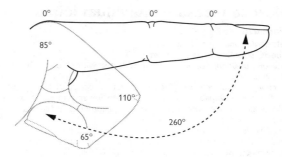

Normal		
Active	**Flexion**	**Extension lag**
MCP	85°	0°
PIP	110°	0°
DIP	65°	0°
Totals	260°	0°
Total active motion (TAM) 260°–0° = 260°		

Fig. 1.1 Total active motion of the finger.

Goniometry

Several types of goniometer are available; choice depends on the type of joint being measured.
- Circular bodied goniometers will permit lateral placement.
- Half-circled goniometers permit lateral, volar and dorsal placement.

There is no strong evidence to indicate the most accurate placement but consistency is essential. Critical points:
- The goniometer axis should be in line with the axis of the joint being measured
- The arms of the goniometer should be parallel to the bones forming the joint.

Recording ROM with goniometry

Typically recorded as extension/flexion, e.g. 15°/85°.
This indicates:
- an arc of movement of 70°;
- either a fixed flexion deformity or an extensor lag of 15°.

If the patient is able to hyperextend this may be recorded as a minus, e.g. − 15°/85°, with 15° of hyperextension achieved.

How to measure individual joints

Forearm

Motion: Pronation and supination
Tool: Goniometer/fluid goniometer
Starting position: Seated, shoulder adducted with elbow at 90°, forearm in mid-position.
Technique: Goniometer—place over dorsal aspect of wrist with pivot mid-carpus. Ask patient to pronate. Keep lower arm static and follow movement through with upper arm of goniometer. For supination place goniometer over volar aspect of wrist.
Fluid goniometer—place over dorsum of wrist and line up water level with 0°. Ask patient to pronate/supinate and follow movement with goniometer. Record position of water level (see Fig. 1.2).

Wrist

Motion: Flexion/extension
Tool: Goniometer
Starting position: Forearm in neutral
Technique: Place goniometer over ulnar aspect of hand—pivot in line with carpal region. Keep proximal arm of goniometer static. Ask the patient to flex/extend their wrist and follow with distal arm in line with 5th metacarpal.
Motion: Ulnar/radial deviation
Tool: Goniometer
Starting position: Forearm in pronation and wrist in neutral
Technique: Place goniometer pivot at mid-carpal region. Line proximal arm up with centre of forearm. Line distal arm up with 3rd metacarpal. Move distal portion in line with movement of 3rd (see Fig. 1.3).

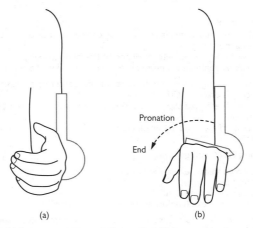

Pronation

End

(a)   (b)

Fig. 1.2 (a) Forearm pronation—starting position; (b) forearm pronation—ending position.

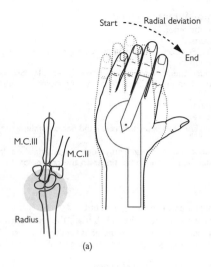

(a)

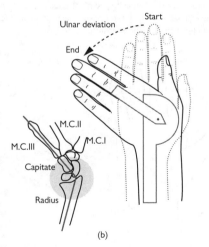

(b)

Fig. 1.3 (a) Wrist—radial deviation; (b) wrist—ulnar deviation.

Thumb: Carpo-Metacarpal joint

MOTION: Palmar abduction

Tool: Tape measure

Starting position: Position hand on table resting on ulnar aspect of little finger, wrist in neutral

Technique: Abduct thumb away from index finger. Measure from the corner of the nail bed on the index finger to the corner of the nail bed on the thumb.

MOTION: Radial abduction

Tool: Tape measure

Starting position: Forearm pronated, rest hand flat on table, wrist in neutral

Technique: Abduct thumb away from index finger. Measure from the corner of the nail bed on the index finger to the corner of the nail bed on the thumb.

MOTION: Opposition

Tool: Kapandji

Starting position: Forearm and wrist in neutral

Technique: Ask patient to touch the thumb tip to the areas shown on the diagram. The number reached by the thumb is recorded (🔲 see Fig. 1.4)

MOTION: Metacarpophalangeal (MP)/ interphalangeal (IP) flexion/extension

Tool: Goniometer

Starting position: Forearm and wrist in neutral

Technique: Place goniometer dorsally with the pivot over the joint and arms flat against metacarpal/phalanx. Keep proximal arm static and follow distal arm of goniometer into flexion/extension.

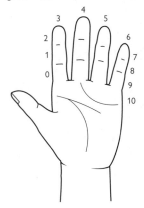

Fig. 1.4 Kapandji's rule of ten (Kapandji 1992).[1]

1. Kapandji IA (1992) Clinical evaluation of the thumb's opposition. *J. Hand therapy.* **2**: 102–6.

Fingers
MOTION: MCP/PIP/DIP flexion/extension
Tool: Goniometer
Starting position: Forearm and wrist in neutral
Technique: Place goniometer dorsally with the pivot over the joint and arms flat against metacarpal/phalanges. Keep proximal arm static and follow distal arm of goniometer into flexion/extension (see Fig. 1.5).

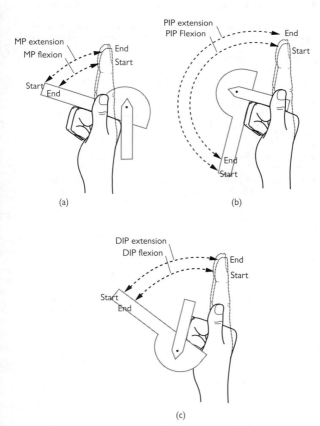

Fig. 1.5 (a) MP flexion/extension; (b) PIP flexion/extension; (c) DIP flexion/extension.

Motion: Hyperextension
- *Tool:* Hyperextension goniometer
- *Starting position:* Forearm and wrist in neutral
- *Technique:* Place goniometer dorsally with the pivot over the joint and arms flat against metacarpal/phalanges. Keep proximal arm static and follow distal arm of goniometer into extension.

Motion: Abduction/adduction of digits (span)
- *Tool:* Ruler/tape measure
- *Starting position:* Forearm pronated, rest hand flat on table, wrist in neutral
- *Technique*: Ask patients to span fingers and measure distance from nail bed on ulnar border of thumb to radial corner of nail bed on little finger.

Motion: Flexion deficit
- *Tool:* Ruler
- *Starting position*: Forearm and hand resting on table in supinate position
- *Technique:* Ask patient to flex fingers as much as possible. Measure flexion deficit from corner of nail beds to distal palmar crease (📖 see Fig. 1.6).

Motion: Extension deficit
- *Tool:* Ruler
- *Starting position:* Forearm and hand resting on table in supinate position
- *Technique:* Ask patients to extend fingers to table top. Measure from corner of nail beds to tabletop.

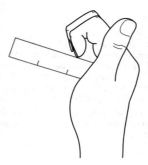

Fig. 1.6 Distal palmar crease.

Oedema

Definition

The presence of excessive fluid in the tissue spaces.

Controlling oedema is the beginning of successful restoration of hand function. It is therefore important that oedema is measured to:

- Establish baselines for comparison
- Evaluate a patient's response to treatment
- Monitor the course of a disease process

There are no normal standards for hand volume, therefore measurements should be compared with the contralateral side or with previous measurements on the treated side.

Tools

Tape measure

Advantages: quick to use, cheap to purchase and able to provide information regarding specific segments. No published studies that examine the reliability of measuring with a tape measure, therefore caution should be exercised.

Accuracy and reliability can be improved by:

- Calibration of tape measures
- Measure over anatomical landmarks
- Use a weighted tape measure (i.e. gluick tape measure to ensure consistency of tension of the tape measure is controlled)

Jeweller's rings

Used to measure the circumference of joints. A range of different-sized jewellers rings are placed over the joints. Quick and easy to use, however expensive to purchase and only allow small joints to be measured.

Volumeter

Provides objective measurements, uses standardized equipment; reliability and validity have been established (📖 see Fig. 1.7)

Based on the Archimedes principle: 'A body partly or completely immersed in a fluid displaces an amount of fluid equal to the apparent volume of that body.'

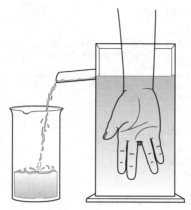

Fig. 1.7 The volumeter.

Contraindications
- Open wounds
- Casts
- External fixators
- Vascular instability

Equipment
- Commercially available hand/arm volumeter
- Collection jug
- Graduated measuring cylinder
- Water source and towels

Technique
- Place the volumeter on a level surface
- Place the collection jug beneath the overflow spout
- Fill the volumeter with room-temperature water just to the point of overflowing
- Remove excess water from collection jug
- Remove all jewellery
- Position the hand with the palm facing the patient and the thumb facing the spout
- Slowly immerse the hand, keeping the hand as vertical as possible
- Rest the web space between the middle and ring fingers on the plastic rod
- Maintain this position until the water has stopped overflowing
- Transfer the water collected into the graduated cylinder and measure amount of water displaced
- If measuring the contralateral side refill the volumeter before use

Muscle testing

Definition of strength

The ability of skeletal muscle to develop force for the purpose of providing stability and mobility within the musculoskeletal system to enable functional movements to occur.

Weakness or disappearance of voluntary movement may be due to:
- Failure of the afferent nerve
- Destruction of muscle tissue
- Ischaemia
- Tendon rupture
- Tendon adhesions

Measurement
- Manual muscle testing
- Grip strength
- Pinch grip

Manual muscle testing (MMT)

Palpating, positioning or the application of resistance through external, manual force to determine whether a group of muscles or an individual muscle is capable of moving through all or part of its range of motion, against gravity or with gravity eliminated, and move against resistance applied.

To test muscle power accurately the examiner must be familiar with the anatomy of the hand and arm, particularly:
- Origins, insertions and slip attachments of muscles
- The general direction and line of pull of each muscle
- The relative positions of muscle and tendons
- Nerve supply and possible anomalies
- Possible trick movements

Indications
- Peripheral nerve lesions
- Tendon transfers
- Neuromuscular conditions

Contraindications
- Where movement or the application of resistance is not recommended (e.g. healing phase of tendon repair)

Muscle group testing

All proximal muscles are tested first, followed by the distal muscles. The patient is asked to move through a full ROM with and without resistance and graded accordingly (normal, slightly weak or extremely weak).

Individual muscle testing

The key to this part of the examination is the study of voluntary movements. Muscle power is graded using the scale adopted by the British Medical Research Council (MRC) (📖 see Table 1.1)

Table 1.1 Grading of muscle power

0	No contraction
1	A flicker of movement (this is usually palpated with the muscle contracting in its middle to outer range)
2	A small range of movement between middle and outer range with gravity eliminated
3	Some movement against gravity, but the muscle is still unlikely to contract through its full range
4	A full range of movement against gravity with some resistance
5	Normal movement and power as compared with the unaffected side

Method of administration

- Ensure the patient is positioned appropriately
- Ensure that the part proximal to the tested part is stabilized
- Select the muscle and joint movement required:
  - Check that the PROM is normal/expected
  - Demonstrate to the patient what is expected
- Observe:
  - Movement at the joint
  - Any contraction of the muscle belly and tendon
- Palpate:
  - Muscle contraction
- Record muscle power:
  - Ensure that the placement of the hand applying pressure is uniform
  - Apply pressure directly opposite the line of pull of the muscle being tested
- Apply pressure gradually

Factors that can affect accuracy include

- Pain
- Swelling
- Joint mobility/ROM
- Sensory loss

Advantages

- No equipment required
- Inexpensive
- Quick to administer

Disadvantages

- Requires skill
- Needs a well-defined protocol
- Subjective
- Difficult to isolate some muscles
- Not sensitive to small change
- No normative data are available

Power grip

Indicator of hand function is measured by isometric grip,

Indications

- To establish a baseline for treatment
- To monitor progress
- To establish final outcome

Contraindications

- Less than 12 weeks after tendon repair or transfer
- Excessive pain
- Patients with active inflammatory disease

Tools

- Jamar dynamometer
- Vigorimeter

Accurate measurement of grip strength depends on reliable test instruments, a standardized administration procedure and access to normative data. All tools should be regularly calibrated.

Jamar dynamometer

The most reliable tool to measure isometric grip strength when calibration is maintained.

Measures grip strength in 5 different grasp positions set at 1.0, 1.5, 2.0, 2.5 and 3 inch spacings. In the normal hand, grip strength varies depending on the position of the handle. Typically the 1st position is the weakest followed by the 5th and 4th. The American Society for Surgery of the Hand (ASSH) state that the 2nd position produces maximal grip strength in women and the 3rd in men.

Administration:

- Arm position:
  - Shoulder adducted and in neutral
  - Elbow flexed to 90°
  - Forearm in neutral
  - Wrist 0–30° extension and 0–15° ulnar deviation
- Seated in a chair without arms and feet flat on the floor
- Ensure the Jamar handle is set in the desired position
- Always use the same Jamar
- The examiner should lightly hold the readout dial at the top and gently support the handle at the bottom
- Explain the purpose of the test to the patient
- Ask the patient to squeeze the handle with maximum strength
- Each hand is tested 3 times to obtain a mean, recorded in either lbs or kgs.

Data collected can be compared with published norms produced by Mathiowetz et al. (1985)[1] using an American population or by Gilbertson and Barber-Lomax (1994)[2] on a UK population.

1. Mathiowetz V et al. (1985). Grip and pinch strength: normative data for adults. *Ach Phys Med Rehabil.* **66**: 69–74.
2. Gilbertson L and Barber-Lomax S (1994). Power and pinch girp strength recorded using the hand-held Jamar dynamometer and B + L hydraulic pinch gauge. Normative data for adults. *Br. J Occ Ther.* **57**: 483–8.

Table 1.2 Grading of muscle 'power grip (pounds): Jamar dynamometer 2nd setting'

Age	20–24	25–29	30–34	35–39	40–44	45–49
R (m)	121	120	122	120	117	110
L (m)	105	111	110	113	112	101
R (f)	70	75	79	74	70	62
L (f)	61	64	68	66	62	56

Age	50–54	55–59	60–64	65–69	70–74	75+
R (m)	113	101	90	91	75	66
L (m)	102	83	77	77	65	55
R (f)	66	57	55	50	50	43
L (f)	57	47	48	41	42	38

(m) = male   (f) = female

Submaximal effort
Some patients, e.g. malingerers and sympathy-seekers, do not exert maximum effort when testing grip strength. An intense grimace suggesting applied effort, contrasting with the low reading obtained, is suspicious.

Bell-shaped curve
When testing in all 5 positions, the normal hand produces a bell-shaped curve with the higher strengths occurring in positions 2 and 3; a less sincere effort produces a flatter or humped curve.

Rapid exchange test
The Jamar is gripped at maximum effort, alternating between both hands, every 2 seconds until the examiner asks the subject to stop. If the results are greater than when compared with the static grip or if the readings rise, then sympathy-seeking or malingering are considered.

Vigorimeter
Measures grip strength using air pressure. Three different-sized rubber bulbs attached via a tube to a manometer. Possibly more comfortable to use than the Jamar dynamometer and due to the ability to vary the sizes, may be better suited for children. Normative data are available both for adults and children.

Pinch grip

Provides a good indication of thumb function. Three different types:
- pure (otherwise known as tip pinch)
- tripod
- key (otherwise known as lateral pinch)

Tools

Several pinch gauges have been marketed; most reliable if regularly calibrated.

Indications for testing

As for grip strength.

Contraindications

- Early tendon repairs
- Early repairs of collateral ligaments
- First 8 weeks after trapeziectomy
- Excessive pain
- Inflamed joints

Tip pinch grip

- The thumb is pinched against the pulp of the index finger whilst the other fingers are flexed
- The gauge is place with dial facing up
- The patient is instructed to place the thumb beneath the gauge and the pulp of the index finger on the top to form an O shape
- Patient squeezes maximally and readings taken
- Repeated 3 times to obtain a mean score

The examiner should observe the patient to ensure that they are not hyperextending the DIP joint and to ensure that they do not use the lateral side of the index finger.

Tripod pinch grip

- Thumb pulp to index and middle finger pulp with remaining fingers flexed
- The gauge should be placed on its side with the dial facing the patient
- The thumb should be positioned on the side of the dial and the index and middle fingers on the underside of the gauge
- Ask the patient to squeeze maximally 3 times and take the mean measurement

Key pinch grip

- Thumb pulp to lateral aspect of proximal interphalangeal joint of the index finger, other fingers flexed
- Place the gauge as for tip pinch
- Instruct the patient to place the lateral side of their index on the underside of the gauge and their thumb pulp on top
- Ask the patient to squeeze maximally 3 times and take the mean

Normative data are available (UK and US) and findings can be compared with the contralateral side.

Sensory testing

The hand is capable of performing many complex tasks and is an important part of skilled hand function. Loss of sensation impacts significantly on the vocational and social aspect of an individual's life.

Sensibility

'The conscious appreciation and interpretation of a tactile stimulus' (Boscheinen-Morrin and Conolly 2004).[1]

Sensibility can be classified into two categories:

* Protective/protopathic sensation which includes temperature, sharp/dull and deep pressure and is mediated by Aδ and C fibres.
* Functional /discriminative/epicritic sensation which includes fine discriminative touch, discrimination of shape and texture and proprioception. These are mediated by Aβ fibres.

Whilst a sensate hand provides protection, tactile input allows the environment to be deciphered.

Sensibility is a consequence of the stimulation of receptors and free-nerve endings within the skin that send an afferent signal to the brain cortex, where the information is interpreted and processed. There are several different types of receptors with specific functional properties that react to different stimuli and vary in number/density and receptive field.

Classification of receptors

Mechanoreceptors are sensitive to mechanical stimulation and have a significant role to play in sensibility. Understanding the role of each of the different receptors and what they respond to is essential to ensure the correct tool is utilized to assess sensibility (see Table 1.3).

1. Boscheinen-Morrin, J and Conolly, W.B (2004). *The Hand: Fundamentals of Therapy.* Butterworth Heinemann, Oxford.

Table 1.3 The role of different receptors in assessing sensibility

Exteroreceptors (in the skin)	Mechanoreceptors (touch, pressure, vibration)
	Thermoreceptors (temperature)
	Nocioceptors (pain)
Interoceptors (in viscera)	
Proprioceptors (within joints and capsules)	Muscle spindles (stretch receptors)
	Golgi tendon organs
	Joint receptors (mechanoreceptors)

There are four types of mechanoreceptor (📖 see Table 1.4):

Table 1.4 The four types of mechanoreceptor

Mechanoreceptor	Pacinian	Meissner	Ruffini	Merkel
Function	Respond to fast mechanical changes in the skin (fast adapting)	Respond to fast mechanical changes in the skin (fast-adapting)	Respond to more static stimuli in the skin (slow-adapting)	Respond to more static stimuli in the skin (slow-adapting)
	Distant moving touch	Moving touch and localization	Control of grip force	Static touch and localization
Density	Low	High in tips of fingers	Low	High in tips of fingers
Receptive field	Large	Small	Large	Small
Responsive to	Vibration 100–300Hz	Vibration 5–40Hz	Skin stretch	Pressure

Types of sensory dysfunction
- Hypoaesthesia: diminished sensation
- Parasthesia: abnormal sensation
- Hyperaesthesia: abnormal sensation
- Anaesthesia: complete loss of sensation

Purpose of sensory testing
- To assist in diagnosis
- To determine the extent of sensory loss
- To determine the level of axonal regeneration (provocative tests, e.g. Tinel's percussion test)
- To evaluate nerve conduction efficiency (threshold tests, electrophysiological tests)
- To evaluate end organ unity/function
- To determine level of somatosensory reorganization (ability to interpret stimuli)
- To identify the need for surgical intervention
- To identify splinting requirements
- To determine when to commence sensory re-education
- To identify level of hand function

Sensory testing is difficult due to:
- Subjective nature of the tests
- Technical difficulties with the tests, e.g. vibration of the assessor's hand during testing, variation in the application of force when utilizing the assessment tools.

Indications for testing sensibility
- Peripheral/digital nerve repair
- Nerve compression
- Nerve replants
- Flaps/grafts
- Brachial plexus injuries
- Crush injuries

Precautions for testing sensibility
- Underlying vascular or neuropathic disease
- Fatigue
- Negative attitude/poor motivation
- Hypersensitivity/pain

Testing guidelines
- Quiet, distraction-free environment
- Prevent inadvertent movement of the hand, support the hand
- Test distal to proximal, following the anatomic course of the nerve
- Same examiner for successive tests

Table 1.5 Classification of tests

Classification	Test
Threshold/innervation tests	SWMT/WEST
	Vibrometry
	Pin prick
	Temperature
Functional tests (localization, discrimination and identification)	2PD
	Point/area localization
	Grating orientation (JVP domes), Moberg pick-up test
	STI
	Tactile gnosis test
Stress/provocative tests	Phalen's wrist flexion test
Objective tests	O'Riann wrinkle test
	Ninhydrin-sweat test
	Nerve conduction studies
	Stereognosis
Tinels percussion test	Tinel's percussion test

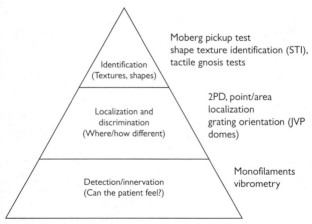

Fig. 1.8 Hierachy for testing sensibility (Jerosch-Herold 2007).[1]

1. Jerosch-Herold C (2007). *Sensory testing and sensory re-education* (handouts). University of East Anglia, Norwich.

Sensibility tests

Tinel's percussion test

Objective: to estimate the level of nerve regeneration.

Design: no equipment required.

Procedure: the examiner gently percusses from distal to proximal along the nerve trunk. The most distal point at which the patient experiences parasthesia (tingling) is the point of a positive Tinel's sign.

SWMT/WEST

Objective: the smallest force, lowest amplitude/frequency that a patient can detect stimuli.

Design: Semmes–Weinstein Monofilaments Test (SWMT) or Weinstein Enhanced Sensory Test (WEST). A pressure aesthesiometer: probes consisting of a nylon monofilament attached to a polymethylmethacrylate rod. Each rod is numbered, ranging from 1.65–6.65, which represents the amount of force that is applied to the skin during testing.

Procedure: the hand is supported and vision occluded. The lightest monofilament is used first and applied perpendicular to the skin until it bows and held in place for 1.5 seconds. Filaments 1.65–4.08 are applied three times to the same spot. Filaments 4.17–6.65 are applied only once. One positive response is required before progressing to the next monofilament. Results are mapped on a hand chart and provide a map showing progression. Kit available as a set of 20 or 5.

Table 1.6 Monofilament values

Monofilament	Level of sensation perceived
1.65–2.83	Normal
3.22–3.62	Diminished light touch
3.84–4.31	Diminished protective sensation
4.56–6.65	Loss of protective sensation
Greater than 6.65	Untestable

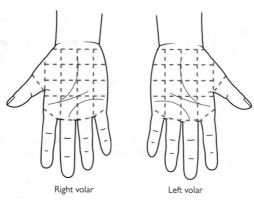

Right volar   Left volar

Fig. 1.9 SWMT mapping chart.

Vibrometry
Objective: detection threshold test.
Design: three clinical tools available: tuning fork, vibrometer and auto-mated tactile tester (ATT).

Tuning fork
Procedure: 30 and 256 CPS tuning fork. Fixed frequency but amplitude not controlled. Tuning fork is struck against a surface and one of the ends of the fork is applied tangential to the tested area. The vibrating fork is ap-plied to the test site and a control site and the patient reports on whether there is any difference between the two sites.

Vibrometer
Procedure: A variable amplitude, fixed-frequency vibrometer and voltage meter. The examiner applies a vibrating head to the denervated area and with eyes occluded the patient is instructed to indicate when vibration is perceived. The threshold level is recorded in volts.

ATT
Procedure: a computer-controlled device that is capable of varying the intensity, rate and duration of the stimulus.

Pinprick
Objective: to establish the presence of protective sensation.
Design: safety pin.
Procedure: vision is occluded and the patient is asked to discriminate between the sharp and dull sides of a safety pin, which are applied randomly by the examiner.

Temperature
Objective: to assess awareness of hot and cold.
Design: test tubes of hot (43°) and cold (4°) water or custom-made ther-mal devices.
Procedure: the patients' hand is randomly assessed using both the hot and cold devices. Responses should be quick in a sensate hand.

Two-point discrimination (2PD)

Static 2PD
Objective: innervation density test that measures overlapping receptive fields.
Design: Dellon-Mackinnon Disk-Criminator™.
Procedure: support the hand fully and occlude vision. Test only the finger-tips, as this is where most tactile gnosis occurs. Start with a 5mm distance between the points and increase or decrease according to the patient's responses. One or two points are randomly applied to the skin to the point of blanching. The points are applied in a longitudinal orientation and perpendicular to the digit. Seven out of ten accurate responses are required for scoring. If less than seven are achieved the distance between the points is gradually increased until 15mm is reached. Results can be compared with the contralateral side and with normative data. This test has better respon-siveness to partial injuries rather than complete nerve injuries.

Normal: less than 6mm
Fair: 6–10mm
Poor: 11–15mm
Protective: one point perceived
Anaesthetic: no points perceived

Static versus moving 2PD
Moving 2PD returns before static 2PD as a nerve recovers. However, moving 2PD is likely to stimulate/recruit several sensory receptors, thereby increasing the patient's chances for achieving a positive response. Static 2PD may or may not stimulate receptors and may provide a more accurate assessment of recovery.

Area localization
Objective: assesses the quality of sensibility.
Design: the locognosia test comprises two copies of the hand map with numbered zones, testing screen, median/ulnar nerve recording sheet and largest monofilament (6.65).
Procedure: the monofilament is applied to a numbered zone and the patient is asked to identify the zone where the stimulus was felt by referring to the map. The stimulus is held on the digit for 2 seconds. Scores are recorded for correct responses.

Point localization
Objective: assesses the quality of sensibility.
Design: pen and ruler.
Procedure: mark on the patients' finger with a pen and ask if the stimulus was perceived and where. The examiner marks on the digit where the stimulus was perceived, and the distance between the dots is recorded.

Grating orientation (JVP domes)
Objective: assesses tactile spatial acuity, alternative to 2PD
Design: The Tactile Acuity Grids (TAG)/JVP domes probe kit is a set of 10 mushroom-shaped probes with progressively greater grid spacing on the dome, up to 3.5 mm.
Procedure: with vision occluded the largest probe is applied to the area to be tested, care must be taken to ensure the probe does not move horizontally on the skin. The patient has to indicate the orientation of the probe. Two correct answers dictate moving to the next smaller probe. As yet not validated for nerve injuries affecting the fingertips.

Moberg pick-up test
Objective: applicable for median nerve injuries. Assesses ability to identify objects.
Design: 10 standardized objects (either all metal or plastic) and one pot.
Procedure: with vision occluded the patient is asked to pick up the objects one at a time and place them in the pot as quickly as possible. Test repeated with contralateral side. No normative data available. Time taken

to perform test and manner of prehension compared with involved and uninvolved hand.

STI (Shape–texture identification) test

Objective: identification of shape and texture.

Design: STI test, test sheet and screen.

Procedure: the patient is asked to touch and identify different shapes (cube, cylinder and hexagon) and simple textures (1, 2 and 3 dots, 1mm in height and 0.5 mm in diameter, placed in a row). The test consists of three assessment disks with shapes (∅ 15, 8, 5 mm) and textures (15, 8 and 5mm apart) that get progressively smaller. The patient starts with the largest shapes. Can be used for ulnar and median nerve lesions.

O'Riann wrinkle test

Objective: to evaluate the sympathetic function of the nerve.

Design: warm water (40°).

Procedure: the patients' hand is submerged in warm water for 30 minutes and examined for evidence of wrinkling. A denervated hand does not wrinkle.

Ninhydrin-sweat test

Objective: to establish is sweating is present in the denervated area

Design: alcohol/acetone, bond paper and spray reagent (N-0507)

Procedure: the patients' hand is cleansed with alcohol/acetone and is placed either under a lamp for 20 minutes or placed in a bag during the exercise to allow it to sweat. The fingertips are then placed on to bond paper for 15 seconds. The paper is sprayed with N-507 (Ninhydrin), which stains the sweat purple. Grading 0–3: 0 = absent, 3 = normal.

Nerve conduction studies

See Neurophysiology tests, 📖 p. 306.

Stereognosis

Objective: object identification.

Design: everyday objects.

Procedure: with vision occluded the patient is asked to identify a variety of everyday objects. Most appropriate for median nerve injuries.

Pain

'An unpleasant sensory and emotional experience associated with actual or potential tissue damage.' (IASP)[1]

Pain is a complex personal experience that is difficult to measure objectively. The clinical assessment of pain can assist with our understanding of its basis and can assist with evaluating the effectiveness of treatment.

General principles for assessing pain

- Obtain a detailed history from the patient
- Use an appropriate and reliable tool

Pain rating scales

Visual analogue scale (VAS)

A 10cm vertical line is drawn with the ends marked with no pain (0) and worst pain imaginable (10cm). The patient is asked to mark on the line the severity of their pain.

Numerical rating scale

The patient is asked to indicate one number on a scale between 0–100 for the severity of their pain.

Pain questionnaire

McGill Pain Questionnaire

Consists of 20 groups of words. Groups 1–10 define the physical characteristics of the pain; 11–15 defines the subjective characteristics; 16 describes the intensity and 17–20 are miscellaneous. The patient is asked to look at each group and where applicable underline no more than one word in a group that best describes their pain.

Charts

Body chart

Used to locate site of pain. Patient also describes the type of pain, depth of pain, severity, whether the pain is constant or intermittent and activities that aggravate or alleviate the pain.

Face chart

Patient is shown a chart with a series of faces that range from smiling to distress. The patient indicates which face best depicts how they are feeling: this is best used with children.

1. IASP (1986). Classification of chronic pain: Description of chronic pain syndromes and definitions of pain terms. *Pain* **27**(suppl): s1–s225.

Scar

A scar is the inevitable result of an injury, composed of disorganized collagen formed during the fibroblastic and remodelling phases of wound healing.

Objective assessment of a scar needs a standardized assessment method:
- Burn scar index (Vancouver)
- Image panel assessment scale (photos)
- Self-rating scale for patients
- Non-invasive measurement of scar and skin pliability (pneumatonometer and Derma-Durameter)
- Numeric scar ratings scale (therapist scored)
- VAS—to measure itching
- High-resolution ultrasound (measures thickness of scar)

The most widely used system is the Vancouver Scar Scale, which provides a standardized, objective and reliable measurement of scars and assists with prognosis and management.

Burn scar index (Vancouver Scar Scale)

Developed based on physical parameters, relating to the healing, maturation of wounds, cosmetic appearance and function of the healed skin.

Equipment
- Plastic ruler
- Clear plastic sheet

Pigmentation
- The skin is blanched with the plastic sheet and compared with a normal area of similarly blanched skin. The scar is rated:
  - 0 = normal, closely resembles colour of rest of body
  - 1 = hypopigmentation
  - 2 = hyperpigmentation

Vascularity
In early phases of healing a scar is hyperaemic, a consequence of increased blood flow which will decrease with scar maturation. Assessed by measuring the amount of redness in the scar.
- Observe the scar
- Blanche the scar and observe the rate and amount of capillary refill
  - 0 = colour and capillary refill are normal
  - 1 = pink, slight increase in local blood supply
  - 2 = red, significant increase in local blood supply
  - 3 = purple, congested, slow refill, cannot be blanched

NB Active scars refill quickly.

Pliability
- Scar is compared with normal skin to compare the elastic nature of the skin (functional mobility):
  - 0 = normal
  - 1 = supple, minimal resistance, flexible
  - 2 = yielding, gives way to pressure
  - 3 = firm, moves as a solid, inflexible unit

- 4 = banding, ropes of scar that do not limit movement
- 5 = contracture, shortening of scar producing deformity or reduced movement

Height

This relates to the amount of collagen within the scar and oedema within the tissue.

- Measure the vertical height of the scar above normal skin
  - 0 = flat skin flush with normal skin
  - 1 = <2mm
  - 2 = 2–5mm
  - 3 = >5mm

Function

Hand function evaluations are an important element in the assessment process. There is a wide range of objective measures of integrated hand function. Some focus solely on dexterity whilst others required the integrated use of the upper limb and hand in a range of activities which represent grip patterns used in activities of daily living (ADL).

Hand function tests:
- Identify causes of functional limitations
- Identify changing health status
- Appropriateness/effectiveness of intervention
- Provide information to the surgeon before and after surgery

No evaluation covers all aspects of hand function, therefore when considering the type of test to choose, assess:
- Types of subtests
- Hand grips used in the test
- If the task is unilateral or bilateral
- If the test is standardized
- Ease of use and fabrication
- Scoring system
- Sensitivity to change

Hand function tests typically fall into two categories:
- Norm-referenced tests
  - Objective grading systems are used, mainly time as the critical measure of hand function. Researchers favour them, as they are quick and easy to administer and produce objective data.
- Criterion-referenced tests
  - Descriptive standards are used to measure a patient's performance. They need an experienced person to interpret the results and to achieve consistency with scoring.

The ultimate choice of test should be dependent on:
- Type of information required
- What use the data are to be put to
- The experience of the assessor
- Time
- Cost

Tests for dexterity and function

Moberg
Objective: dexterity and sensibility (timed).
Design: board with 1 pot containing 9 standardized objects.
Procedure: objects are picked up one at a time and placed in the pot. Unilateral task, both hands tested. Test can be repeated with vision occluded.

Nine-hole peg test
Objective: measure of finger dexterity (timed).
Design: wooden base with 9 holes and 9 pegs.

Procedure: to place the pegs into the 9 holes in any order as quickly as possible. A quick and cheap measure of finger dexterity but with poor test–retest reliability.

Purdue pegboard

Objective: measure unilateral and bilateral fine manual dexterity (timed).
Design: a board comprising of pins, collars and washers.
Procedure: divided into 4 subtests:

- First 3 tests involve the subject placing the maximum number of pins, right, left and both simultaneously into the board within 30 seconds.
- The fourth test. Alternate hands are used to make assemblies comprising pins, collars and washers within 60 seconds.

The patient has a demonstration and practice before each subtest.

Developed in the 1940s (Tiffin 1948)[1] as a test of dexterity for use to select personnel in industries. Its administration procedure is well standardized and its subtests involve varying degrees of difficulty.

Assessors need to be aware of practice-effect.

Minnesota Rate of Manipulation Test

Objective: measures manual dexterity involving arm and hand function (timed).
Design: wooden board with counters.
Procedure: involves the rapid manipulation of objects.

Five subtests involve:

- Placing,
- Turning

It is claimed that each subtest provides a reasonably comprehensive scale to assess hand impairment. The test correlates well with the American Medical Association guide to the evaluation of impairment.

The Serial Occupational Dexterity Assessment (SODA)
(Van Lankveld et al. 1996)[2]

Objective: measures dexterity, which is defined as a complex of bimanual functional abilities in ADL (ability scored).
Design: 12 standardized tests are performed:

- Write a sentence
- Pick up an envelope
- Pick up coins
- Hold a telephone receiver to the ear
- Unscrew a toothpaste cap
- Squeeze out toothpaste
- Handle a spoon and knife
- Button a blouse
- Unscrew a large container
- Pour out water
- Wash hands
- Dry hands

Procedure: scores patients on their ability to perform the above standardized tasks that involve unilateral and bilateral tasks.

The test incorporates 6 out of the 8 handgrips as outlined by Sollerman (1978).[3] The test has proven to be reliable and valid with good test–retest reliability, is internally consistent and sensitive to change. Unfortunately to date it has only been validated in RA patients.

Sollerman Hand Function Test (Sollerman 1995)[4]

Objective: measure unilateral and bilateral hand function (time and ability scored).

Design: 20 ADL tasks, based on 7 of the 8 most common handgrips as defined by Sollerman (1978). The article provides clear instructions on how to make and administer the test.

Procedure: the patient is scored on their ability to perform the tasks and the time taken to complete the tasks.

The test has proven to be both reliable and valid and correlates well when compared with other tests. The tests main criticism is its lack of portability.

Jebsen Hand Function Test (Jebsen 1969)[5]

Objective: measures hand function (timed).

Design: activities designed to represent various hand activities.

Procedure: test involves 7 subtests:

- Writing
- Turning over cards
- Picking up small objects
- Simulated feeding
- Stacking chequers
- Picking up light objects
- Picking up heavy objects

A unilateral assessment that measures the dominant and non-dominant hand separately. Does not consider the quality of prehension patterns and does not assess hook/power grip.

Baltimore Therapeutic Equipment (BTE) (Curtis, Clark Syder 1984)[6]

Objective: to simulate ADL/work task.

Design: work simulator.

Procedure: the patient carries out tasks with a variety of tools/handles attached to the BTE. ROM, time, resistance and force can be modified to individual need.

The BTE can be used as a treatment method or as an assessment tool. Normative data are available although unfortunately this equipment is extremely expensive and not portable.

1. Tiffin J (1948). The Purdue Pegboard Norms and studies of reliability & validity. *Journal of Applied Psychology*. **32**, 234–47.
2. Van Lankveld W *et al.* (1996). Sequential Occupational Dexterity Assessment (SODA) A new test to measure hand disability. *Journal of Hand Surgery.* **9**, 27–32.
3. Sollerman C and Sperling L (1978). Evaluation of ADL function – especially hand function *Scar J. Plastic Recon Surgery*. **6**: 139–43.
4. Sollerman C, Ejeskär A (1995). Solleman hand function test. *Scan J Plastic Recon Surg.* **29**, 167–76.
5. Jebsen RH *et al* (1969). An objective and standardised test of hand function. *Arch Physic Med Rehab*. **3**, 11–19.
6. Curtis, Clark and Syder (1984). The Work Simulator. In: Hunter, Mackin and Callahan. *Rehabilitation of the Hand: Surgery and Therapy*, 2nd edn. Mosby, St. Louis, pp. 905–908.

Outcomes

Why use outcome measures?

To provide objective evidence of:
- Patients' status:
  - Functional level
  - Level of disability
- Progress/change
- Effectiveness of our interventions

Outcomes may be assessed against various different standards, for example:
- Anatomic:
  - Goniometers
  - Dynamometer
- Objective function:
  - Jebsen
  - Sollerman
- Subjective function:
  - Disability of the Arm, Shoulder and Hand (DASH),
  - Patient Evaluation Measure (PEM),
  - Michigan
- Cost:
  - Unit of currency
- Radiological:
  - Change in density

The tools used to measure depend largely on what we need to measure:
- Subjective: patient-derived, e.g. functional score
- Objective: assessor-derived, e.g. radiological angle

Properties of outcome measures

- Test reliability:
  - The test must be consistent at producing the same results with the same rater, different rater and at different time intervals
- Test validity:
  - Does it measure what it intends to measure?
  - It must be relevant and clear
  - Must measure the concept comprehensively
  - Must correlate well with other tools that measure the same concept
- Responsive to change:
  - Ability to measure small changes over time

Scoring

Outcome measures can be scored in several ways:
- Nominal scales:
  - Numbers assigned to different characteristics or different items, e.g. 1 = male, 2 = female
- Ordinal scales:
  - Verbal description on a continuum, e.g. easy to impossible
- Interval scales
  - Intervals between any two numbers on the scale are known, e.g. numbers on a thermometer

- Ratio scales:
  - Similar to interval scales, however the starting point is zero, e.g. a stop watch

Measuring

Different methods of measuring are available:
- Observation
- Self-rating
- interview

Checklist for choosing a questionnaire

Is the measure:
- Standardized?
- Valid?
- Reliable?
- Applicable?
- Condition specific?
- Profession specific?
- Sensitive to change?
- Cost-effective?
- Quick and easy to use?
- Easy to score?

Does the measure:
- Require specialist training?
- Require specialist training to interpret the scoring?
- Have a ceiling or floor effect?

Types of outcome measures:

- Global questionnaires:
  - SF-36,
  - HAQ
- Region-specific (e.g. upper limb):
  - DASH
  - PEM
  - Michigan Hand Questionnaire
- Joint-specific:
  - Patient-rated wrist evaluation
- Disease-specific:
  - Levine (carpal tunnel syndrome)
- Condition-specific:
  - Arthritis Impact Measure Scales (AIMS)

Specific questionnaires

SF-36 (Short-Form 36)

Originally developed in the USA. Measures general health status. Comprises 36 questions designed to be easy to understand and relevant to everyday lives. Measures all aspects of health, a person's functional level and general psychological status. The test is both reliable and valid.

Health Assessment Questionnaire (HAQ)

Comprises 20 questions relating to activities of daily living (ADL), which include self-care, eating, grip and walking. The patient scores each questionnaire according to how they have performed the tasks in the last week:

- Without difficulty
- With some difficulty
- With much difficulty
- Unable

This test is well validated.

Disability of the Arm, Shoulder and Hand (DASH)

Thirty-item self-reported questionnaire. Measures physical function and symptoms in patients with single or multiple upper limb disorders. Designed to measure the level of disability experienced by a patient and to monitor changes in symptoms and functional ability. The DASH also includes two optional modules that focus specifically on athletes, performing artists and patients who are involved in physically demanding jobs. These modules are scored separately.

The **QuickDASH** is a shortened version of the DASH that uses 11 items. Like the original DASH the shortened version also includes two optional modules.

The QuickDASH and the full DASH are valid and reliable and are responsive to change.

Both questionnaires can be downloaded from http://www.dash.iwh.on.ca and include instructions on scoring.

Patient Evaluation Measure (PEM)[1]

Three sections:

- Treatment
- How is your hand?
- Overall assessment

consisting of a series of questions using a visual analogue format to score. The score is calculated by summing up the values for each item in section 2 and 3 and expressing the result as a percentage of the maximum score possible. The PEM is internally consistent, has validity, reliability and is responsive to change. The form is quick and easy to use.

Michigan[2]

A hand-specific outcome questionnaire consisting of six categories that focus on overall hand function, activities of daily living, pain, work, aesthetics and patient satisfaction with hand function. In addition there are also questions referring to age, ethnic background and hand dominance. In total there are 72 questions. Outcomes are considered for both the dominant and non-dominant hand, unlike the DASH, which assesses outcomes for the person as a whole rather than a specific hand. The Michigan is reliable, valid and responsive to change. The questionnaire takes approximately 15 minutes to complete and calculation of the score is complex.

Boston Carpal Tunnel Questionnaire (BCTQ)[3]

Self-administered questionnaire to assess the severity and functional status in patients who have carpal tunnel syndrome.

Two scales:
- Symptom Severity Scale (SSS)—11 questions and uses a 5-point rating scale
- Functional Status Scale (FSS) which contains 8 items rated for degree of difficulty on a 5-point scale.

Each scale generates a final score (sum of individual scores divided by number of items) with a higher score indicating greater disability. The BCTQ has been used as an outcome measure in clinical studies, and has also undergone extensive testing for validity, reliability and responsiveness.

1. Macey AC and Burke FD (1995). Outcomes in hand surgery. *Journal of Hand Surgery* **20B:** 841–55.

2. Chung KC et al. (1998). Reliability and validity testing of the Michigan hand outcomes questionnaire. *Journal of Hand Surgery* **23A:** 575–85.

3. Levine DW et al. (1993) A self-administered questionnaire for the assessment of severity and functional status in carpal tunnel syndrome. *Journal of Bone and Joint Surgery* **75A:** 1585–92.

Rehabilitation

Introduction

Rehabilitation of the hand is critical to ensure the best outcome after hand surgery or injury. Whilst surgical and therapeutic interventions have progressed, the principles of treatment have remained much the same.

Principles of rehabilitation

- To provide early intervention
- Minimize the risk of complications
- Promote healing
- To restore function
- Promote independence
- To be patient-centred
- Multidisciplinary
- Evidence based

Role of the hand therapist

A hand therapist is either an occupational therapist or a physiotherapist who has specialized in the rehabilitation of patients with injuries/conditions affecting the upper limb/hand.

The clinical expertise of a hand therapist enables a patient to maximize their potential following an injury or as a consequence of disease or deformity.

A hand therapist is capable of evaluating and identifying complex problems and can provide advice and treatment.

A hand therapist often works alongside surgeons, planning and implementing postoperative care in order to hasten patients' recovery following surgery.

Treatment modalities

- Exercise
- Splinting
- Oedema control
- Scar management
- Hypersensitivity/desensitization
- Pain management
- Sensory re-education
- Psychological support

Exercise

The unique anatomy of the hand and the ability of its structures to glide relative to each other enable us to use our hands for a variety of tasks ranging from simple to complex. However, stiffness, contractures and tendon adhesions, consequences of injury or disease, can significantly impair hand function. Early mobilization programmes to maintain or restore gliding surfaces are an essential part of a rehabilitation programme.

Aims of mobilization:
- Maintain/restore gliding surfaces
- Maintain/restore joint range of motion
- Reduce oedema
- Reduce pain
- Maintain/improve functional ability

Whilst mobilization programmes should commence as early as possible, the exact timing and nature of the exercises will depend on the type of injury/condition. The decision to commence mobilization should be based upon:
- Diagnosis
- Medical/surgical management
- Surgeon's preference
- Evidence

Types of exercise
1. Active exercise
2. Passive physiological movements
3. Passive stretching
4. Accessory mobilizations

1. Active exercise
Normal physiological movements performed by the patient with or without resistance. Aim:
- Maintain mobility
- Reduce oedema
- Reduce pain
- Produce tendon glide
- Maintain bone integrity
- Patients should be taught exercises in a systematic manner to ensure optimal results—finger wiggling is not enough

Contraindications
- Tendon and nerve repair (check postoperative protocol)
- Unstable fractures
- Circulation problems
- Skin grafts
- Acute inflammatory disease

Active-assisted exercise
A type of active mobilization with external force (manual or mechanical) applied to assist with movement.

Resisted exercise
Commenced at an appropriate time to increase muscle power throughout the available range of motion.

2. Passive physiological movement
Performed by a therapist or by a CPM (continuous passive motion device). Aim:
- To maintain range of motion
- Prevent loss of motion
- To prevent pathological changes occurring

Knowledge of normal joint range of motion is essential when performing passive mobilizations.

Performed by a therapist:
- The proximal bone is stabilized whilst the distal bone is mobilized
- The joint is mobilized through a full range of motion, in all directions
- Where stiffness is present the joint is oscillated in a small range of motion at the end of the available range
- Jerky movements should be avoided to prevent tissue trauma

Performed by CPM device
- Patient can control the CPM
- Portable versions are available and may permit use at home

Contraindications
- Recent fractures
- Tendon injuries/repairs
- Swollen/inflamed/infected joints
- Intracapsular damage
- Painful joints
- Mechanical joint blocks
- Reduced sensation

3. Passive stretching
Useful where stiffness is associated with soft tissue adhesions/injury.
Performed by the therapist or splinting.
Performed by a therapist
- Proximal portion is supported firmly
- The distal part is slowly and gradually stretched into the stiff range
- The stretch is sustained
- Slight traction can be applied at the same time
- Tension should be released slowly
- Follow with strong active exercises
- Any discomfort should disperse once the tension has been released

Contraindications
- Tendon repairs until week 8
- Recent fractures
- Articular surface damage
- Inflammatory disease

Splinting
- Gutter splint
- Plaster of paris
- Capener
- Joint jack
- Flexion strapping/glove

4. Accessory mobilizations
Defined as small glides, slides and rotations that are essential for normal movement, which a patient is unable to isolate. The shape of a joint surface will determine the direction and type of mobilization possible.
Technique
- Firmly fix the joint proximally with one hand
- With the opposite hand mobilize the distal bone on the proximal bone in the required range of motion.

Movements are graded from 1–4 (Maitland 1986):[1]
1. Small amplitude oscillatory movement out of resistance
2. Larger amplitude oscillatory movement out of resistance
3. Large amplitude oscillatory movement at end range with some resistance
4. Small amplitude oscillatory movement at the end of range with resistance

Types 1–2: used for pain relief
Types 3–4: used to increase range of motion

1. Maitland GD (1986). *Peripheral manipulation*. Butterworth-Heinemann, UK.

Splinting

Definition

Orthopaedic device for immobilization, restraint or support.

Purposes of splinting

- Protection
- Immobilization
- Support
- Positioning
- Correction
- Gain optimum hand function
- Mobilize stiff joints
- Prevent contractures
- Substitute for absent muscle power or to assist weak muscles
- Overcome soft tissue tightness/adhesions

Categories of splints

Static/resting

Static splints have no moving component. They are used to improve function and inhibit increased tone. In addition they may be:
- Supportive
- Corrective
- Protective

Static progressive

Provides a low-load, prolonged stress at end range. Used to increase range of motion and correct contractures

Serial static

Holds tissues at end range until they adapt to new length at which point the splint is remoulded to increase passive range of motion.

Dynamic

Consisting of a static portion to which a lever or spring may be attached. Used to:
- Prevent muscle imbalance
- Substitute for lost/weak muscles
- Increase range of motion
- Reduce adhesions

Splint classification system

The American Society of Hand Therapists published the Splint Classification System in 1989[1] (SCS); 4 descriptive levels:

Anatomic focus

- The primary joints or segments affected by the splint, e.g. MCP

1. American Society of Hand Therapists (1989). *Splint classification system*. Chicago.

Kinematic direction
- The direction that the primary joints are moved, i.e. flexion–extension

Primary purpose
- Whether the splint intends to mobilize, immobilize, or restrict the primary joint or segment

Inclusion of secondary joints
- The number of joints other than the primary joints that are included in the splint

For example, middle finger PIP extension immobilization type 0.

Points to consider when making a splint

Theory
- Anatomy
- Physiology:
  - Understanding the response of tissues to injury
  - Understanding the normal phases of wound healing
  - Understanding the consequences of prolonged immobilization
  - Understanding tissue response to application of stress through the use of splints
- Normal hand function:
  - Hand grips
  - Arches
- Pathology:
  - Of different conditions
- Biomechanical principles of splinting:
  - Application of force
  - Levers

Evaluation
- Origin of injury/disability
- Surgical/non-surgical management
- Complications
- Physician's recommendations
- Patient awareness

Planning
- Function of the splint
- Design:
  - Ease of don/doffing
  - Durability
- Weight of splint construction:
  - Patterns/precuts
  - Choice of equipment/tools

Implementation
- Positioning the patient
- Moulding
- Aesthetic appearance of the splint
- Patient education
- Provision of splint information leaflet
- Wearing regime

- Correct application
- Care of splint
- Precautions

Re-evaluation
- Is the splint serving its purpose?
- Is it comfortable?
- Does the patient understand the wearing regime?

General principles for making forearm-based splints
- The splint should follow the contour of the hand and forearm and maintain the arches of the hand
- Even distribution of pressure
- The length should be determined by the joint whose movement should be maintained
- Add contour

Optimum position of the hand: position of safe immobilization (POSI) (📖 see Fig. 2.1)
Immobilizing:
- Wrist—neutral or few degrees of extension
- Thumb CMC Carpo-metacarpal joint—abduction and opposition
- Thumb IP—extension
- MCPs—60–90° flexion
- IPs—extension

General principles of dynamic splinting
- Static portion should fit well
- The bone proximal to the joint being mobilized should be well stabilized
- The line of pull should be at a right angle to the axis of the skeletal segment being moved
- During flexion fingers converge to the scaphoid
- Ensure the elastic bands are of the correct tension

Splinting precautions
- Skin
- Bony prominences
- Friction
- Pressure
- Oedema

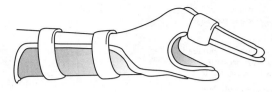

Safe position splint

Fig. 2.1 Optimum position of the hand in splinting.

Materials: what is on the market?
- High-temperature thermoplastics
- Plaster of Paris
- Metal strips and wire
- Neoprene
- Low-temperature thermoplastics
- Fibreglass
- Elastomer

Properties of splinting material
- Resistance to stretch
- Thickness
- Perforation
- Padded or non-padded

Choosing a material
Dependent upon:
- Function of the splint
- Therapist's ability and preference
- Ability to position the patient
- Required amount of rigidity and support
- Degree of ventilation
- Level of patient compliance
- Budget

Straps
- Consider:
  • Position
  • Angle of application
  • Width
- Materials:
  • Velcro
  • Ready-made
  • Rivets
  • Taping

- Bandages
- Cohesive bandages

Padding
- Use only when required
- Increases pressure
- May increase comfort

Splinting regimes
Dependent upon:
- Diagnosis
- Acuity/chronicity
- Goals of the splint
- Patient's tolerance to wearing the splint
- Importance of active movement
- Number of splints involved in the treatment plan
- Patient's need to use the hand 'normally'

As a general rule
For collagen to realign plastic deformation must occur, therefore wearing a splint for a couple of hours each day may not be sufficient; consider gentle force for a prolonged period to effect permanent changes in length of tissues. The amount of force required to elicit this change is unclear.

Oedema control

Definition

Excessive accumulation of fluid in the body tissue spaces.

Injury to the hand causes disruption of capillary integrity, culminating in a protein-rich fluid leaking into the interstitial spaces.

One of the commonest problems that a therapist will encounter, oedema has the capacity to inhibit wound healing, increase the risk of infection, reduce range of motion and cause fibrosis.

Types of oedema

Acute (transudate)

An inflammatory response consisting of mainly water and electrolytes. Soft on palpation and easily reducible. Temporary displacement of fluid referred to as 'pitting oedema'.

Chronic (exudate)

Present in the fibroplastic and remodelling phase. The fluid is high in protein content, more viscous and stagnant.

Assessment of oedema

See Chapter 1, p. 12.

Appearance of oedema

- Puffy
- Shiny
- Dull skin
- Stiff joints on movement
- Tightness of skin and loss of skin creases

Oedema over the dorsum of the hand causes the skin to tighten, forcing the MCPs into hyperextension and the IP joints into flexion. As a consequence the MCP collateral ligaments and the volar plate over the volar aspect of the PIP joints shorten. In addition the arches of the hand flatten and the thumb becomes adducted and extended. Without early management the persistent oedema may result in fixed contractures (📕 see Fig. 2.2).

Management of oedema

Elevation

The first line of treatment unless contraindicated due to vascular insufficiency. Enhances venous and lymphatic flow.

Active range of movement

Results in muscles pumping, soft tissue movement and compression of veins and the lymphatic system.

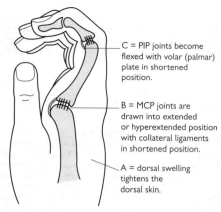

C = PIP joints become flexed with volar (palmar) plate in shortened position.

B = MCP joints are drawn into extended or hyperextended position with collateral ligaments in shortened position.

A = dorsal swelling tightens the dorsal skin.

Fig. 2.2 Typical oedematous hand position.

Retrograde massage
Performed with the hand in elevation, the hand is massaged distal to proximal producing a mild pressure gradient and thus reducing oedema.

Compression
- Intermittent—external pressure is applied using a compression pump and sleeve. Air is pumped in and out of the sleeve producing a pumping action. Thus increasing the pressure gradient.
- Continuous—either through pressure gloves/sleeves (whole hand/individual digits) or coban wrap (applied to the digit distal to proximal).

Cold therapy
Ice is applied to the limb producing vasoconstriction, a reduction in metabolic rate and blood flow culminating in reduced membrane permeability and capillary filtration.

Contrast bathing
The affected limb is submerged into hand-hot and ice-cold water (alternating) to encourage both vasodilatation and vasoconstriction, producing a pumping action.

String wrapping
Cord/string is applied to the digit distal to proximal and immediately removed, repeated several times.

Scar

Scars are the inevitable result of injury to the skin. The final scar that forms secondary to the reparative process is variable and never completely predictable. Scars are classified by colour, texture, pattern and overall presentation.

Types of scar

Mature scar
Light-coloured, flat scar.

Immature scar
A red, itchy or painful and slightly elevated scar in the process of remodelling. Will usually mature with time, become flat and assume pigmentation similar to the surrounding skin. Produced during the normal healing process. Abnormal immature scar shows a proliferation of fibroblasts in a loose myxoid stroma running parallel to the skin surface. Blood vessels are prominent. As the scar matures over a few weeks mature collagen is laid down and fibroblasts decrease in number. The number of blood vessels begins to rapidly decrease in size and numbers during the final repair process. The thickness, colour and size of the scar all diminish as maturation continues

Linear hypertrophic scar (surgical/traumatic)
Red, raised, sometimes itchy scar confined to the border of the original incision. Usually occurs within weeks after surgery. These scars may increase in size rapidly for 3–6 months and then fade. They mature slightly elevated with a rope-like appearance. Maturation can take up to 2 years. Hypertrophic scars exhibit nodular structures containing fibroblastic cells and collagen. These nodules are not observed in normal dermis, other scars or the majority of keloids. Hypertrophic scar fibroblasts respond normally to growth factors and demonstrate only a modest increase in collagen production.

Widespread hypertrophic (burn) scar
Widespread red, raised, sometimes itchy scar that remains within the borders of the burn.

Minor keloid
Focally raised, firm, mildly tender, itchy scar extending over normal tissue, usually worse in areas where the skin is under tension or is thickest. The borders are usually well demarcated but are irregular or bizarre in outline. May develop up to 1 year after injury and does not regress on its own. Simple surgical excision is often followed by recurrence. Keloids are usually hyperpigmented with red to purple colouration. They show an increased level of histamine, which may contribute to the itching and pain. Dark-skinned individuals and patients with blood group A are more susceptible to keloid formation. The response to treatment varies depending on the anatomical location and from patient to patient. Fibroblasts in keloids respond abnormally to stimulation, show a greater capacity to proliferate and produce high levels of collagen, elastin, fibronectin and proteoglycan.

Major keloid

A large raised scar possibly painful or itchy extending over normal tissue. Often results from minor trauma and can continue to spread for several years.

Grading

📖 See, p. 32.

Prevention

- Careful wound repair
- Avoidance or minimization of risk factors:
  - Smoking
  - Poor nutrition
  - Infection
  - Foreign bodies
  - Venous insufficiency
  - Arteriosclerosis
  - Renal and pulmonary disease
  - Radiation damage
  - Steroid therapy
  - Diabetes

Treatment

Therapy

Many techniques, little evidence. Cutaneous scar management relies heavily on the experience of practitioners. Techniques include:

- Hydrotherapy
- Massage
- Ultrasound
- Pulsed electrical stimulation
- Desensitization

Corticosteroid injections

Dermal injection of triamcinolone is efficacious, 1st-line therapy for the treatment of keloids and 2nd-line for hypertrophic scars if other treatments have not been effective. Flattens and softens scar. Mechanism of action remains unclear, probable suppression and modulation of collagen synthesis. Complications:

- Significant injection pain
- Skin atrophy
- Hypopigmentation
- Necrosis
- Ulceration

Topical steroid creams

Used with varying success but limited absorption through an intact epithelium into the deep dermis.

Silicone gel sheeting

Effective improvement in size, texture, colour, level of itchiness, range of motion and thickness of keloid and hypertrophic scars. Few complications or side-effects. Mechanism involves hydration and occlusion: by decreasing evaporation of water silicone gel reduces collagen deposition, induces scar regression and provides symptomatic relief. Occlusion may alter proinflammatory cytokine expression. Silicone gel products vary considerably in composition, durability and adhesion. No consensus on exactly when to start treatment.

Silicone elastomers

Purpose:
- Reduce scar formation and provide protection
- Work hardening (to absorb vibration/shock)
- Achieve proper positioning in the splint/web spaces or concave areas
- Desensitize hypersensitive stumps
- Varieties of elastomers include:
  - Elastomer 121 (NCM)
  - Soft putty elastomer (NCM)
  - Rolyan 50:50 (Homecraft Ability One)
  - Putty elastomer (NCM)
  - Otoform K (NCM)
  - Rolyan silicone elastomer (NCM)
  - Rolyan ezemix elastomer putty (Homecraft Ability One)

Pressure therapy

The mechanism by which continuous pressure decreases the size and thickness of hypertrophic scars and keloids is not completely understood. Probably continuous pressure produces tissue ischaemia, decreasing tissue metabolism and increasing collagenase activity. Other theories include pressure-induced release of metalloprotinase-9 or prostaglandin E2 that may effect scar softening by the induction of extracellular matrix remodelling. It is standard therapy for hypertrophic burn scars. Recommended that pressure be maintained between 24–30 mmHg for 6–12 months to be effective. Scars older than 6–12 months often respond poorly and it may be difficult to achieve the required pressure particularly over joints.

Radiotherapy

Difficult to evaluate, as most studies are retrospective and use a variety of radiation techniques with varying follow-up. The inhibition of fibroblast proliferation and angiogenesis during the exaggerated wound healing process is the proposed mechanism of action. The use of a potentially carcinogenic treatment for the treatment of a benign process is controversial. Infrequently used as only treatment: reserve for adults with scars and keloid resistant to other treatment.

Laser therapy

Laser-induced tissue hypoxia leads to decreased cellular function and laser-induced heating leads to bond disruption with subsequent remodelling of the fibres. Role for laser therapy emerging : recent use with flashlamp-pumped pulsed-dye laser showed improved scar erythema, texture, height and pliability.

Cryotherapy

Freezing-induced ischaemic damage to the microcirculation. Cryotherapy alone results in keloid flattening in 51–74% of patients after two or more sessions. When combined, use of cryotherapy and injection has been reported to be superior to either freezing or injection alone. The scar is frozen with liquid nitrogen applied with a swab or cryosurgical instrument until it turns white. As the lesion thaws it turns pink and becomes oedematous. During the thaw phase each segment of the lesion is injected. Successful injection is seen by blanching of the scar, 3 or 4 injections are required at 4–6 week intervals. Side-effects include:

- Permanent hypopigmentation
- Hyperpigmentation
- Moderate skin atrophy
- Pain

Surgery

Excision alone of keloid results in high recurrence rates (45–100%) within 4 years after surgery. Combining it with steroid injections reduces the rate of recurrence.

Hypertrophic scarring can be treated effectively with surgical excision in conjunction with surgical taping and silicone gel with a low recurrence rate.

Surgical options:
- Primary excision and closure
- Z-plasty
- W-plasty scar revision
- Dermablasion
- Skin grafts
- Pedicled and free flaps

Hypersensitivity

Definition

Condition of extreme discomfort or irritability in response to normally non-noxious stimulation. Mechanisms that cause it or the physiological changes that produce the symptoms poorly understood. Hypersensitivity may develop after traumatic hand injuries including:

- Amputation
- Scarring
- Crush injury
- Neuroma
- Burns

Terminology

Allodynia

- Pain secondary to a stimulus that is not normally painful

Anaesthesia dolorosa

- Pain in an insensitive area/region

Causalgia

- Severe incapacitating pain after a traumatic nerve lesion

Dysaesthesia

- Any unpleasant abnormal sensation either spontaneous or evoked. Allodynia and hyperpathia are examples of dysesthesia

Hyperalgesia

- Increased sensitivity to noxious stimuli

Hyperpathia

- An extreme form for hyperalgesia and allodynia characterized by the intensity of the pain, faulty localization, radiating pain and over-reaction and after-sensation

Hyperaesthesia

- Otherwise known as hypersensitivity; increased sensitivity to all stimuli. Usually described as tactile and thermal stimuli. May be caused by scar tissue, neuromas, amputation and regenerating nerves.

Neuralgia

- A nerve lesion causing intense and pain felt maximally in the nerve distribution

Pain

- A subjective sensation recognizable to the patient but difficult to define by the observer

Evaluation of hypersensitivity

Hypersensitivity is subjective and thus difficult to quantify.

Treatment

Aim to lessen reactivity to an external stimulus through the use of a graded series of modalities and procedures. Desensitization techniques are identical in concept to sensory re-education. The patient learns to filter out unpleasant sensations to perception of the more meaningful sensory input. Desensitization may inhibit the development of permanent pain pathways in the central nervous system.

Desensitization techniques

- Capsaicum cream (used 3–4 times daily)
- Haemorrhoid cream (soothes)
- Percussion
- Vibration
- Massage
- Heat
- Stroking
- Trans-cutaneous electrical nerve stimulation (TENS)
- Acupuncture
- Compression
- Distraction
- Graded textures
- Ultrasound
- Opsite flexigrid (vapour permeable dressing)
- Electromyography (EMG)
- Patient education

Choice depends on patient presentation and therapist experience. Desensitization may be more effective if done throughout the day instead of the prescribed 3–4 times daily. A multifaceted approach should incorporate not only physical modalities but also cognitive and psychological techniques. Outcome assessment following desensitization should not only focus on the reduction of hypersensitivity but also a patient's functional status.

Pain

'An unpleasant sensory and emotional experience associated with actual or potential tissue damage'.[1]

Physiology of pain

Pain receptors in the skin, muscle and joints (nociceptors) detect the sensation of pain and relay the information to the spinal cord and onto the brain via Aβ fibres and C-fibres.

Aβ fibres
- Myelinated
- Fast acting
- Concentrated at the point of stimulation
- Superficial
- Respond to mechanical and thermal stimulation

C-fibres
- Unmyelinated
- Slow acting
- Present in deeper parts of the skin
- Large well-defined receptive field
- Found in all tissue except the spinal cord and the brain
- Sensitive to damage
- Respond to thermal and mechanical stimulation
- Longer-lasting pain
- Secondary aching pain

Characteristics of pain

Transient
- Short-lived
- Localized

Acute
- Immediate onset
- Sharp
- Localized

Chronic
- Insidious onset
- Long duration
- Cause may not be known
- Poorly localized
- Affects behaviour
- Prognosis unpredictable

Pain may also be
- Superficial/deep
- Localized/referred/projected
- Intractable
- Psychogenic

1. IASP (1979). Pain terms: A use with definitions and notes on usage. *Pain* **6**: 249–252.

Influencing factors
- Severity and extent of injury
- Cognitive factors:
  - Previous experiences
  - Culture
  - Gender
  - Expectations
- Circumstances and emotions
  - Stress
  - Environment
  - General health
  - Social support
  - Compensation

Assessment of pain
📖 See, p. 29.

Management of pain

Analgesics
- Simple analgesics
  - Paracetamol
- Opiates
  - Codeine, dihydrocodeine (weak)
  - Tramadol (alternate)
  - Morphine (strong)
- Non-steroidal anti-inflammatories
  - Diclofenac
  - Ibuprofen, etc.

For nerve pain
- Antidepressants
  - Amitriptyline
- Anticonvulsants
  - Gabapentin and its pro drug Pregabalin

Therapy
- Oedema control
- Reducing the distension of tissue spaces reduces the chemical irritation of the nocioceptors
- Rest:
  - To reduce inflammation
  - To reduce muscle spasm
- Mobilization:
  - To reduce oedema
  - Alter the sensory input from joints and muscles
  - Prevention of scar tissue
- Function
- Electrotherapy
  - Alter the sensory input to the nervous system

- Thermal
  - Relieve local ischaemia
  - Alter sensory input
- Acupuncture
  - Altering the energy flow
- TENS:
  - Stimulates large nerve fibres and closes the pain gate, and
  - Stimulate the production of endorphins
- Massage
- Relaxation
- Education

Sensory re-education

'A process in which a person learns to interpret the abnormal sensory impulses that are generated at the periphery following an interruption in the peripheral nervous system' (Dellon 1981).[1]

Factors affecting sensibility

Quality of sensibility that returns to the hand after nerve repair in adults is poor; better results in children. Several factors are associated with this poor outcome:

Peripheral factors
- Level of injury
- Scar tissue
- Distal stump atrophy
- Regenerating axons enter different endoneural sheaths
- Delay to repair
- Health of tissue bed
- Quality of repair

Cortical modelling

The central nervous system representations of the body surface are constantly remodelled by tactile experiences throughout life. After nerve repair and regeneration this cortical representation changes. Some of the observed changes after nerve repair and regeneration are:

- The regenerating nerves may reactivate only a fraction of their normal cortical space, suggesting only partial recovery of sensibility in the hand.
- Enlarged cortical representations of the skin adjacent to denervated skin, which may account for hypersensitivity of adjacent skin.
- A point in the skin is commonly represented in several cortical locations after injury explaining false localization.
- The normal adjacent skin site to adjacent cortical site relationship, which enables us to recognize objects, is lost.

Sensory re-education programmes

Timing

Typically introduced in the rehabilitation phase after nerve repair when some degree of nerve regeneration can be demonstrated. The hypothesis is that sensory re-education reorganizes central connections, attempting to retrain the patient so that they may use their reinnervated sensory mechanisms to their advantage. More recent theory (Rosen et al 2003)[2] suggests that very early sensory re-education should be introduced in the early rehabilitation stage when no axons have yet arrived in the asensible hand; if the vacant area of the denervated hand after nerve repair could be given relevant information at an early stage it may help to minimize the synaptic reorganization, hypothetically making the brain better prepared for the relearning training once the nerve has regenerated and reinnervated the peripheral targets.

Types

The most common programmes are:

- Desensitization
- Protective education
  - As the patient experiences no pain/discomfort and is susceptible to blisters and bruises, the purpose is to teach the patient to compensate for the lack of protective sensory input, i.e. to avoid exposure to extreme heat/cold and to avoid excessive pressure (avoiding skin attusion)
- Correction of faulty localization
- Recognition of materials and objects

Dellon (1974)[3]

Dellon based his programme on observed recovery patterns. He observed that order of recovery as:

- Pain and temperature
- Followed by 30cps vibration
- And quickly after by moving touch
- Much later by constant touch
- Finally by 256 cps vibration

This was then used as a timetable for treatment.

Early phase

initiated when patients could perceive 30 cps vibration. Programme focused on moving and light touch and localization of those perceptions.

Late phase

initiated when moving and constant touch could be perceived at the fingertips, with good localization. Focused on size and shape discrimination and object recognition using objects familiar to the patient.

Wynn Parry (1976)[4]

- Patients are blindfolded
- A number of different shapes are put into the patient's hand and they are asked to recognize them. If they are unable to do so the patient then compares the abnormal sensation with the normal hand and also relates this with their eyes open
- Once successfully recognized the patient progresses to texture recognition
- Finally onto everyday objects
- The ability to localize a touch accurately to the correct part of the hand is also re-trained

Nakada and Uchida (1997)[5]

Proposed a programme classified into 5 stages specific to hand function based on neurophysiological findings.

Stage 1: feature detection and recognition of objects

Before we hold an object we try to distinguish the characteristics of the object:
- Volume/form:
  - Visual perception
- Height/quality of the surface:
  - Tactile sensation
- Compressibility/flexibility:
  - Tactile sensation
- Thermal characteristics:
  - Tactile sensation

Finger motion is essential to perform these tasks. Patients with no cutaneous sensation will use proprioception to recognize the objects through a sense of force using the whole hand. The task is completed with vision occluded.

Stage 2: correction of the pattern of prehension in the hand
With normal sensibility and motor function the hand precisely fits the form of an object it is holding. The pattern of prehension depends on the detection of the differing characteristics of that object. The hand outlines the form through touching the surface and then judges the axis and gravity of the object. This stage encourages the patient to choose different objects of different size and shape using the vision-occluded technique.

Stage 3: control of precise force for grasping
With normal sensation we hold an object without crushing or dropping it. A hand with a loss of sensibility tends to apply excess pressure for grasping. Use a strain gauge for pressure feedback during re-education patients learn how much pressure they are applying.

Stage 4: maintenance of grasping force during movement of more proximal joints
During prehension we use more proximal joints. For patients who have lost sensation it is common to drop objects as soon as proximal joints are moved. Patients are asked to move more proximal joints whilst holding an object in the hand.

Stage 5: manipulation of fine objects
To manipulate an object it is necessary to perform sensory as well as fine motor functions. A hand that has sensory function and adequate motor function might reach this level.

Rosen et al. (2003)[2]
Phase one: maintenance of the cortical hand map
- Patient is asked to think about how touch normally feels by observing someone touching something
- The area of denervation is touched in combination with watching
- The area of denervation is touched at the same time as the corresponding area on the contralateral side is touched, whilst watching
- Mirrors training: placed vertically in front of the patient to reflect the non-injured hand. Creating an illusion that there is movement/activity in the injured hand.
- Sensor glove system: acoustic signals are used from microphones mounted on the fingertips of a glove worn on the injured hand,

providing the somatosensory cortex alternative sensory input. The stimuli generated by active touching of various structures can be picked up and amplified and transposed to stereophonic acoustic stimuli. Pilot studies show good results.

Phase two: cortical retraining
- An area on the regenerating hand is touched. The patient is encouraged to focus on how, where and what this feels. The area is compared with the non-injured contralateral side. The patient repeats the task with their eyes open and closed until they are familiar with the location and character of the touch.
- Once protective sensibility has started to return the patient is asked to differentiate between different objects, shapes and textures, with eyes open and then closed.
- Selective cutaneous anaesthesia: using EMLA cream in weekly intervals the volar aspect of the forearm of the injured hand is anaesthetized. This area becomes vacant in the body map, allowing sensory re-learning in the hand. This technique can significantly improve tactile discrimination.

1. Dellon AL (1981). *Sensibility and Re-education of Sensation in the Hand.* Baltimore, Williams-Wilkins.
2. Rosen B, Balkenius C and Lundborg E (2003). Sensory re-education today and tomorrow: a review of evolving concepts. *British Journal of Hand Therapy.* **8**: 48–56.
3. Dellon AL *et al* (1974). Re-education of sensation in the hand after nerve injury and repair plast. *Reconstr Surg* **33**: 297–305.
4. Wynn Parry CB and Slater M (1976). Sensory re-education after median nerve lesions. *Hand* **8**: 250–7.
5. Nakada M and Uchida H (1997). Case study of a five-stage sensory re-education program. *Journal of Hand Therapy* **10**: 232–239.

Psychological implications of hand problems

The hands and face are the most sociably visible portions of a person's body. Injuries to the hand are common and are often accompanied by a variety of perceived psychological reactions. The hand is a strong component of a person's self-image. A large proportion of the cortex of the brain is dedicated to the hands.

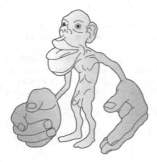

Fig. 2.3 Homunculus man.

When injury occurs it affects a large proportion of the patient's neurological activity and consequently their psychological state. As the hand is a major receptor and activator of stimuli, when it is out of action the normal level of stimulus is greatly reduced, the patient thus suffers neurological and psychological deprivation, which may lead to depression, anxiety and varying degrees of psychosomatic symptoms.

Use of the hand
- Gesture
- Feel
- Stabilize
- Manipulate
- Give
- Take
- Express
- Caress
- Sooth
- Welcome
- Protect
- Aggress
- Signal

The hands are also used to:
- Maintain independence
- Maintain personal hygiene

Psychological effect of hand Injury

The way in which a person responds and copes with disruption of an injury varies.

- ↓ Self-esteem
- ↓ Motivation
- Emotional instability—dependency
- Lack of control
- Alteration of routine
- ↓ Concentration
- Employment/financial concerns
- Altered social life
- ↑ Isolation
- Loss of appetite
- Depression
- Alteration of sleep pattern
- Guilt
- ↓ Libido/avoidance of close interpersonal relationships
- Altered body image/body preoccupation
- Loss of roles
- ↑ Self-consciousness/cosmetic concerns
- High levels of anxiety
- Fear of death
- Hypervigilance for any event in which they may hurt themselves
- Impulsive behaviours

Three stages in response to injury

1. Shock
2. Growing awareness
3. Acceptance

Shock

Acute shock caused by loss of health, independence and anticipation of permanent incapacity and disfigurement. Few patients will have had comparable experience of such an injury.

Growing awareness

Of the implication of the injury.

Acceptance

Rehabilitation and recovery of independence and self-respect cannot be achieved until final acceptance is achieved.

Emotions expressed

During the above stages the patient may experience and display a variety of feelings that include:

- Anger
- Denial
- Repulsion
- Guilt
- Fear and anxiety
- Misery and depression
- Defeatism

Behaviours expressed

In response to these feelings the patient may react in the following way:
- Withdrawal
- Dependence
- Regression
- Non-cooperation
- Complaint
- Violence
- Control

Coping strategies will depend upon

- Severity of injury
- Personality traits
- Previous traumatic experience
- Social situation
- Work situation
- Pre-existing psychological problems

Acute stress disorder

One of the earliest psychological manifestations is acute stress disorder. The patients often experience a variety of psychological symptoms, the most prevalent being intrusive thoughts, flashbacks and nightmares. Early treatment is important with structured re-exposure to the thoughts and memories of the trauma.

Post-traumatic stress disorder (PTSD)

A combination of symptoms that can occur after a specific traumatic event. Diagnosis is made by the presence of:
- Intrusive thought
- Avoidance of stimuli associated with the injury
- Physiological arousal
- Symptoms persisting for at least 30 days after the injury.
- The hallmark of PTSD is persistent re-experiencing of the traumatic event.

Role of the hand therapist

The therapist is often the only person that sees the patient frequently, helping them to return to a functioning level. The therapist needs to be proactive in this phase of physical and emotional healing. The therapist can elicit pertinent information from the patient regarding:
- The injury
- The patient's support system
- Understanding the patients perception of injury
- Avoidance/denial

Techniques
- Be honest
- Be supportive
- Provide a safe environment
- Reassure the patient that many of the initial responses that are experiencing are normal

- Non-judgemental/reactive: the patient will observe a therapists reaction, i.e. to the disfigurement
- Provide education—needs to be sensitively delivered. Education is the basis for compliance and will empower the patient to make decisions.
- Involve the patient's family and carers
- Provide patient-centred treatment
- Make decisions with the patient
- Focus on the entire extremity—to ensure the patient incorporates the injured part back into their total body image.
- Teach coping strategies—for pain relief (relaxation/distraction/pacing).
- Assist acknowledgement and adaptation—long-term prospects of physical recovery, disfigurement and scarring
- Monitor mental state

Treatments
- Stress management
- Anxiety management
- Relaxation
- Achievement and creativity—to build self-esteem and confidence
- Physical fitness
- Leisure restoration
- Work hardening
- Humour

Other treatments

Some treatments are outside the scope of the therapist. Therapists may have counselling skills but are not counsellors. Therapists need to be aware of when to refer to more suitable professionals.

Stiffness

The definition of stiffness is rigidity and inflexibility. Stiffness in the hand significantly reduces function.

Causes
- Oedema
- Infection
- Fibrosis
- Anatomical factors (damage to joint dynamics)
- Prolonged immobilization
- Delayed treatment
- Poor splintage
- Complex Regional Pain Syndrome
- Patient anxiety

Preventative measures
- Elevation
- Adequate pain relief
- Promote good wound healing
- Early mobilization (where possible)
- Appropriate splinting (i.e. POSI)
- Achievement of good early passive and active ROM (where appropriate)
- Patient education
- Early functional use (where appropriate)

Assessment of stiffness

Prior to commencing treatment it is essential that the therapist assesses the patient and obtains a full history, including mechanism of injury, exact location of injury and management. This will enable the therapist to gain an understanding of the potential physiological changes that may have occurred and to be able to formulate an appropriate treatment plan.

Manual examination of the tissues is necessary to determine what structures are limiting motion.

Assessment should include:
- Oedema evaluation:
  - Volumeter
  - Tape measure
  - Jeweller's rings
- Joint tightness evaluation:
  - Examine the passive range of motion of the joint and then move both proximal and distal joints. If the ROM does not change joint tightness is the cause of stiffness
- Skin tightness:
  - A stretch is applied to the area of scar/tight skin. Blanching of the skin is observed or increased tightness is noted
- Muscle–tendon tightness:
  - Occurs along the course of the muscle–tendon unit anywhere between the origin and insertion. Tightness is indicated when ROM at distal joints is altered when more proximal joints are mobilized.

Intrinsic tightness is observed when ROM at the IP joints is less and resistance is greater when the MCP joints are held in extension/hyperextension rather than when they are flexed. The contralateral side should also be tested.

Therapist's treatment of stiffness

- Oedema reduction:
  📖 see p. 54.
- Pain reduction
  📖 see p. 62.
- Exercise programmes:
  - Active
  - Passive
  - Accessory mobilizations
- Splinting:
  - Serial static
  - Dynamic
  - Casting motion to mobilize stiffness (CMMS)
- Wax
- Patient education
- Functional activities

Priorities when improving range of motion:
- A hand that flexes is functionally more useful than a hand in extension
- A functional hand requires good MCP and PIP flexion
- Function and grip require the wrist to be in some extension
- Ulnar deviation is more functional than radial deviation
- The thumb can tolerate stiffness better than the fingers
- The thumb needs to retropose and the MP joints need to extend in order to prepare the hand for prehension
- A mobile thumb CMC joint is more important than a stiff MP joint

Surgery for stiffness

Prerequisites

- Pain-free joint
- Congruous joint
- Good muscle function
- Cooperative patient
- Communication with hand therapist to plan postoperative rehabilitation (active movement, passive movement, splintage)

Distal radioulnar joint

Loss of supination usually due to contracture of the anterior capsule. Released through an anterior approach between flexor digitorum profundis (FDP) and ulnar neurovascular bundle. Joint identified under image intensifier. Anterior capsule divided longitudinally. Anterior limb of triangular fibrocartilage complex (anterior radioulnar ligament) preserved. Splint in supination for two weeks then begin active supination, held by a supination strap.

Metacarpophalangeal joints

Usually stiffen in extension due to contracture of the collateral ligaments. Dorsal approach. Extensor tendon divided in midline. Dorsal capsule elevated longitudinally, then elevated to each side, scooping the proximal insertion of the collateral ligament from its recess. Tendon repaired with interrupted sutures. Splint with MCP flexed to 90°. Begin early active movement, supported by a dorsal blocking splint at rest.

Proximal interphalangeal joints

Usually stiffen in flexion due to contracture of the accessory collateral ligaments and contraction of the proximal attachment of the palmar plate alongside the metacarpal neck. Palmar Brunner approach. Neurovascular bundles swept aside and sheath exposed. The proximal extension of the thickened palmar plate ('check rein ligament') divided on each side and the attachment of the accessory collateral ligaments divided. Splint in extension but start very early active and passive movements.

Thumb carpometacarpal joint

In severe stiffness, particularly adduction, joint release may fail. Trapeziectomy can restore functional abduction and opposition. May need ligament reconstruction to maintain abduction/extension.

Complex regional pain syndrome (CRPS)

Introduction

CRPS is a debilitating condition that has been recognized for more than a century. First observed in 1864 by American Silas Weir Mitchell amongst war veterans in the American civil war. Patients presented with burning pain and trophic changes after penetrating limb injuries, which he described as causalgia.

Alternative terms

- Reflex sympathetic dystrophy (RSD)
- Post-traumatic dystrophy
- Causalgia
- Algodystrophy
- Sudek's atrophy
- Shoulder–hand syndrome

Definition

RSD became the popular term as described by Evans (1946)[1] following sympathetic blockades being used to relieve pain. This taxonomy became problematic as the activity of the sympathetic nervous system is not the only likely causative factor.

In 1986 the International Association for the Study of Pain (IASP) redefined RSD and changed its name to CRPS, subdividing into type I and type II, distinguished by the presence of a nerve lesion in type II, although both present with the same signs and symptoms.

CRPS I	CRPS II
Initiated by a noxious event or a cause of immobilization	Initiated by nerve injury
Continuing pain, allodynia or hyperalgesia with which the pain is disproportionate to the inciting event	Continuing pain, allodynia or hyperalgesia after a nerve injury, not necessarily limited to the distribution of the injured nerve
Presence of oedema, changes in blood flow to the skin or abnormal sudomtor activity in the region of the pain	Presence of oedema, changes in blood flow to the skin or abnormal sudomtor activity in the region of the pain
Diagnosis is excluded by the existence of conditions that would otherwise account for the symptoms	Diagnosis is excluded by the existence of conditions that would otherwise account for the symptoms

Some authors describe a third category CRPS-NOS (not otherwise specified) to include patients who do not exhibit the symptoms specified in type I or II.

Harden et al. (1999)[2] suggested that the current criteria are not sufficiently specific, may lead to over diagnosis and fail to consider motor

---

1. Evans JA (1946). Reflex sympathetic dystrophy. *Surg Clin North Am* **26**: 780–790.
2. Harden RN et al. (1999). Complex regional pain syndrome: are the IASP diagnostic criteria valid and suficiently comprehensive? *Pain* **83**: 211–9.

and trophic signs and symptoms. Modified diagnostic criteria have been proposed:
1. Continuing pain, which is disproportionate to any inciting event.
2. At least one symptom in each of the four following categories:
    a. Sensory: hyperaesthesia
    b. Vasomotor: temperature asymmetry and /or skin colour changes and/or skin colour asymmetry
    c. Sudomotor/oedema: oedema and/or sweating changes and/or sweating asymmetry
    d. Motor/trophic: decreased range of motion and/or motor dysfunction (weakness, tremor, dystonia) and/or trophic changes (hair, nail, skin)
3. Must display at least one sign in two or more of the following categories:
    a. Sensory: evidence of hyperalgesia (to pin prick) and/or allodynia (to light touch)
    b. Vasomotor: evidence of temperature asymmetry and/or skin colour changes and/or asymmetry
    c. Sudomotor/oedema: evidence of oedema and/or sweating changes and/or sweating asymmetry
    d. Motor/trophic: evidence of decreased range of motion and/or motor dysfunction (weakness, tremor, dystonia, neglect) and/or trophic changes (hair, nail, skin)

Epidemiology

Usually follows trauma but can develop after surgery with immobilization of a limb.
- 1–2% limb fractures
- 22–37% Colles' fracture
- 5% myocardial infarction
- 12% Cerebro-vascular accident
    1. More prevalent in the upper limb
    2. Female 3:1 male
    3. Mean age 40–50 years
    4. May occur in children

Pathophysiology

The underlying mechanisms of CRPS are still not clearly understood and many factors contribute to the generation and maintenance of CRPS.

Trauma
- Link remains unclear
- Trauma and mechanical injury activate mast cell production, which releases tryptase in tissue and blood. Patients with CRPS have an elevated level of tryptase, which correlates with pain intensity. Mast cell derived tryptase can activate nociceptors that are in part responsible for peripheral pain mechanisms

Limb immobilization
- Linked to the production of free radicals which increases during immobilization
- Osteoclast differentiation is promoted leading to possible osteoporosis
- Mast cell activity is promoted (see Trauma)

Tight bandages
- Underlying oedema associated with CRPS may cause tight casts/bandages. The opposite is not necessarily true.

Ischaemia/reperfusion
- Some cases of CRPS may be due to injury occurring during ischaemia–reperfusion.
- Associated with the production of reactive oxygen species (ROS), including free radicals

Genetic
- There may be some correlation between CRPS and human leukocyte antigen (HLA). HLA-DR13 was associated with progression to multifocal dystonia in patients with CRPS.

Mechanisms of pain
Current theories include:

Neuroimmunoinflammatory factors
- Pain is normally caused following tissue damage, which results in the production of chemicals such as substance P, bradykinins, certain antihistamines and prostaglandins, which in turn activate nociceptors. It is believed that these chemical mediators can sensitize nociceptive fibres resulting in an increased response to a range of thermal, mechanical and chemical stimuli.
- In addition, sensitized spinal cord neurons can excite sympathetic efferent activity that causes norepinephrine (NE) to be released. NE further excites the pain afferents thereby perpetuating the pain and oedema cycle.

Abnormal sympathetic nervous system
- Sympathetically maintained pain (SMP) may be a symptom of CRPS in some patients, although the overall prevalence is unknown
- It is possible that the sympathetic nervous system may be involved in the pathophysiology of CRPS in several ways:
  - Sympathetic outflow is not normally responsible for the activation of nociceptors whereas in CRPS, SMP may likely be a mechanism of pathogenesis. Studies suggest that there is a coupling between sympathetic neurons and efferent neurons. Sympathetic fibres are thought to mediate the effects of inflammatory compounds which sensitize nociceptors and may be a factor in the inflammatory pain of CRPS I
  - Acute injury is a stimulus for sympathetic arousal. Sympathetic nerve regeneration occurs rapidly to reinnervated capillaries and bring them under vasoconstrictive control. This normally occurs 2 weeks after injury to bring the inflammatory phase to a close, but may not occur in CRPS

- It has been suggested that some people are hypersympathetic reactors, they have a sympathetic dominance possibly making them more susceptible to CRPS after injury

Central sensitization
- The intense/prolonged bombardment of substance P and excitatory amino acids sensitizes the dorsal horn pain-transmitting neurons and causes central sensitization. This may be an important factor in the development of mechanical allodynia and hyperalgesia

Spinal cord microglia
- Recent evidence suggests that the activation of spinal cord microglia may be a factor in the hyperexcitability of pain-transmitting neurons in the dorsal horn.

Cortical reorganization
- It is believed that some patients with CRPS have dysfunctional processing in the somatosensory and motor cortices, which may contribute to the perpetuation of CRPS.
- In the motor cortex changes occur in cortical representation when comparing subacute and chronic CRPS to healthy individuals.
- Patients with CRPS may develop hyperexcitability of the motor cortex. It has been suggested that downregulation of the cortical excitability may improve symptoms.

Psychosocial factors
- There is no evidence that psychological factors may lead to the development of CRPS. However, psychological stress and prolonged pain may lead to behavioural changes and may influence the perception and response to pain.

Diagnosis
Symptoms and signs
- Pain:
  - Aching, burning, pricking or shooting
  - Localized deep in somatic tissue
  - Aggravated by mechanical stimulation or joint movement
  - Usually located in the distal part of an extremity but can spread proximally and can involve the entire limb and occasionally the ipsilateral quadrant of the body
- Sensory disturbances:
  - Hyperesthesia
  - Hyperalgesia to mechanical or thermal stimuli
  - Allodynia
  - Temperature sensitivity
  - Hypoesthesia
  - May affect the entire extremity or complete body side
- Autonomic dysfunction:
  - Swelling
  - Colour changes (red and mottled)

- Temperature changes (usually warmer but may turn cold in the later course of the condition)
- Sweating abnormalities
- Motor function impairment:
  - Weakness
  - Reduced ROM
  - Tremor
  - Dystonia
  - Myoclonus
- Trophic changes:
  - Altered nail growth (brittle and grooved)
  - Altered skin growth (thin and shiny progressing to hyperkeratosis and palmar fibrosis)
  - Altered hair growth (increased)
  - Bone demineralization

Patients with CRPS typically adopt a protective posture, cover the affected limb and may dislike the limb being examined or touched.

Tests

No single test confirms the diagnosis of CRPS. History, clinical examination and laboratory tests assist. Useful diagnostic tools include:
- Blood tests—to exclude other diseases
- X-ray: osteopaenia
- Triple phase bone scan: alteration in perfusion phase
- Quantitative Sensory Testing (QST):
  - Assesses quantitatively function of small fibres
  - May show hypothermaesthesia to warm stimuli with reduced pain thresholds
- Infrared thermography:
  - 90% of patients with CRPS demonstrate temperature side differences
- Pressure pain thresholds (using a dolorimeter)

Natural course of CRPS

CRPS may pass through three continuous stages

Stage 1: hours to weeks
- Onset of severe pain
- Localized oedema
- Stiffness and limited joint ROM
- Skin warm, red and dry to touch (progressing to cold, sweaty and cyanosed)
- Increased sensitivity to touch and pressure
- Muscle cramps

Stage 2: weeks to months
- Pain more severe and diffuse, spreading proximally
- Oedema spreads and becomes brawny
- Skin cools
- Hair becomes course
- Nails grow faster then slow and brittle
- Early muscle wasting
- Osteoporosis commences

Stage 3: months +
- Pain becomes intractable and may involve the entire limb
- Contractures
- Limited joint motion
- Marked wasting
- Osteoporosis
- Psychological and emotional problems
- May last indefinitely

Management
- Management must be multiprofessional and should involve the patient.
- Early diagnosis and prompt treatment are essential to:
  - Restore function
  - Relieve pain
  - Provide psychological support

Pharmacological
- Antidepressants:
  - Established efficacy for the treatment of neuropathic pain
  - Tryciclic antidepressants (TCAs): amitryptilene, nortriptyline, desipramine
  - TCAs have poorly tolerated adverse reactions (urinary retention, nightmares, weight gain, drowsiness, dry mouth and constipation)
- Anticonvulsants:
  - Established efficacy for the treatment of neuropathic pain
  - Gabapentin, pregabalin
- Non-gabapentinoid anti-epilepsy drugs (AEDs):
  - Topiramate
  - Other AEDS may have an adjuvant analgesic effect in neuropathic pain
- Steroids:
  - Efficacy limited
- Non-steroidal anti-inflammatory drugs (NSAIDs):
  - Trials are lacking
  - Effect may be limited
- Opioids:
  - May have a peripheral analgesic affect during painful inflammatory states
  - Chronic pain may require the use of long-acting agents (methadone) or controlled release preparations (morphine)
  - Tramadol has been shown to be effective in the treatment of neuropathic pain
- Bone metabolism modulators:
  - Biophosphonates: studies have revealed a dose-dependent analgesic effect on inflammatory, neuropathic and cancer pain
  - Calcitonin: indicated for patients with bone pain. Reduces resporption by inhibiting osteoclastic activity
- Alpha blockers (prozocin, phenoxybenamine)
- Clonidine:
  - Intraspinal clonidine for controlling neuropathic pain
  - Found to potentiate intrathecal opioid analgesia

- Capsaicin:
  - Natural substance present in hot chillis
  - Produces a prolonged deactivation of capsaicin-sensitive nocioceptors
  - Analgesic effect is dose-dependent
  - May last for several weeks
- GABA (neurotransmitter):
  - GABA-B agonist: baclofen—effective in the treatment of CRPS related dystonia
  - GABA-A agonist: benzodiazepines—clinical use for chronic pain is controversial
- Mannitol 10%:
  - 1000mls/day, continuous infusion for 7 days
- DMSO 50% in water (anti oxidant)
  - Topical for 5 days
- Vitamin C:
  - Free radical scavenger
  - Used prophylactically to prevent CRPS

Interventions
- Intravenous regional anaesthesia (IVRA):
  - Local anaesthetic into the venous system (Biers block)
  - Depletes post-ganglionic noradrenaline (NA)
  - May be considered to facilitate hand therapy
- Chemical sympathetic nerve block (stellate ganglion block, guanethidine block):
  - Randomized trials suggest very limited effect except probably for those with marked cold intolerance as part of their symptomatology. Much less widely used than before.
- Surgical sympathectomy:
  - Not all patients respond
- Spinal cord stimulation:
  - Implantable devices used successfully to provide symptomatic relief
  - Produces sympathetic outflow inhibition
  - Research has demonstrated that spinal cord stimulation provides an analgesic effect even to those patients that have a sympathectomy, suggesting that its mode of action may not mediated by inhibition of the sympathetic function
  - Evidence suggests that it should be considered relatively early in the treatment (3–4 months) from onset of symptoms
- Dorsal root procedure/dorsal root entry zone (DREZ):
  - Uses electric current to remove nerves by heating them to disrupt pain signals
- Infusion techniques:
  - Intrapleural catheters/epidurals
  - Requires inpatient admission
  - Requires intensive hand therapy

Surgery

- If the CRPS is being promoted by neurogenic pain (e.g. neuroma, compression) then that stimulus may need surgery to achieve resolution of the CRPS.
- Otherwise, one should beware surgery whilst the CRPS is still active, lest the painful stimulus of surgery aggravates the CRPS.
- Once the CRPS has resolved, residual joint contractures (distal radio-ulnar joint, PIPJ) can be addressed by surgery if hand therapy has not achieved an adequate range.

Hand therapy

Hand therapy is the main treatment for CRPS. The therapist often has most input with patients and may be the first to recognize the signs and symptoms. With careful assessment and a good rapport with the patient, a treatment programme can be devised that is patient-focused and achievable.

To ensure optimal results adequate education, support and pain relief are essential for the patient to maximize their potential and to ensure the successful application of treatment modalities.

Specific treatments:

- Pain:
  - TENS
  - Acupuncture
  - Splints (splinting that results in immobility is counterproductive, although splinting overnight might be useful)
  - Desensitization
  - Mobilization of the nervous system
  - Continuous passive motion (CPM)
  - Wax baths (this may have an adverse effect in early CRPS)
- Oedema:
  - Elevation
  - Retrograde massage
  - Active ROM
  - Contrast bathing
  - Pressure garments
- Joint stiffness:
  - Gentle exercise within the patient's tolerance
  - Contraindicated in an insensate area
  - Commence with gentle active and active assisted exercises
  - Avoid aggressive or passive exercises
  - Focus on postural normalization, stabilization and balanced use of limbs
  - Hydrotherapy may be beneficial
- Hypersensitivity:
  - Desensitization programme
  - Opsite flexifix
- Stress loading programme, weight-loading of joints through the affected limb:
  - Progressive programme
  - Patient required to scrub using a scrubbing brush on all fours
  - Placing weight on the arm as the patient scrubs in circles

- Patient is also required to carry small objects progressing to a handled bag that can be loaded with heavier weights
- Mirror therapy:
  - Congruent visual feedback of the moving unaffected limb via a mirror reduces the perception of pain and stiffness
  - When normal somatosensory feedback is missing mirror therapy restores the information flow from the posterior parietal cortex to the premotor cortex, thereby reducing pain and facilitating limb movement
  - Technique: Patient is seated and asked to visualize both limbs. A non-reflective board is placed perpendicular to the patient's midline with the unaffected limb facing the non reflective surface, with the affected limb hidden. The patient is asked to concentrate on the non reflective surface and for 5 minutes exercise their non-painful and if possible painful limb (flexion and extension exercises). A mirror is then positioned so that the unaffected limb is reflected in the mirror. Patients are asked to focus on the reflection and exercise both limbs for 5 minutes (same exercises). Patients are encouraged to use the mirror as often as they wish
- Functional restoration:
  - Emphasis on normalization of function
  - Home assessment
  - Vocational rehabilitation
  - Work hardening
  - Return to school
  - May require the use of adapted equipment
- Psychological problems:
  - Counselling
  - Behaviour modification
  - Relaxation
  - Imagery
  - Hypnosis
  - Coping skills

Prognosis

The prognosis is for CRPS is variable and seems to be partly dependent upon the severity of symptoms. Studies have reported resolution with a few months whereas others report symptom duration up to 5 years after diagnosis. Early diagnosis and prompt treatment are key to symptom relief and restoring function.

Anaesthesia

Local and regional anaesthesia

Local and regional anaesthesia is widely used in hand surgery due to its favourable attributes. These are mainly:

- Prevention of pain from reaching the central nervous system (CNS)
- Usefulness for emergency procedures as no need to starve
- Avoidance of intra- and postoperative complications of general anaesthetic (GA)
- Ideal for outpatient procedures
- Provision of postoperative pain relief
- Enables faster hospital discharge

Regional anaesthesia requires a trained anaesthetist. Complications include iatrogenic injury and failure to obtain anaesthesia with subsequent need to switch to GA.

Pharmacology of local anaesthetics

Chemical composition

Local anaesthetic agents (LA) are organic amines with an esther or amine linkage between the lipophilic head and hyrdrophilic tail of the molecule.

Mechanism of action

Anaesthesia is achieved by inhibition of the function of voltage-gated sodium channels in the axonal membrane. LA's bind to the channel molecule to prevent conformational changes inhibit opening of the channel. This leads to:

- Blockade of generation of action potentials
- Blockade of propagation of action potentials

And results in nerve conduction block.

Minimum concentration (Cm)

This is the drug concentration that stops electrical discharge of the nerve. It is specific for each LA and dependent on environment, i.e. pH, temperature etc.

Table 3.1 Examples of two chemical types of LA

Amines (metabolized in liver)	Esters (hydrolysed in plasma)
Lidocaine	Procaine
Mepivacaine	Amethocaine
Bupivacaine	
Prilocaine	

Differential action of LA drugs:

LA action on different types of nerve fibres is variable and dependent on
- Variations of diffusion
- Lipid solubility
- Fibre size (A–α motor least sensitive unmyelinated C and A–δ most sensitive)
- Degree of myelinization
- Internodal distances
- Irritability

Table 3.2 Potency and duration of action for some commonly used LA agents

	Potency	Duration of action
Procaine	Low	Short
Lidocaine Mepivacaine Prilocaine	Intermediate	Intermediate
Bupivacaine Ropivacaine Etidocaine Amethocaine	High	Long

Dosage

Nerves exhibit phasic or 'frequency-dependent inhibition' in response to LA agents. This means that a resting nerve is less sensitive to the effect of LA than stimulated nerve.

Toxicity of local anaesthetics

Toxic effects depend on injection site and total dose administered. Adding adrenaline at a concentration of 1:200 000 (5 µg/ml) decreases peak plasma concentration due to vasoconstriction and reduced absorption. This effect is variable between types of LA. Adrenaline has very little effect when mixed with prilocaine, etidocaine and bupivacaine. Usage of adrenaline for hand surgical anaesthesia is highly controversial, and therefore best avoided.

Local toxicity is extremely rare, hence nerves recover full sensation once the action is reversed. However, all LA's are toxic to the CNS and heart at high plasma concentrations. Constant alertness for signs of neurotoxicity and/or cardiotoxicity is required during administration. Direct injection into a blood vessel or intrathecal injection are the usual culprits. These may precipitate convulsions and coma. Allergy is rare to amine type LA's. Allergy to esters is often associated with known allergy to para-aminobenzoic acid (PABA).

Recommended maximum doses

- Bupivicaine 2mg/kg
- Bupivicaine with adrenaline 2mg/kg
- Lidocaine 3mg/kg
- Lidocaine with adrenaline 6mg/kg
- Prilocaine 6mg/kg
- Prilocaine with adrenaline 8mg/kg

Symptoms and signs of systemic toxicity

- Mild:
  - Headache
  - Ringing in the ears
  - Tingling and numbness around mouth and tongue
  - Blurred vision
  - Slurred speech
  - Muscle twitching
  - Restlessness
- Severe:
  - Convulsion
  - Bradycardia
  - Hypotension
  - Respiratory arrest

Treatment of toxicity

- Stop administration
- Establish airway
- Give oxygen
- Establish IV access and give fluids
- Midazolam to reduce risk of convulsions
- Prevent injury during convulsions
- Benzodiazepines, thiopental or propofol for convulsions
- Vasopressors (ephedrine/dopamine) or cardiotonics (milrinone) for reduced cardiac output
- Treat arrhythmias (amiodarone)

Peripheral nerve blockade

These are convenient and effective for limited surgery and avoid the risks of a full GA.

Advantages
- Can be performed by surgeon
- Minimal complication rate
- Provides postoperative analgesia

Disadvantages
- Unsuitable for extensive surgery
- Little or no effect on tourniquet pain

Local infiltration anaesthesia

Effective for small areas and minor surgery such as excision of small lumps of skin and subcutaneous tissue.

Anaesthetic injection technique
- Freeze skin with ethyl chloride or apply topical anaesthetic prior to inserting needle.
- Sterilize skin with alcohol, chlorhexidine or iodine.
- Do not move the injection needle at an angle whilst in tissue: the hypodermic needle tip has a slanted cutting edge and can easily sever nerves and vessels. The needle should be introduced in a straight line, the injection delivered and withdrawn in the same direction. If the needle needs to be redirected this should be done after withdrawal to the skin level.

Elbow block

Simple to perform, however infrequently used as it involves multiple injections for the radial, median, ulnar as well as medial and lateral antebrachial cutaneous nerves. It does not cover the area of tourniquet application. Same amount of anaesthetic yields a better result if used as a brachial plexus block, as long as this skill is available.

Wrist block

Median, ulnar and superficial radial nerve is blocked. Simple to perform, but does not cover tourniquet pain. Limited motor block (because long flexors and extensors still active).

Technique
- *Median nerve* (MN): lies between palmaris longus (PL) and flexor carpi radialis (FCR) tendons. For safer injection, avoiding injury to the nerve, the needle is inserted just ulnar to PL and directed at 30° in frontal and sagittal planes
- *Ulnar nerve*: infiltrate just radial to flexor carpi ulnaris (FCU) tendon.
- *Superficial radial nerve*: infiltrate subcutaneously about 3cm proximal to the radial styloid.

Digital block

Both proper digital nerves (palmar) and both dorsal primary branches need to be blocked for complete anaesthesia.

Technique
- *Dorsal approach*: Insert needle to one side of the extensor tendon at MCPJ level. Block dorsal nerve then advance needle volarly and block volar digital nerve. Withdraw needle just short of exiting skin and redirect transversely across the dorsum superficial to extensor. Block contralateral dorsal nerve. Withdraw and remove needle, reinsert on contralateral side to block volar nerve.
- *Volar approach* (single injection technique): Insert needle at MCP joint level in the midline. Inject LA in the fatty plane anterior to the joint. Redirect the needle to inject around dorsal digital nerves at each side.
- *Flexor tendon sheath technique*: Start as above with a volar midline insertion and advance the needle to enter the flexor sheath. Inject LA into the sheath from where it will disperse to the digital nerves via the microcirculation.

Complications of peripheral nerve blocks
- Unexpected extension of block to neighbouring area
- Damage to neighbouring structures
- Toxicity
- Nerve damage

Accidental injection of LA into a peripheral nerve may occur especially when the patient is unconscious, such as when under GA. The damage is increased in the presence of adrenaline. If numbness or a radiating sensation is reported by the patient, the needle should immediately be withdrawn and redirected.

Regional anaesthesia

IV regional anaesthesia (Bier's block)

This technique entails emptying the extremity's veins with the use of compressive bandage , inflation of a tourniquet to prevent further arterial inflow followed by injection of a sufficient volume of LA to fill the empty venous bed. The LA then diffuses into the surrounding tissues to effect anaesthesia.

Advantages
- Versatile
- Easy to perform, requires little training
- Effective
- Can be done on both sides simultaneously (beware overdose)
- Rapid return of motor function

Disadvantages
- Special double-cuff tourniquet required
- Cuff pain limits useful anaesthesia to 1hr
- Systemic toxicity possible on release of tourniquet
- No muscle relaxation obtained

Technique
Establish venous access with a large bore canula (14–16G) and secure. Apply double-cuff tourniquet to upper arm. Use pneumatic exsanguinator, or Esmarch bandage to exsanguinate limb. Inflate proximal cuff only. Inject prilocaine at the dose of 6mg/kg or lidocaine 3mg/kg. Test for anaesthesia, normally 5 minutes is sufficient. Inflate distal cuff of the tourniquet and deflate proximal cuff. The distal cuff should now lie within the area already perfused by the LA.
DO NOT DEFLATE for at least 15 minutes (prilocaine) or 20 minutes (lidocaine). Otherwise risk of a systemic bolus at toxic dose.
DO NOT USE bupivicaine as more risk of toxicity.

Brachial plexus block

This is the most common and versatile regional anaesthetic technique for the upper limb. There are four approaches covering different levels of the upper limb:
- Interscalene
- Supraclavicular
- Infraclavicular
- Axillary

The intrascelene and supraclavicular technique provides anaesthesia for the shoulder, upper arm, elbow, forearm and hand. Infraclavicular and axillary approaches are used to cover the forearm and hand. Good knowledge of the applied anatomy is essential for appropriate utilization of these techniques. A nerve stimulator and ultrasound are helpful in locating the appropriate trunks and divisions.

Table 3.3 Characteristics of anaesthesia in brachial plexus block

	Anaesthetic volume (ml)	Onset	Duration	Complications
Interscalene	20–25	20–30	8–12	Uncommon but significant, may be fatal
Supraclavicular	25–40	20–30	8–12	Uncommon but significant, may be fatal
Infraclavicular	30–40	25–35	12	
Axillary	30–40	25–35	12	Insignificant

Complications of regional anaesthesia

- Central extension (subarachnoid, subdural, epidural), rare but dangerous
- Needle misplacement into intervertebral foramen
- Phrenic nerve paralysis (35–100%)
- Intra-arterial injection (vertebral or axillary artery), this is rare but potentially lethal
- Stellate ganglion block (Horner's syndrome)
- Recurrent nerve block
- Pneumothorax (0.6–6%)

Topical anaesthesia

Useful prior to venpuncture.

Ethyl chloride
Freezes skin, temporary numbness.
Highly flammable!

EMLA (eutectic mixture local anaesthetic) cream
Lidocaine, prilocaine + emulsifier + thickener + water.
Apply 2 to 5 hours prior to use

Ametop
Topical amethocane.
Apply 30 minutes prior to use. Remove after one hour. Lasts 4 to 6 hours

Tourniquet

The tourniquet is an essential tool in hand surgery, enabling a blood-free field. This, together with loupe, or occasionally microscopic magnification, allows proper visualization of the complex anatomy on which the surgeon operates.

History

1674 Morell: field garotte
1718 Jean Petit: *tourner* (to tighten)—screw device over an artery
1864 Joseph Lister: first to use a bloodless field for surgery
1877 Henry Martin: flat rubber tourniquet bandage
1904 Harvey Cushing: pneumatic tourniquet—major innovation as much safer

Types

Finger

- Rubber tube and clamp: this is to be abandoned. There is an uncontrolled pressure over a narrow area. Risk of nerve damage and skin necrosis.
- Rolled-glove. A glove finger is at its base. The tip of the glove finger is also cut off to result in a cylinder open at both ends. The residual glove is then rolled from distal to proximal, left as a cuff at the base of the finger. This elegantly exsanguinates the finger and acts as a tourniquet. Pressure damage is possible, but unlikely with a generous-sized glove and relatively short (<30 minutes) time.

Forearm

Limited by the conical shape of the forearm which precludes a good fit and even distribution of pressure.

Above elbow

- Do not use Esmarch bandage. Uncontrolled pressure (900mmHg possible), skin necrosis, compartment syndrome, nerve crush
- Exsanguination:
  - Mark ganglions prior, otherwise may burst!
  - Rubber exsanguinator—check latex status. Need servicing.
  - Elevate only if some arterial definition needed, e.g. revision Dupuytrens, flaps
  - Do not exsanguinate in case of infection or malignancy to avoid metastasis
- Use device with alarm timer, pressure gauge, default settings 60 minutes, 250mmHg
- Set tourniquet pressure:
  - 50 to 75mm Hg above systolic pressure (BP can vary during procedure)
  - Slightly higher for obese patients
  - Lower for narrower cuffs
  - Lower for children
  - If set too low, may act as venous tourniquet—blood in but not out
- Observe tourniquet time:
  - Painful after 20 to 30 minutes, c-fibre activation due to ischaemia. Not reliably relieved by axillary blockade; scalene blockade better

- Direct pressure changes to skin, muscle, nerve
- Reperfusion injury to general circulation from metabolic toxins and free radicals causing systemic acidosis
- Less than 2 hours
- Mimimize inflation time:
  - Shave, sterilize, and mark skin prior to inflation
  - Plan surgery. Delay parts of procedure that do not need bloodless field—definitive fracture fixation, extensor tendon repair etc.
  - Regular reminders from theatre staff, set alarm
- Avoid re-inflation too soon as this will incur a second reperfusion injury:
  - Guidelines for re-inflation (based on Wilgis, pH returning to normal)

1hr	5 to 10 minutes
1½hrs	10 to 15 minutes
2hrs	15 to 20 minutes

- Deflate tourniquet before closure:
  - Confirm arterial perfusion (Dupuytren's, sympathectomy, dissection near major vessels)
  - Avoid haematoma
  - Reflex hyperaemia (may reduce risk of venous thrombosis. Clotting time increases as pH falls; bipolar diathermy to persistent bleeding points)
  - Avoid tight dressings. Volume of arm swells up to 10% after deflation so dressings could occlude.

Bone and joint injuries— wrist and forearm

Bone and joint injuries—wrist and forearm

Anatomy

The wrist and elbow together with the forearm constitute a quadrilateral functional unit. This includes the proximal radioulnar joint (PRUJ) including the stabilizing annular ligament, the radius and ulna held together by the interosseous membrane (IOM) and the distal radioulnar joint (DRUJ) with its stabilizing ligaments unified as the triangular fibro-cartilage complex (TFCC).

Biomechanics

The proximal and distal radioulnar joints (PRUJ, DRUJ) move together with the interosseous membrane as the stabilizer to simulate a ginglymus joint of which one condyle is the radius and the other the ulna. The axis of rotation is between the centre of the radiocapitellar joint and the fovea of the ulna. The DRUJ both rotates and glides during rotation. The ulna is the stable joint of the forearm; the radius is merely suspended by the IOM, annular ligament and TFCC. Stability is maintained by the tone of muscles passing transversely or obliquely across the radius and ulna, as well as the articular congruity of the PRUJ and DRUJ. The ulna head should never be excised as it destabilizes the entire forearm joint.

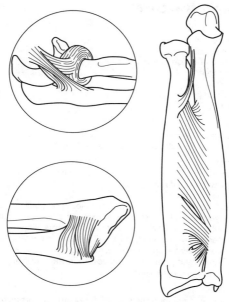

Fig. 4.1 Anatomy of proximal and distal radioulnar joints and the interosseous membrane.

Forearm fractures

Classification

- One bone
- Both bones
- Fracture dislocation of forearm joint
  - Monteggia
  - Galeazzi
  - Essex–Lopresti
- Children's

One bone

It is an unusual injury pattern to just break one bone in the ring. More common to have a dislocation at one end or another.

Ulnar shaft

Due to the subcutaneous position of most of the ulnar shaft, these injuries normally result from direct impact, such as falls or being hit (e.g. night stick injury). Always check PRUJ alignment.

If undisplaced, can be treated in above-elbow cast but risk of displacement, delayed union, stiffness and weakness or arm. Open reduction and anatomical fixation (under compression if fragments allow, if not bridging plate), is generally recommended to allow early movement and secure anatomical alignment. If open fracture, thorough wound debridement, rigid internal fixation and primary wound cover. Consider primary bone grafting if high energy or comminuted.

Radial shaft

Apart from the distal third the shaft of the radius, well protected by overlying muscular tissue. Isolated fracture rare. Treatment similar to isolated ulna fracture. Always check DRUJ alignment.

Radial nerve particularly vulnerable in fixation of proximal third. Henry approach, holding forearm supinated to protect nerve.

Both bones

Usually displaced and unstable. Often high energy—watch for compartment syndrome. Unless undisplaced or contraindications for surgery, recommend open reduction-internal fixation (ORIF).

Fracture dislocation of forearm joint

Monteggia fracture dislocation

This injury involves fracture of the proximal ulna together with dislocation of the PRUJ. Anatomical reduction of the ulnar fracture and rigid fixation is required.

FOREARM FRACTURES **103**

Table 4.1 Bado classification of Monteggia fracture-dislocations

Type	Description	Percentage*
I	Fracture of middle or proximal third of ulna and anterior dislocation of radial head	65
II	Fracture of the middle or proximal third of ulna and posterior dislocation of radial head	18
III	Ulnar fracture distal to coronoid process with lateral radial head dislocation	16
IV	Fracture of proximal or middle third of ulna with an anterior dislocation of radial head and fracture of the proximal third of radius	1

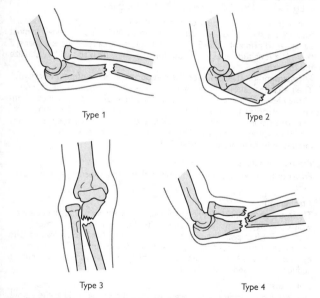

Type 1

Type 2

Type 3

Type 4

Fig. 4.2 Monteggia variants. The same injury mechanism produces various patterns of injury.

Galeazzi fracture

This injury involves fracture of the distal third of the radial shaft with subluxation or dislcation of the DRUJ.

Treatment is surgical—accurate reduction and rigid fixation of the radius fracture. The DRUJ is usually reduced and stable; if not it may need temporary stabilization with a K-wire across the DRUJ in mid-rotation; if irreducible, the DRUJ should be opened, the obstructing elements removed and then repaired, followed by K-wire across the DRUJ.

Essex Lopresti lesion

Longitudinal force transfer through the wrist, forearm up to the elbow. May affect a number of structures, most notably:
- Radial head
- Central band of IOM
- Ligaments of the DRUJ including TFCC attachment.

The most important aspect of treatment is to maintain the radial head. If fractured it should be repaired; if it is too comminuted for repair it must be replaced primarily. NEVER remove the radial head and leave a space: if there is a longitudinal injury of the forearm joint then this will destabilize the forearm.

Treatment for an established Essex–Lopresti injury is often unsuccessful. The radial head should be replaced if still feasible (after time the alignment of the neck with the capitellum and radial notch of the proximal ulna cannot be restored). Distal ulnar shortening osteotomy will reduce symptoms of ulnacarpal impaction and may stabilize the distal forearm by tightening the interosseous membrane. There is no established reliable technique for interosseous membrane reconstruction.

Forearm fractures in children

Forearm fractures are very common in childhood. Open injuries are also seen.

Mechanism

These are commonly low-energy injuries, e.g. falls from a bike, direct impact whilst playing ball sports etc. Due to its thickness, the periosteum has a protective effect against displacement far beyond that it provides in adults. Fractures of the greenstick type have one cortex intact. This makes reduction difficult. Also, fractures of only one forearm bone are difficult to reduce with closed manipulation.

Diagnosis

Swelling and deformity. X-rays are diagnostic and should include the elbow as well as wrist joint.

Treatment

Closed manipulation is possible for most, normally under GA. Suspension in finger traps can help.The fracture is immobilized in an above-elbow plaster with three-point fixation. If the fracture is proximal to pronator teres, the forearm is held in supination: if it is distal to pronator teres, then the forearm is held in neutral. If satisfactory, splintage is retained until both fractures are united (depends on age). Fractures that are impossible to reduce or keep reduced require fixation. Flexible nails are preferred, avoiding the growth plate. Alternatives are K-wires or plates.

The acceptable malalignment (angulation, translation or rotation) depends on the location of the fracture as well as the age of the child. As a rule of thumb a minimum of 2 years of growth potential is required for satisfactory remodelling. Table 4.2 shows the maximum acceptable malalignment for different fractures.

Table 4.2 Acceptable limits of malalignment for children's forearm fractures

Age	Location	Translation	Angulation (degrees)
<9	Any level	Complete	15
>9	Forearm	Unicortical	10
	Wrist	Complete	15

Children may also sustain a Galeazzi or Monteggia fracture. The PRUJ and DRUJ must be carefully checked. A proximal ulna fracture in a child (Monteggia) is challenging. The fracture must be perfectly reduced to secure a congruous PRUJ, which is difficult in a greenstick fracture or if there is plastic deformation. Incomplete ossification of the elbow epiphyses also confuses reduction.

In these cases significant length difference between radius and ulna may ensue. The presence of an Essex–Lopresti injury is an indication for anatomic reduction and internal fixation of the radial fracture, as well as the DRUJ.

Ulnar corner injuries

Dislocation of the DRUJ

Fractures of the distal radius may be accompanied by dislocations of the DRUJ due to injury to the TFCC. The TFCC includes dorsal and volar radiocarpal ligaments and is a powerful stabilizer of the joint together with the interosseous membrane. The clinical sign is described as 'piano keying' which is painful in the acute state. Prono-supination is painful and limited. Other causes of DRUJ have been described, such as fractures of the ulnar head and incarceration of the ECU tendon in the joint. The DRUJ may dislocate without a fractured radius.

Fractures of the distal ulna

Fractures of the distal ulna may be grouped into:
- Ulnar styloid fractures
- Ulnar head fractures
- Ulnar neck fractures

Ulnar styloid fractures
- Common with distal radial fractures.
- If at the tip, stable. Treat symptomatically.
- If at base, associated with DRUJ instability, because it involves a large fragment including the fovea to which the TFCC attaches. If displaced, secure with a headless compression screw or tension band wiring if displaced to ensure normal tension of the TFCC.

Ulnar head fractures
- Uncommon, they may be seen with high energy or open injuries.
- Fixation is difficult. If good bone, fixation with buried screws. If poor bone or too comminuted, consider primary ulnar head replacement.
- Poor results with Darrach's.

Ulnar neck fractures
- Common with distal radius fractures.
- These should be surgically treated at the time of the fixation of the distal radius to prevent deformity and limitation of prono-supination.
- A low-profile blade plate or better still locking plate is used in order to gain adequate unicortical purchase in the ulnar head.

TFCC injuries

Anatomy
- Anterior and posterior radioulnar ligaments
- Meniscal homologue
- Ulnocarpal ligaments
- Underside of extensor carpi ulnaris (ECU) sheath.

Function
- Aid the transfer of force across the ulnocarpal articulation. This constitutes about 35% of the total load going through the wrist joint with 65% going through the radiocarpal articulation.
- Connect ulnar head to sigmoid notch of radius.

Injury
- Central perforation from longitudinal compression
- Avulsion from base of fovea
- Pulling off large fragment of ulnar styloid
- Radial avulsion
- Tear of anterior or posterior limb

Table 4.3 Classification of traumatic TFCC tear according to Palmer

Palmer Type 1 traumatic TFCC tear	
A	Central perforation
B	Ulnar avulsion (with or without ulnar fracture)
C	Distal avulsion
D	Radial avulsion (with or without sigmoid notch fracture)

Symptoms
- Depends on type of injury.
- Pain accentuated by ulnar deviation of the wrist, particularly with loading (e.g. tasks such as hard gripping of a tool handle, lifting a kettle or a saucepan, pushing oneself up from a sitting position etc.), pain on rotation, DRUJ instability, frank dislocation
- Clicking or clunking on rotation

Signs
- Again, depends on type of injury
- Tender over ulnar head
- Pain on rotation
- Instability on balloting ulnar head
- Pain on ulnocarpal compression

Investigation
- Standard X-rays (views at mid-rotation, elbow 90°, shoulder 90°) may show a narrowing of the ulnocarpal gap (this predisposes to central perforation).
- Fracture of base of styloid or sigmoid notch.
- MRI scan enhanced by gadolinium provides accurate information in doubtful cases.
- A diagnostic arthroscopy may be performed to verify the diagnosis and to treat a tear.

Treatment
Depends on type of injury
- Rest in splint (minor symptoms and signs)
- Repair fracture ulnar styloid base
- Arthroscopic debridement of central perforation
- Reattachment of avulsion (open or arthroscopic)
- Later reconstruction for chronic instability (see p. 478)

Fractures of the distal radius in adults

Types of fracture

The distal radius is prone to various patterns of injury
- Low-energy Colles'
- High-energy fractures
- Smith's
- Barton's
- Radial styloid

Classification

There are multiple classification systems for distal radius fractures. These are shown in Figs 4.3, 4.4 and 4.5.

Frykman classification of distal radius fractures
see Fig. 4.3.

Table 4.4 Frykman classification

Type I:	Extra-articular
Type II:	Type I with ulnar styloid fracture
Type III:	Involvement of the radiocarpal joint
Type IV:	Type III with ulnar styloid fracture
Type V:	Involvement of the distal radioulnar joint
Type VI:	Type V with ulnar styloid fracture
Type VII:	Involvement of the radiocarpal and radioulnar joints
Type VIII:	Type VII with ulnar styloid fracture

Melone classification
see Fig. 4.4.

Fernandez–Jupiter classification.
see Fig. 4.5.

Table 4.5 Fernandez–Jupiter classification

Type I:	Metaphyseal bending fracture (Colles' and Smith fracture)
Type II:	Shear fracture of the joint surface (Barton fracture)
Type III:	Compression fracture of the joint surface
Type IV:	Avulsion fracture associated with ligamentous injury
Type V:	High-energy injury (combination of mechanisms)

AO classification

The AO classification is organized into three groups—A, B, and C which are subdivided into numbered subsets on the basis of joint involvement If the full AO classification is used, there are 27 potential fracture patterns. The interobserver agreement for this classification is poor.

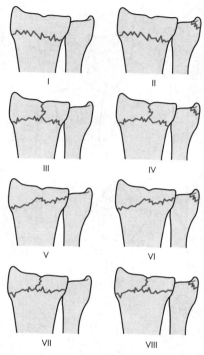

Fig. 4.3 Frykman classification of distal radius fractures.

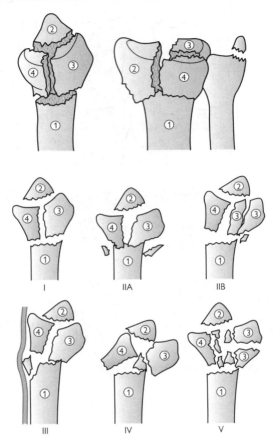

Fig. 4.4 Intra-articular fracture classification of Melone. The four fragments are:
① radial shaft, ② radial styloid, ③ dorsal-ulnar facet, ④ volar ulnar facet.

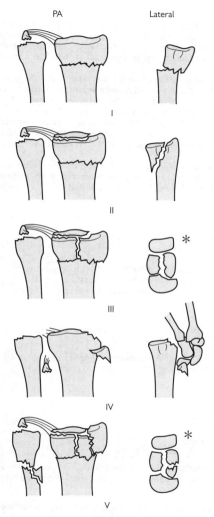

Fig. 4.5 Fernandez–Jupiter classification.

Normal values

The quality of reduction can be assessed by the following measurements:

Distal radial inclination: This is measured on the postero-anterior film and is the angle between the longitudinal axis of the radius and a line drawn through the ulnar corner and the tip of the radial styloid. The normal average angle is 22°.

Distal radial tilt: This angle is measured on the lateral film and is the angle between the longitudinal axis of the radius and a line drawn through the dorsal and volar lips of the distal radius. The normal average angle is 11°.

Distal radial height: The radius shortens down as a result of bone comminution and impaction caused by the fracture. The radial height is measured on a PA film and constitutes the distance between the tip of the radial styloid and the distal articular surface of the ulna. The normal average is 11mm.

Ulnar variance: The vertical difference between the distal articular surface of the radius and ulna, measured on an X-ray centred on the carpus, mid pro-supination, elbow 90° flexed, shoulder abducted 90°.

Rule of 11's

22 degrees radial inclination
11 degrees radial tilt
11 degrees distal radial height

Colles' fracture

Colles fracture (Abraham Colles, Irish surgeon, 1814) is predominantly seen in the above-50 age group and consists of a distal radial fracture with dorsal displacement with or without an avulsion fracture of the ulnar styloid.

Mechanism

The most common mechanism is a fall on the outstretched hand.

Diagnosis

Classical 'dinner fork' deformity. PA and lateral radiographs are required to show the amount of shortening, displacement and comminution.

Treatment options

- Plaster cast
- K-wires
- External fixation
- Locked volar plate
- Intramedullary locked nail
- Dorsal plate

No clear guidelines or randomized controlled trial (RCT) data. Match treatment to personality of fracture, surgeon's skill and facilities available

Undisplaced fractures

Plaster immobilization for 4 weeks. Check X-ray at one week to exclude displacement.

Displaced fractures

- Can usually be manipulated into a good position under haematoma block or regional anaesthesia but maintenance of the achieved alignment in plaster-of-Paris (POP) is extremely difficult.
- The plaster is moulded to keep the wrist volarly flexed by about 30° volar flexion and 10° ulnar deviation. No more angulation, otherwise risk of carpal tunnel syndrome and CRPS. Plaster may be below or above the elbow, the latter controlling brachioradialis pull.
- Due to osteoporosis especially in females the fracture is prone to bone impaction (= loss of bone volume and hence length). Redisplacement is therefore extremely common, particularly in cases of severe osteoporosis and lacking dorsal bone stock.
- Acceptance of a displaced position is appropriate for low-demand individuals. If anatomical reduction is preferred then various options are available, as listed above.
- Primary K-wiring after manipulation is preferred in such cases, although displacement is still possible as fixation can 'cheese-wire' through the soft bone.
- Dorsal buttress should therefore be reconstructed using bone substitute through a mini dorsal incision in addition to K-wire fixation.
- ORIF with a locking plate (dorsal or volar) is the preferred alternative for fit and functionally demanding individuals.
- Alternative is K-wire fixation and neutralization of longitudinal compressive force with an external fixator, plus supplementary percutaneous bone substitute into dorsal defect.

Outcome

The outcome determinants for extra-articular fractures are:
- Restoration of radial length
- Restoration of the distal radial inclination
- Restoration of distal radial tilt
- Technique of conservative treatment (position of POP, tightness)
- Technique of operative treatment (metalwork complications, surgical mishaps)
- Compliance with rehabilitation

Poor outcome is associated with:
- Loss of radial length by more than 5mm
- Distal radial tilt of more than +20° dorsiflexion
- Distal radial inclination of less than 15°

Technique of dorsal plate fixation

Under tourniquet and antibiotic prophylaxis, a dorsal midline incision is made. Lister's tubercle is palpated to locate the third extensor compartment. The compartment is opened and extensor pollicis longus (EPL) tendon retracted. From this point a subperiosteal approach is made under the 2nd and 4th compartments. The fracture is thus exposed, reduced and held using low profile plates. The EPL tendon is left outside the compartment and the retinaculum is closed underneath to provide separation from the fracture and plate. Complications include tendon rupture, intra-articular penetration of screws, non-union, infection, stiffness, and dystrophy.

Technique of volar plate fixation

Under tourniquet and antibiotic prophylaxis a volar incision is made along the FCR tendon. FCR is retracted ulnarwards and the floor of the tunnel is incised to expose pronator quadratus (PQ). The PQ is sharply elevated off the radius and the fracture is exposed. Buttress or locking plates are used depending on fracture type. Only skin is sutured. Complications include dorsal screw protrusion with tendon rupture, joint penetration, fraying of flexor pollicis longus (FPL) or abductor pollicis longus and extensor pollicis brevis (APL/EPB) tendons, non-union, infection, stiffness, dystrophy and median nerve traction palsy.

Technique for highly comminuted fractures

An external fixator is applied to the wrist with pins in the radius and second metacarpal. The bolts are not tightened. The hand is suspended using an arthroscopy tower and fingertraps. A countertraction bar may also be used. The C-arm image intensifier is brought in from the side and fragments of suitable size are fixed using K-wires. When satisfactory reduction is obtained the external fixator is tightened to neutralize the pull of muscles. The hand is taken off the tower and final X-rays are taken to ensure that the fracture is not overdistracted. Complications include pin tract infection, pin pullout, damage to nearby tendons, nerves and vessels, overdistraction of the fracture, joint stiffness and dystrophy.

High-energy fractures

Mechanism

These fractures are generally seen as a result of falls from a height and road traffic collisions. The hallmarks of these injuries are comminution and intra-articular involvement. They may also present as compound injuries. They are found in younger high-demand individuals and should be treated more aggressively than Colles' fractures.

Diagnosis

These injuries may be seen as part of a polytrauma patient. X-rays taken in the resuscitation room may be of poor quality but they should guide the initial management of the injury.

Treatment

- Life- and limb-threatening injuries take precedence and the advanced trauma life support (ATLS) protocol should be followed. Treatment of the injury should not be unduly delayed.
- Fracture-dislocations should be reduced expeditiously and splinted in the best possible position pending definitive treatment.
- Special attention should be given to:
  - Compound injuries
  - Median nerve compression
  - Compartment syndrome
- *Undisplaced fractures:* treat in plaster for 5 weeks, check X-rays at 7 and 14 days for displacement
- *Displaced extra-articular fractures:* closed reduction. Plaster if stable, if not percutaneous wires or locked volar plate.
- *Intra-articular fractures:* need anatomical reduction. Treatment matches fracture configuration, surgeon skills, and implants available. If the fragments are of sufficient size closed reduction and K-wire fixation is recommended if reduction can be achieved closed. ORIF with a locking plate is preferred if this is not possible. In case of extensive comminution with insufficient fragment size for K-wire or screw purchase, an external fixator is chosen to hold the fracture out to length (neutralization). K-wires are used to fix large size fragments, bone graft to fill defects. Traction tower and arthroscopic guidance may be helpful.

Outcomes

The outcome determinants for intra-articular fractures are:
- All of the factors discussed above plus
  - Restoration of the articular congruency to within 2mm

Smith's fracture (□ see Fig. 4.6)

Smith's fracture is an extra-articular distal radius fracture with volar displacement of the distal fragment. It is therefore sometimes referred to as a 'reverse Colles' fracture'. The treatment for this injury is usually accomplished by volar plating, although conservative treatment in a cast with wrist dorsiflexion is possible.

Barton's fracture (📖 see Fig. 4.7)

Barton's fracture is an intra-articular lip fracture of the distal radial surface. There can be a dorsal lip or a volar lip fracture. The fracture is prone to displace volarly and proximally by the 'weight' of the carpus. This in turn causes a subluxation of the radiocarpal joint. Non-operative treatment of this injuriy is difficult, particularly for the volar type, and the results are unsatisfactory. Volar buttress plating is the preferred treatment.

Volar buttress plating of distal radius

The distal radius is approached through a volar approach, as described above. The fracture is reduced by traction and dorsiflexion of the wrist. A stout plate is applied in 'buttress mode', i.e. by putting in the proximal screws to allow the plate to abut against the fracture fragment, thereby compressing it down. No screws are required in the fracture fragment as this would interfere with the buttressing effect. The wound is closed and the wrist is rested in slab. Rehabilitation may commence after suture removal.

Radial styloid

The fracture of the radial styloid takes place by dorsiflexion and ulnar deviation of the wrist. It may be the first stage of a perilunate fracture-dislocation described below. Fully undisplaced fractures are amenable to conservative treatment in a cast, however being an intra-articular injury any displaced fracture should be fixed to restore the articular congruency of the distal radius. Furthermore the styloid bears the origin of radiocarpal ligaments, hence its non-union or malunion causes instability of the wrist. Surgical treatment can be accomplished by percutaneous fixation with a cannulated screw. This could be facilitated by arthroscopic visualization of the joint surface during fixation. These fractures are associated with a high rate of post-traumatic arthritis.

Salvage of malunited distal radius fractures

In cases of symptomatic malunion distal radial osteotomy is indicated. The timing of this operation is best no earlier than 6 months but also no later than 18 months from the fracture date. A dorsal or volar approach may be used. The operation involves dividing the distal radius at the malunion site using a cooled saw. The distal fragment is distracted and angled to achieve a relationship as close as possible to the anatomical parameters described above. Corticocancellous iliac bone graft is used to fill the gap, which may be supplemented with bone substitute in the absence of good-quality iliac bone. The construct is plated from dorsal or volar; the current standard is to use locking plates. It may be necessary to perform an ulnar shortening osteotomy at a later date, in cases where satisfactory restoration is not achieved. However, these two procedures should never be performed at the same time to avoid cross-union.

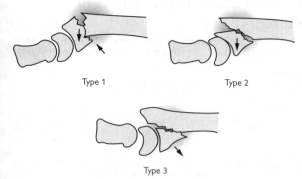

Type 1

Type 2

Type 3

Fig. 4.6 Smith's fracture. Modified Thomas classification. Type 1, extra-articular, transverse; type 2, extra-articular, oblique with palmar carpal displacement; and type 3, intra-articular palmar displacement of the carpus. Type 3 is equivalent to a palmar Barton fracture-dislocation.

(a)   (b)

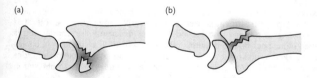

Fig. 4.7 Barton's fracture dislocation (a) palmar Barton; (b) dorsal Barton.

Fractures of the distal radius in children

These are very common and are usually the result of low-energy trauma. Due to the thickness and protective nature of the periosteum extreme displacement is unusual. Fractures may be:

- Undisplaced
- Displaced: 📖 see Fig. 4.8, Salter–Harris (S-H) classification
- Greenstick variety (also called torus)
- Adult-type displaced

Usual mechanism is a fall on the outstretched hand, the non-dominant wrist is injured more commonly.

Diagnosis

Some fractures are not obviously deformed. Swelling and non-usage may be the only sign. PA and lateral X-rays are diagnostic.

Injury to the growing wrist

The presence of the physis is the main determinant in the differential pathogenesis of these fractures. This is because the physis has reduced resistance to trauma compared with the adjacent metaphyseal or epiphyseal bone. The ulna can also sustain growth plate injuries although it is less common than the radius.

Treatment

Before any treatment is commenced it is important to explain to the parents (and the child) that growth disturbance may occur regardless of the type of treatment chosen. Residual displacement may be tolerated according to the age of the child. Younger children will remodel better than older ones due to the time left for growth. POP application in babies and toddlers requires special attention as retention is a problem, therefore above-elbow POP is preferred. Undisplaced fractures are immobilized in a POP cast for comfort. Displaced fractures of the greenstick type and of the adult type are reduced closed under GA and immobilized in a plaster. Only in cases of frank instability is fixation with K-wires indicated. Fixation is preferably achieved using smooth pins (Kirschner wires). Any surgical trauma to the growth plate should be kept at a minimum to lessen the chance of physeal arrest. This is achieved by reducing the number of passes, going through at 90° and by restricting to a maximum of 2 K-wires. Screws may be used to fix the bony fragments in S-H type II-IV injuries. Joint or physeal incongruity is mostly seen in type III and IV injuries.

Outcome of growth plate injuries

Contrary to the caveats, growth disturbance is uncommon considering the frequency of these injuries. S-H type I and II injuries rarely cause growth disturbance. S-H type III and IV (and V) have greater propensity to cause growth disturbance. Accurate closed or open reduction is required for these injuries

Treatment of physeal arrest

This is a serious problem ensuing from trauma, but also infection. The relationship of forearm bones is affected leading to shortening, deformity and instability of the limb. If the bony bridge is less than 50% and the child has growth potential, a physiolysis can be performed to enable continuation of growth. In cases where the deformity has already set in, an osteotomy is preferred after conclusion of growth.

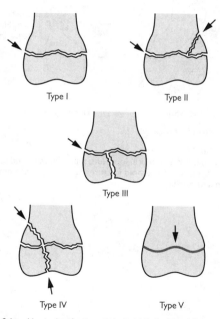

Fig. 4.8 Salter–Harris classification of physical injuries. Type I: Fracture through the physis (growth plate); Type II: a type I including metephyseal fragment; Type III: fracture of the epiphysis; Type IV: fracture through epiphysis, physis and metaphysic; Type V: crush injury to the physis.

Fractures of the scaphoid

Anatomy and physiology

The scaphoid is the most commonly fractured carpal bone. Because it is situated in a key position between the two carpal rows and helps to transfer significant loads from the hand to the forearm, fractures of the scaphoid present a challenge for diagnosis and management. The reasons for this are mainly its anatomical configuration and the blood supply. The main blood supply to the scaphoid enters the bone distally and dorsally. For this reason, the proximal pole of the bone is prone to be cut off from the circulation in very proximal fractures.

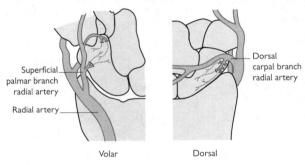

Superficial palmar branch radial artery

Radial artery

Dorsal carpal branch radial artery

Volar   Dorsal

Fig. 4.9 Blood supply of the scaphoid.

Location of injury

Fractures occur in three anatomical locations; tubercle, waist and proximal pole. Herbert has classified scaphoid fractures according to the time from injury, location and stability.

Type A
Stable acute fractures

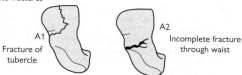

A1
Fracture of
tubercle

A2
Incomplete fracture
through waist

Type B
Unstable acute fractures

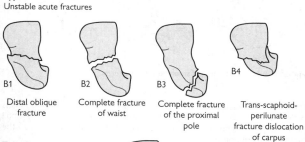

B1
Distal oblique
fracture

B2
Complete fracture
of waist

B3
Complete fracture
of the proximal
pole

B4
Trans-scaphoid-
perilunate
fracture dislocation
of carpus

Type C
Delayed union

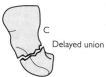

C
Delayed union

Type D
Established nonunion

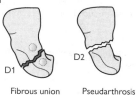

D1

D2

Fibrous union   Pseudarthrosis

Fig. 4.10 Herbert classification of scaphoid fractures.

Tubercle fractures are usually benign injuries. Due to the excellent blood supply of the area and the low mechanical demands, most fractures heal without any noticeable problems with minimal or no immobilization.

Waist fractures are the most common type of scaphoid fractures. The mechanical demands on this part are significant and blood supply is variable depending on the exact location. Nevertheless 85–90% of these fractures consolidate with conservative treatment. Russe has classified these fractures into three patterns namely horizontal oblique, transverse, and vertical oblique (📖 see Fig. 4.11).

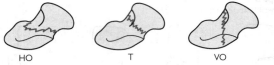

HO   T   VO

Fig. 4.11 Russe classification of scaphoid waist fractures.

Proximal pole fractures have the highest incidence of non-union. This is mainly due to lack of dedicated blood supply to this region. Very small proximal pole fragments may be extremely difficult to fix and have the highest rates of non-union.

Mechanism

Fractures of the scaphoid are sustained following a fall on the dorsiflexed outstretched hand.

Diagnosis

Symptoms

Pain is on the radial side of the wrist joint in the area between the FCR and extensor carpi radialis brevis (ECRL)/ extensor carpi radialis brevis (ECRB) tendons. Sometimes reduced movement and second dorsal compartment tendons.

Signs

Tender in the anatomical snuffbox and over the scaphoid tubercle. Sometimes swollen.

X-rays

Due to the paucity of reliable clinical signs one is reliant on good-quality radiographs. PA and lateral X-rays are not sufficient in visualizing scaphoid fractures; additional scaphoid views are needed, namely a PA radiograph centred on the scaphoid with the wrist in ulnar deviation and a pronation view, also called external oblique. A PA of a clenched ulnarly deviated fist with the tube angled proximally, i.e. towards the elbow, accentuates scaphoid extension and may help to show hidden fractures.

If there is no radiographic confirmation of the fracture at the initial stage but clinical suspicion of a fracture is strong, other imaging modalities, including bone scans, CT and MRI may be used.

Treatment

Uncertain fractures

As explained above, radiological visualization of the fracture is difficult in some cases. However, plaster treatment should be started even if the X-rays are normal. Repeat X-rays after two weeks, when—due to the initial bone resorption at the fracture site and hence widening fracture gap—it may be easier to see the injury. If this is not the case and the symptoms have disappeared there is no justification to continue plaster immobilization. If the symptoms are present but radiological proof is still lacking, the options are:

- Continue POP and further X-rays taken in 2 weeks
- CT
- MRI
- Isotope bone scan

Tubercle fractures

Cast for 6 weeks. Usually heal without any complications in the vast majority of cases. Occasional symptomatic non-union treated by excision of small fragment or grafting of large fragment.

Undisplaced waist fractures

The treatment of choice is a scaphoid type plaster worn for 8 weeks. X-rays then taken. If united, begin mobilization in splint. If not united, plaster for a further 4 weeks and repeat X-ray. If in doubt, CT scan. If on the CT scan, signs of non-union are present, treat as below. An X-ray or CT scan 3 months later is wise to exclude an overlooked persistence of fracture.

Percutaneous fixation should be offered to those who cannot tolerate plaster, e.g. sportsmen and light workers who may wish to resume work as soon as possible. Expertise and special screws needed. Risk of surgical complication.

Technique of percutaneous screw fixation

A cannulated headless screw system is used. A guide wire is laid along the skin under image intensification (II) and skin marked. Small incision is made over the scaphoid tubercle, Guide wire passed from the scapho-trapezoid (ST) joint along the medullary canal of the scaphoid. Position checked meticulously from several directions with II. After guide wire placement, cannulated drill and tap is used by hand followed by placement of the screw of appropriate length. A bulky bandage is sufficient and POP is not needed. Complications include infection, dystrophy and misplaced metal.

For proximal pole fragments, screw can be passed from proximal to distal. Wrist fully flexed and guide wire passed with II control.

Displaced waist fractures

These are unstable and prone to non-union. Attempt closed reduction and percutaneous fixation; if still displaced, then open reduction and cannulated screw fixation.

Proximal pole fractures

Plaster treatment: may need 4 or 5 months in plaster to unite; 30–40% will not unite.

Consider early screw fixation if skills and equipment available for those who cannot tolerate this prolonged time and uncertainty.

Non-union of the scaphoid

- About 10–15% of waist fractures and 30–40% of proximal pole fractures go on to non-union when treated conservatively. It is critical not to misdiagnose non-union too early as some fractures may progress to union at a late stage, i.e. beyond 12 weeks.
- The diagnosis of non-union may not be straightforward in some cases and requires CT.
- MRI is not useful as it does not define the cortex well and the medullary signal does not predict the outcome of surgery.

Patterns of non-union

- Persisting cortical breach, cystic resorption, alignment of scaphoid preserved. Affects proximal pole and waist.
- Humpback collapse—loss of palmar cortex, flexion of distal pole, compensatory extension of the lunate through the intact scapholunate ligament. Usually in the waist, preceded by cystic change.
- Increased density and fragmentation of proximal pole.

Predisposing factors

- Proximal pole fracture
- Delay in diagnosis more than 3 weeks
- Unstable or displaced waist fractures
- Smoking
- Inadequate in immobilization
- Poor fixation (e.g. distraction from inappropriate screw length)

Treatment

Once a firm diagnosis of non-union is established, a detailed discussion with the patient is needed to outline the treatment options. These are:

- Benign neglect. This approach is justifiable in patients who are above 50 years of age and do not have a manual occupation. The risk of osteoarthritis (OA) in particular SNAC wrist should be carefully explained to the patient.
- Percutaneous fixation and bone grafting. For those with preserved alignment. Compression fixation, and injection of bone graft into the cannulated drill space, a technically demanding option
- Wedge. Bone grafting and internal fixation (Fisk–Fernandez). For those with a humpback deformity. This option is preferred in young male patients whose occupation is mainly manual. This approach is aimed at achieving bony union, or at least fibrous union in the presence of mechanical stability between fragments so as to ensure concerted

movement of the scaphoid bone. Complications include infection, stiffness, and persisting non-union. About 80% union rate.

Surgical technique for structural bone grafting and compression screw fixation (Fisk–Fernandez)

The involved upper limb and one iliac crest is prepped and draped. Under tourniquet a volar hockey stick-type incision is made starting over the FCR tendon and curving onto the thenar eminence. Through the bed of the FCR the wrist capsule is incised and the scaphoid exposed. The non-union site is cleaned of fibrous scar tissue. The non-union is excised with a cooled saw with each surface pepedicular to the axis of the proximal and distal pole respectively. The medulla is curetted down to bleeding bone using hand-held instruments to avoid thermal injury. K-wires may be inserted as joysticks to distract the fragments. This will demonstrate the size of the graft required. A cortico-cancellous graft is taken from the iliac crest and inserted with the cortex facing volarly. A (headless) compression screw or, if insecure, 2 K-wires, is used to hold the construct together. The wrist capsule is closed using strong absorbable sutures. A plaster is worn for 6 weeks.

- Inlay graft and internal fixation:
  - For those with preserved alignment.
  - Palmar approach for waist, dorsal approach for proximal pole.
  - A rectangular trough excavated across front of scaphoid and medulla excavated with curette to bleeding bone. Packed with cancellous graft from radial styloid. Held with double-pitched screw.
  - In proximal pole fractures, if no punctuate bleeding from proximal fragment then very low chance of union; consider vascularized graft.
- Vascularized bone grafting:
  - The indications are not clearly defined but usually performed for proximal pole fractures, revision surgery, avascular necrosis diagnosed preoperatively or intra-operatively. Reported union rate for various techniques 15–100%. The following techniques have been described:
  - 1,2 Intercompartmental supraretinacular artery (1,2 ICSA) (Zaidemberg)
  - Pronator quadratus pedicle graft
  - Base of second metacarpal
  - Volar carpal artery
  - Free iliac crest
  - Bundle implantation of superficial radial artery or 2nd dorsal metacarpal artery

Vascularized bone graft using the 1,2 ICSA (Zaidemberg)

The extensor retinaculum is exposed through a dorsal-radial incision. The 1,2 ICSA is identified. A block of cortico-cancellous bone is raised from the radius with care not to injure the pedicle containing the vessel. The pedicle is dissected to ensure an adequate length to reach the non-union site. The wrist capsule is incised to expose the scaphoid. The non-union is freshened up using hand-held instruments. Cancellous graft from the distal radius may be used. A trough is made on the scaphoid to accommodate the pedicled bone flap. The construct is carefully fixed using a headless screw. The wrist capsule and skin are closed. Postoperative management includes a cast period of 6–8 weeks and X-rays at 8 weeks and 3 months.

Fractures of the other carpal bones

Lunate

Fractures of the lunate are thought to be infrequent, however they are difficult to diagnose which may have contributed to this perception. The following types are described.

- Fractures of the body (usually coronal)
- Fractures of the dorsal pole
- Fractures of the palmar pole
- Fractures of the corners

Mechanism

Fractures of the body occur with forces acting along the longitudinal axis of the limb, such as falls on the hand, punching etc. Dorsal and volar pole fractures of the avulsion type occur with hyperflexion and hyperextension respectively. The dorsal pole may also fracture with hyperextension of the wrist.

Diagnosis

Clinical examination and suspicion are paramount. Plain X-rays have poor sensitivity for body fractures and CT scans are required.

Treatment

POP immobilization for undisplaced fractures. For displacement more than 1mm ORIF is recommended.

Triquetrum

Fractures of the triquetrum are common, and usually easy to diagnose and treat. Three types are recognized:

- Avulsion fractures of the dorsal radiotriquetral or ulnotriquetral ligament
- Dorsal impaction fractures from hyperextension against ulnar styloid
- Fractures of the body
- Palmar fractures seen in conjunction with perilunate dislocations

Mechanism

Forced hyperflexion of the wrist or direct impact.

Diagnosis

These fractures require a careful clinical examination and PA and lateral wrist X-rays. An oblique view is helpful. CT sometimes required for body fractures.

Treatment

POP immobilization is generally adequate. Displaced fractures may need fixation. Non-union of the triqetrum has not been reported.

Capitate

Isolated capitate fractures are rare, and if seen involve the proximal pole. They are generally seen as part of a trans-scaphoid transcapitate fracture (= scaphocapitate syndrome).

Mechanism

Either direct trauma or hyperextension, e.g. holding handlebars of a motorcycle.

Diagnosis

Fractures are visualized on the wrist films, caution is needed with perilunate injuries as the anatomy is heavily distorted with these injuries. CT scans if in doubt.

Treatment

Unless a simple undisplaced fracture, ORIF is required, particularly in scaphocapitate syndrome. This involves displaced fractures of both bones.

Hamate

Fractures of the hamate can be grouped into:
- Fractures of the body
- Fractures of the hook
- Fractures of the articular surfaces

Mechanism

Fracures of the body are associated with direct impact, or ligamentous avulsion. The hook may fracture with a fall on the outstretched hand or hitting with the hypothenar eminence such as seen in ulnar hammer syndrome. Fractures can be caused by certain sports such as golf, hockey and to a lesser extent cricket. Fractures of the articular surfaces, e.g. fracture-dislocations of the 4th and 5th CMC joint are commonly sustained after punching an object or person, less commonly they may be result of falls as well as injury with power tools or heavy machinery. They may be accompanied by other injuries such as dislocation of the rest of the CMC joints, carpal, metacarpal or phalangeal fracture dislocations.

Diagnosis

Careful clinical examination is essential, especially in chronic discomfort involving weak grip. Ulnar nerve palsy, thrombosis of the ulnar artery or flexor tendon rupture should be excluded. Even good-quality radiographs are often insufficient to appreciate the extent of the injury. A carpal tunnel view may show a fracture of the hook. CT is preferred if there is uncertainty, particularly concerning the integrity of the articular surfaces, or where the hook is fractured due to the difficult of visualization on plain films.

Treatment

- Any dislocation needs to be reduced swiftly under anaesthetic.
- Fractures of the body may be treated with POP immobilization if undisplaced.
- K-wiring or open reduction internal fixation with screws may be chosen depending on the fragment size and displacement.
- Hook fractures closer to the base of the hook heal more reliably than ones further to the tip. Hook fractures can be treated in a below-elbow POP, alternatively with ORIF using a screw for a fracture sufficiently large and displaced to warrant this. Surgical excision is the preferred option for symptomatic non-unions.

Pisiform

The pisiform is an intratendinous sesamoid bone, akin to the patella. Its main function is to help the FCU tendon to track along the groove of the triquetrum to enable flexion and extension of the wrist. Intra-articular fractures are mostly symptomatic and cause post-traumatic OA.

Mechanism

Fractures of the pisiform are usually the result of a direct blow, such as a fall onto the hypothenar eminence.

Treatment

Plain X-rays difficult. 30° supinated lateral or CT scan often needed. The sesamoid has plenty of cancellous bone and healing is usually achieved within 4–6 weeks in a below-elbow POP with neutral or semi-flexed wrist. Total pisiformectomy is indicated for painful OA uncontrollable with intra-articular steroid injections or in case of non-union. Good outcome with no apparent functional deficit.

Trapezium

Fractures of the trapezium are uncommon. Two types are recognized:
- Tuberosity
- Body

Mechanism

The tuberosity (the site of the origin of the transverse carpal ligament) fractures with direct impact, such as fall or a blow onto the thenar eminence. In contrast, a longitudinal impact through the axis of the thumb is responsible for fractures of the main body of the bone.

Diagnosis

Difficult to diagnose due to its superimposition with the trapezoid, scaphoid or with the base of the thumb seen on routine wrist films. A carpal tunnel view or CT scan will may give more information.

Treatment

- Undisplaced fractures: short Bennett's cast for 4 weeks.
- Displaced fractures: need fixing, either closed or open using a K-wire or mini compression screw fixation.

Trapezioid

These are very rare. Usually CT is needed for diagnosis. Large fragments can be fixed, especially if intra-articular. Otherwise plaster 5 to 6 weeks is adequate.

Carpal ligament rupture and dislocations

Subluxation or dislocation of the carpus dorsally or volarly usually occurs in the presence of a distal radius fracture. Isolated dislocation of a single carpal bone is rare. The lunate can fully dislocate into the space of Poirier, however in the majority of cases a perilunate type applies, in which the carpal bones 'peel off' from the lunate. A rare dorsal lunate dislocation has been described as well as dislocations of the scaphoid, triquetrum, trapezium, trapezoid, hamate and pisiform.

Peri-lunate and lunate dislocations and fracture-dislocations

This is a spectrum of injuries, which have a common sequence of development. These injuries are caused by high energy such as a fall from a height or motor vehicle accidents. To result in this pattern the forces in action should cause:

- Hyperextension of the wrist
- Ulnar deviation
- Intercarpal supination

As described by Mayfield and colleagues, based on their experimental work on cadaveric wrists, the injury may disrupt either the lesser arc, i.e. the ligaments stabilizing the lunate; or the greater arc, i.e. bony structures stabilizing the lunate (see Fig 4.12). The injury starts disruption on the radial side and work its way towards the ulnar side of the wrist. The first step of the injury pattern involves a scapholunate ligament rupture (Stage I). This may be followed by the separation of the lunate from the capitate (Stage II). Should the acting force continue at this stage the lunotriquetral ligament gives way (Stage III). The final stage is reached if the lunate is ejected volarly with the rest of the carpus dislocated dorsally (Stage IV) (see Fig. 4.13).

Perilunate fracture dislocations

The injury pattern may run in a number of ways through the wrist. This may be either in form of ligamentous (as described above) or bony failure. The following three types are well recognized:

- Trans-scaphoid
- Trans-capitate
- Trans-styloid

It is customary to fix the fracture in the acute stage to allow primary healing of the fractures and to prevent instability.

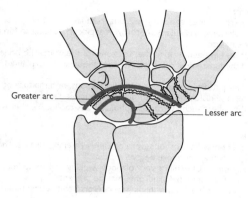

Fig. 4.12 Diagram of the lesser and greater arc.

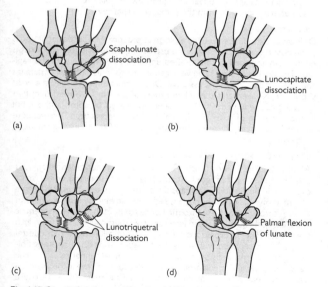

Fig. 4.13 Stages of perilunate dislocation. (a) Stage I: perilunate dissociation at scapholinate joint; (b) Stage II: dissociation at lunocapiate joint; (c) Stage III: dissociation at lunotriquetral joint. (d) Stage IV: complete lunate dislocation.

Mechanism
- High-energy injuries, generally resulting from fall from a height or road traffic collisions, particularly motorcycle accidents, leading to forced hyperextension.
- The lunate has been termed the 'keystone' of the wrist. The bones around the lunate peel off from it in a set sequence as explained above.
- The injury pattern may involve pure dislocations, or a mixture of fractures and dislocations. The fractures are named according to the bone they affect such as 'trans-scaphoid', 'trans-capitate' or 'trans-styloid'.

Diagnosis
- The patient may have other severe or life-threatening injuries. The carpal injury may therefore be overlooked.
- Clinically, the wrist exhibits very obvious swelling and sometimes deformity. Carpal tunnel syndrome may be present.
- X-rays seem at best overwhelming to interpret to the uninitiated eye, and at worst may seem to be normal.
- The key to diagnosis is to look for the critical relationships between the lunate and its neighbouring carpal bones, most notably the capitate. The lunate itself may appear triangular due to volar flexion and sometimes extrusion from the proximal carpal row.

Treatment
Dislocations should be reduced as soon as practicable. Closed reduction is often possible, sometimes with the use of fingertrap traction. The wrist is dorsiflexed and the lunate is pushed upwards to articulate with the capitate. The manoeuvre must be very gentle not to inflict additional damage and radiographic imaging is essential. Once reduction is achieved the wrist should be X-rayed and the relationships of the carpal bones identified. Closed treatment with POP has been advocated by some authors but in the presence of extensive instability this is unpractical. Percutaneous K-wire fixation may be used, but open repair of torn wrist ligaments is preferable.

Technique of open ligament repair
A dorsal midline incision is used. The 3rd dorsal compartment is opened and EPL tendon is retracted. At this stage the tear in the dorsal wrist capsule will be obvious. The capsule is opened as described by Berger. The relationships of the bones are reduced and held by inserting 1.6mm K-wires through the radius into the lunate (to hold the lunate concentric in its fossa), through scaphoid into capitate and through triquetrum into the lunate. The interosseous ligaments Scapho-lunate luno-triquetral (S-L, L-T) are repaired with transosseous sutures or bone anchors. Following this, a volar incision is made and the carpal tunnel released. The flexor tendons and median nerve are retracted to reveal the (usually) transverse tear in the volar wrist capsule. This is repaired. Skin closure and immobilization in a plaster slab follows. The wires are removed 8 weeks postoperatively.

Scapholunate ligament injury

📖 See p. 500.

Lunate-triquetrum ligament injury

📖 See p. 476.

Salvage procedures for failed treatment of wrist injuries

Late presentation of wrist injury or presentation after failed treatment constitutes a sizeable proportion of a hand surgeon's work. The aim with this type of treatment is no longer to restore the anatomy of the wrist. It can be seen as a compromise to preserve as much function with as little residual discomfort as possible. Procedures of this type described in Chapters 14 and 15.

Bone graft and bone substitutes

Definitions

Osteoinductive
The property of a material which promotes the formation of new bone from mesenchymal cells

Osteoconductive
The property of a material which promotes the formation of new bone through that material, by acting as a scaffold.

Osteogenic
Stimulating the formation of new bone from bone-producing cells

Autograft
Bone from the patient

Allograft
Bone from another person

Xenograft
Bone from another animal

Demineralized bone matrix

Allograft treated with acid to remove minerals. Contains various osteo-inductive growth factors—bone morphogenetic proteins (BMPs).
Many formulations available commercially. May be delivered as putty, granules, powder, or gel.

Bone morphogenetic proteins

Can be extracted from bone (poor yield) or recombinant gene production. Very expensive. Effective doses and combinations of BMP not yet known.

Allograft

Risk of disease transmission so rigorous screening is essential. Sterility is also very important. Freeze-drying allows subsequent storage but degrades osteogenetic and osteoconductive properties.

Calcium phoshpate

Osteoconductive but no osteo-inductive properties. Presented as granules, cement or putty. Hydroxyapaptite is a type of calcium phosphate.

Bone and joint injuries of the hand

Thumb dislocations and ligament injuries

CMC joint dislocation

Mechanism

Associated with sports and motorcycle injuries. The mechanism of this injury is controversial, however likely to be axial loading of semiflexed thumb. Base of thumb metacarpal dislocates dorsally, rupturing the palmar oblique ligament ('beak' ligament). May reduce spontaneously.

Presentation

Deformity and painful inability to move the basal joint of the thumb. Instability in case dislocation was reduced before hospital. Late presentation in cases of missed diagnosis or if primary treatment was inadequate.

Diagnosis

Deformity and tenderness of thumb base. Instability if stressed (may need local anaesthesia into joint).

PA and lateral views of the thumb aid diagnosis. In case of spontaneous reduction comparative X-rays are taken either under manual stress or both thumb radial aspects pushing against each other.

Treatment

- Non-operative treatment in plaster cast. Must check at 7 and 14 days to exclude subluxation. If unstable (and these injuries usually are!) K-wire across reduced joint supplemented by POP.
- Inadequate treatment predisposes to ongoing symptoms from instability. Continuing instability requires operative reconstruction of the palmar oblique ligament using FCR tendon (Eaton–Littler). FCR is split distally and half passed through a drill hole across the base of the first metacarpal and then across the front of the joint, attached back to the insertion into the base of the 2nd metacarpal. Can be performed acutely if very unstable. 75% good results for chronic instability. Alternative is *joint fusion* but not recommended due to loss of movement, technical difficulties, and complication rate.

Fracture dislocation of the first metacarpal (Bennett's)

This is a fracture dislocation of the first metacarpal with a volar ulnar fracture fragment and a proximally-dorsally displaced metacarpal shaft under the pull of the APL tendon. As the fracture is intra-articular, significant step-off can be produced by the displacement.

Treatment
- Non-operative treatment in plaster cast may be tried but displacement may occur within the plaster making future treatment difficult. Not recommended.
- Closed manipulation under anaesthetics (MUA) and K-wiring (Wagner) is the method of choice to prevent displacement in the POP.
- If the fragment does not reduce or if there is late presentation, then open reduction is required. (Palmar curved incision described by Moberg). A larger fragment can be held with a small screw.

Acute injuries of the thumb MCP joint

Injury to the MCP joint of the thumb is common. It is seen across a spectrum from a minor partial tear ('sprain') to full dislocation.
   The injury can occur in various directions:
- Radial wards or ulnarwards (injuring the ulnar collateral or radial collateral ligament).
- Dorsal dislocation of the proximal phalanx on the metacarpal (injuring the palmar plate).
- Palmar dislocation of the metacarpal on the proximal phalanx.

Presentation and diagnosis
- History of fall or direct blow. Pain in the joint aggravated by movement.
- Examine for tenderness over each collateral ligament and palmar plate. Examine for instability with local anaesthetic (LA) into joint. Flex the MPJ to 30° (to negate the secondary collateral stabilization provided by the palmar plate) and then test collateral ligaments.
- X-ray may show incongruity of joint, subluxation, or accompanying fracture component. Avulsion fractures occur mainly at the insertion site of the ulnar collateral ligament (UCL) into the proximal phalanx. These may affect joint congruity in case of larger fragments.
- Stress X-rays with LA into the joint aids diagnosis in case of spontaneous reduction.

Stener lesion
- Displacement of the distally avulsed UCL proximal and superficial to the adductor aponeurosis preventing spontaneous healing of the ligament onto bone.
- Variable incidence reported, 20–80%.
- Ultrasound scan or MRI helpful in diagnosing Stener lesion, however accurate diagnosis is difficult. Surgery is therefore the preferred option in suspected complete UCL rupture.

Treatment
- **Dorsal dislocation:** Reduction with traction is successful in the majority of dorsal dislocations. If irreducible, palmar plate may be trapped in joint and dorsal exposure is required. These injuries are usually stable but can be rested in a dorsal blocking splint for 3 weeks.
- **Palmar dislocation** (rare): Reduction with traction may fail if palmar plate, sesamoid or FPL interposed. Open reduction through a dorsal approach needed. Splint 4 to 6 weeks.

- **Radial and ulnar collateral ligament sprains** (i.e. mild tenderness and stable) treated symptomatically in a splint for 3 or 4 weeks. Most do well but can take months to settle.
- **Radial collateral rupture**: if completely unstable then surgical repair. Otherwise, plaster 6 weeks, DIP free.
- **Ulnar collateral rupture:** in the presence of a Stener lesion or a displaced bony fragment surgery is recommended.

Repair or reinsertion of ulnar collateral ligament

Slightly curved incision on dorsal ulnar aspect of thumb MCP joint. Carefully protect the primary dorsal branch of digital nerve. Adductor aponeurosis is incised and retracted. This reveals the ulnar collateral ligament. Look for Stener lesion. The ligament is sutured together if there is enough material proximally and distally. Alternatively a bone anchor or drill holes are used for re-insertion. Late reconstruction is best achieved using a tendon graft, e.g. PL. After surgery, immediate movement of the IPJ is essential to avoid loss of IP flexion as otherwise the adductor aponeurosis adheres to the repair. The MP joint can be moved in the flexion–extension plane immediately as the ligament is isometric and so the repair will not be stressed.

Chronic instability of the thumb MCPJ or CMCJ

Gamekeeper's thumb

Chronic attrition rupture of the ulnar collateral ligament of the thumb MCPJ from repeated wringing of bird's necks. Painful instability treated by ligament reconstruction but if osteoarthritis supervenes or if symptoms persist, then MCP fusion (low-profile plate) gives excellent durable result.

Late-presenting ulnar collateral ligament rupture

- Reefing of ligament if intra-substance tear and good tissue
- Excision of avulsion fragment and reattachment of ligament with anchor
- Reconstruction with tendon graft through drill holes
- Fusion if secondary OA or very high demand on thumb

Chronic dorsal instability of the thumb MCPJ

- Seen after trauma or usually generalized ligamentous laxity.
- Sesamoid arthrodesis. The abductor sesamoid is fused to the underside of the metacarpal neck. This preserves some flexion yet prevents hyperextension. An alternative is formal arthrodesis. The use of a low-profile compression plate allows early mobilization. The functional result is usually very good.

Chronic instability of the thumb CMCJ

- FCR tenodesis (described above)
- CMC fusion especially if multidirectional, e.g. Ehlers–Danlos.

Rheumatoid arthritis

📖 See Chapter 12, p. 361

Finger dislocations and ligament injuries

CMC joint dislocation

These are high-energy injuries following punching or forceful landing. They are also frequently seen as fracture dislocations involving same or adjacent carpal bone. Dislocation of more than 2 CMC joints at one time is rare and results from extremely forceful impact.

Mechanism

Various mechanisms have been suggested:
- Direct impact from volar to dorsal (e.g. handlebars of a bike)
- Axial loading (punching with clenched fist)
- Leverage with fulcrum at dorsum of wrist (e.g. watch)

Presentation

Grossly swollen hand with painful inability to form a composite fist.

Diagnosis

- Clinical diagnosis possible, however easy to miss. Palpation should elicit tenderness and reveal the prominence of the dorsally dislocated metacarpal bases. If instability is present the base can be relocated and dislocated with ease, a phenomenon called 'piano keying'.
- True lateral views are needed as PA's and obliques are particularly difficult to interpret. The same may apply to true lateral view due to superposition of the metacarpal bases in which case the key to diagnosis is recognition of the diverging angle of the dislocated metacarpals in relation to the normal ones. These views should also confirm the nature of any accompanying fracture(s).
- CT is very helpful in cases of doubt.

Treatment

- Closed reduction with K-wiring of the dislocated CMC joints with plaster immobilization is the choice in the acute phase. Wires removed at around 5 weeks.
- Missed and irreducible dislocations and those with significantly displaced fracture components require open surgery to relocate the joint and reconstruct the joint surfaces.
- K-wires or low-profile plates/screws are used for fixation.

Complications

Joint damage can lead to painful osteoarthritis. Salvage procedures include joint excision and fusion 📖 see p. 253.

The high-energy impact can lead to early compartment syndrome; later stiffness or intrisic tightness.

Complete dislocations are uncommon due to the extensive soft tissue envelope, ligament injuries are frequently seen.

Mechanism

The main stabilizers of the MCP joints are the collateral ligaments and palmar plate. The palmar plate acts as a stabilizer with the joint in full extension. Laterally directed force with the joint in flexion is constrained by the collateral ligaments which are already taut in this position. The impact is usually directed ulnarwards in the case of the ring and little fingers thereby causing a radial collateral ligament (RCL) injury. In case of the index and middle fingers the reverse is true, however RCL injuries to the index do occur.

The joint can dislocate palmarwards, dorsally or sideways.

Diagnosis

- **Collateral ligament injury/avulsion fracture:** these injuries present with swelling and tenderness over the MCP joint(s) with varying degrees of instability. The stability of the ligament should be tested in full flexion
- **Simple dorsal dislocation:** the finger is extended about 7°.
- **Complex dorsal dislocation:** The avulsed palmar plate and sometimes index sesamoid sits in the joint, blocking reduction. Furthermore, the metacarpal head can be clasped between the flexor tendon and lumbrical tendon. The finger is extended only about 30° and there is usually a tell-tale dimple in the palm.
- **Volar dislocation:** rare. Dorsal indentation, finger extended.

X-rays

PA and lateral views as well as Brewerton views should be obtained to visualize any avulsion fragments. Sesamoids appearing in joint on lateral view implies volar plate interposition.

Treatment

- **Simple dorsal dislocations** are usually easily reducible with traction, hyperextension then flexion of the joint. The finger is strapped to its neighbour and early mobilization is encouraged.
- **Complex dorsal dislocations:** For irreducible dislocations try inflating the joint by injecting LA (1–2% lidocaine) into the joint; this may push the interposed soft tissues out. Surgical reduction may be required preferably through a dorsal approach. Palmar approach risks damage to the digital nerves. Usually unstable. Immobilization in semi-flexion required only if instability is noted. Otherwise commence early movement.
- **Volar dislocations** may reduced closed but tend to be unstable. If so needs surgical repair of the ruptured collateral ligament to restore stability.
- **Fractures:** Large displaced fragments should be fixed. A volar approach gives best access to the fragment. Bony avulsions are fixed back using a screw or tension band suture if a sizeable fragment is present. Otherwise the fragment is excised and the ligament re-inserted either using a bone anchor or transosseous sutures.

- **Ligament tears:** If *partial tear* (slight laxity on flexion, good end point) then splint in mid-flexion 3 weeks then mobilize with neighbour strapping. *Unstable complete tears*—primarily repaired or reattached using non-absorbable sutures. The ligament is exposed preferably through a dorsal incision.
- **Children:** In children, there may be a Salter–Harris Type III fracture through the physis. This should be reduced and fixed with smooth K-wires which should not cross the growth plate.

PIP joint

These injuries are extremely common and appear with or without a fracture. Ball games are a particular hazard for these injuries.

Mechanism

Most dislocations (90%) are dorsal, the rest are palmar (5%) and sometimes purely lateral (5%). The direction of the force has an axial component together with a force vector directed either dorsally, palmarly or laterally (📖 see Figs 5.1–5.3). The following structures may be injured:

- At least one of the collateral ligaments
- Volar plate
- Central slip of extensor tendon

Presentation

Swollen and deformed finger with painful inability to move the PIPJ

Diagnosis

Clinical diagnosis with X-ray to confirm the additional components of the injury, i.e. fracture, avulsion

Treatment

- **Pure dorsal dislocations** (often with an insignificant avulsion fragment of the volar plate) are treated with reduction under LA and a mixture of rest and active ROM exercises. The collateral ligaments are intact. Fixed flexion deformity, rather than instability in extension, is the more likely outcome, therefore early movement is paramount. If there is hyperextension instability, dorsal blocking splint 2 to 3 weeks is recommended.
- **Pure volar dislocations** reduce easily. The central slip is ruptured, so treat in extension for 4 weeks (splint or K-wire) leaving DIP and MCPJ free.
- **Rotatory volar dislocation:** one condyle caught between central slip and lateral band—difficult to reduce due to soft tissue interposition. Try flexing MCPJ and PIPJ to lengthen lateral band. If stable reduction, hold extended at PIP for 4 weeks. If not reducible, open reduction (dorsal approch) repair central slip. Splint or K-wire with extended PIPJ 4 weeks.

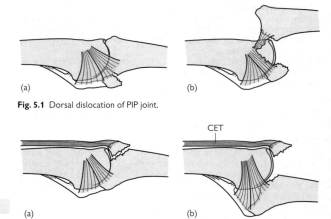

Fig. 5.1 Dorsal dislocation of PIP joint.

Fig. 5.2 Volar dislocation of PIPJ.

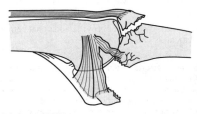

Fig. 5.3 Axial dislocation of PIPJ.

- **Ligament repair:** The palmar plate does not need repair. A slightly unstable collateral ligament will heal with splintage against collateral stress and movement at 3 weeks. However, a completely unstable collateral ligament should be repaired acutely. In late presentation, either repair or reconstruction with a tendon graft is needed.
- **Late presenting dorsal dislocations** have a poor prognosis. Through a palmar approach, palmar plate is reattached to the base of the proximal phalanx with a bone anchor, the avulsion fragment having been excised (palmar plate arthroplasty).
- **Dorsal fracture dislocation:** see below

Mallet finger

Mechanism

The injury follows a sudden flexion injury (e.g. stubbing the finger on a ball). Can be very low energy (e.g. tucking in a bed sheet). The terminal phalanx droops and cannot be straightened actively. There are three types of mallet finger:

- a tendinous avulsion
- tendinous avulsion with a small flake of bone
- a large dorsal bone fragment, sometimes with subluxation of the joint

Presentation

Deformity of the end of the finger. May be painless or painful inability to extend the DIP joint. A secondary swan-neck deformity may develop in delayed cases.

Diagnosis

X-rays show a flexed fingertip. There may be no, a small or large bone fragment, with or without incongruity of the joint.

Treatment

- **Tendon rupture**: splint DIP in extension for 8 weeks constantly and for a further 4 weeks at night. 80–90% good results. This works even if presentation delayed for up to 3 or 4 weeks.
- **Bone fragments** should be treated by splintage for 6 weeks. The outcome of surgical fixation is not always good—wound failure; stiffness, loss of fixation. Therefore avoid unless a large fragment with joint subluxation. Closed transarticular K-wiring with DIPJ extension, alternatively ORIF (screw).
- **Late presentation**: if symptomatic extensor lag then tendon can be reconstructed followed by prolonged splintage, alternatively, joint fusion. If secondary swan neck and passively correctible deformity is present, a central slip tenotomy can rebalance the finger effectively.

Jersey finger

Avulsion of the FDP tendon from the distal phalanx. It occurs with forceful passive extension of the DIPJ when the FDP is contracted (e.g. player's finger is caught in the 'jersey' sportswear of another player). Usually the non-dominant ring finger.

Leddy and Packer classification of FDP tendon avulsion

I: Tendon in palm
II: Tendon at PIPJ level (held by vinculum)
III: Tendon at A4 pulley (held by bone fragment)
IIIa: Fracture of distal phalanx and avulsion

Diagnosis

DIP joint held in hyperextension. No active flexion. Tender swelling may present in palm. Lateral X-rays may show bone fragment. Ultrasound or MRI if doubt.

Treatment

- Best results with repair in first few days. Tendon reattached into distal phalanx (bone anchor or transosseous sutures). Bone fragment reattached with small screws and plate.
- Delayed presentation: a large bone fragment should be reattached and good result still possible even after a few weeks. A retracted tendon, after 10 days or so, cannot be reattached easily; a flexion deformity develops. Two-stage tendon grafting is considered, but this is complex and risks losing some PIP flexion (which restricts hand function more than loss of similar DIP flexion). Alternative is joint fusion.

Metacarpal fractures

Mechanism

Direct trauma such as punching, heavy impact (fall of heavy object, stampede, forceful fall) or indirect trauma (twisting movement).

Presentation

Painful dorsal swelling and deformity commonly with inability to extend involved digit.

Diagnosis

Clinical diagnosis, confirmed by X-ray.

Anatomical considerations

There are four anatomical areas of the metacarpal bone that can be involved in the fracture: head, neck, shaft, base.

Head

- Fractures of the head are by definition intra-articular injuries. The amount of displacement dictates treatment.
- Surgery is difficult but is required to reconstruct the joint surface in cases of significant displacement.
- Brewerton view (MCPJ flexed 60°, beam from 30° ulnar.) and CT scan may be needed. In destroyed joint, primary arthroplasty considered.

Neck

- Neck fractures are the most common type of metacarpal fractures. These are usually associated with punching object or person.
- In the presence of a tooth injury it is treated as human bite. Contamination with oral flora poses significant risk of bone/joint infection.
- In the absence of such exposure, conservative treatment is the mainstay of treatment as significant angulation (up to 70°) is usually well tolerated in the little finger (due to flexibility of the CMC joint and the hyperextension available at the MCP joint); in the index only about 20° is tolerated (as no mobility at the base).
- Beware shaft fractures misinterpreted as neck!
- MUA followed by a splint in position of safe immobilisation (POSI). Do not flex PIPJs to maintain position.
- Surgery reserved for persistent gross angulation or rotation. See below for surgical techniques.

Shaft

- Fractures should be treated more aggressively as angulation or rotation is much more likely to have a detrimental effect on hand function.
- Shortening of more than 5mm will alter balance of intrinsic and extrinsic muscles. Reduced grip and extensor lag ensue.
- Rotation of only a few degrees will cause finger overlap on flexion.
- Palmar angulation will cause protruding metacarpal head in the palm (index and middle); in little and ring, the movement at the CMCJ will compensate. There is virtually no movement in the CMCJs of the index and middle fingers.

- After closed reduction, the fracture can be rested for a few days in a splint in the POSI. Early mobilization is encouraged as this tends to reduce and hold any slight rotation due to tension in the intermetacarpal ligaments.

Base

- Fractures occur due to high-energy injury (motorbike accident) in the younger group, however in the elderly a simple fall is sufficient.
- Diagnosis is difficult; 30° pronated X-rays and CT may be required to define the injury.
- Treatment of simple undisplaced base fractures is conservative.
- In complex injuries, e.g. fracture dislocations, MUA with K-wiring is indicated.
- Major intra-articular step-off in the young patient may need ORIF.
- The little finger can sustain a 'reversed Bennett's' fracture with a triangular fragment aligned normally with the distal hamate and the main metacarpal shaft pulled proximally by the ECU.
- X-ray helpful. If displaced, treated with closed reduction and percutaneous pinning, then 4 weeks plaster.

Thumb metacarpal base fractures

- The thumb has a high degree of omnidirectional mobility at the CMC joint. Angulation of up to 30° can therefore be accommodated. Extra-articular fractures with less angulation than this are treated with a thumb spica worn for 4 weeks.
- Intra-articular fractures (Bennett and Rolando) types are treated with MUA and K-wiring or ORIF in case of significant step-off.
- Highly comminuted displaced Rolando fractures are best treated by external fixation–distraction.

Surgery for metacarpal fractures

- **Neck fractures.** Intramedullary wiring. Single or multiple K-wires are inserted through a bone window at the base of the MC. ('Bouquet') Less invasive than ORIF and has low complication rate. Wires may be subsequently removed or left *in situ* if fully buried in bone.
- **Head fractures.** can be treated by elevation of small fragments and fixation with buried or headless screws, Graft may be needed. Occasionally primary joint replacement.
- **Shaft fractures.** Plate and screw fixation using low profile 2.0–2.4mm titanium implants. *Transverse fractures* dynamic compression through a pre-bent plate. *Long oblique fractures* with two or three lag screws; screw diameter less than a third of the spike width. Plates act as a dorsal tension band only if dorsal cortex intact. If not, consider locking plate and anterior graft. Early movement is essential: tendon adhesions are a common problem necessitating subsequent tenolysis for restoration of MCP flexion. Over-enthusiastic soft-tissue stripping may predispose to non-union.
- **Percutaneous transverse K-wiring.** This is a straightforward technique particularly suitable for fracture dislocations of the base of the metacarpal. However, it should be used judiciously for shaft and neck fractures and avoided if the surgeon has the skills to perform one of the two techniques described above as it does not provide very stable fixation, and is associated with stiffness and infection.

Finger fractures

Principles of treatment

There are many different ways to treat finger fractures, from simple neighbour or 'buddy' strapping to an adjacent uninjured digit, to complex internal fixation using plates and screws. Factors which determine the choice of treatment method include the type of injury, experience of the surgeon, the facilities available and the likely needs and compliance of the patient.

Phalangeal fractures take approximately 6 weeks to unite. The visible radiographic changes may lag behind the clinical state of the fracture.

Fractures in concave surfaces in the hand (and distal radius) often do better than expected even with residual displacement.

Conservative (non-surgical)

- Manipulation under anaesthetic (ring block usually sufficient) if required
- Immobilization using plaster of Paris, Zimmer (aluminium and foam), or thermoplastic splints
- Controlled mobilization by therapists, with appropriate splintage

Conservative treatment is cheap, simple and non-invasive. It avoids swelling and the potential complications of surgery, but requires longer periods of splintage and immobilization with the risk of stiffness.

The type of splint depends on the fracture configuration.
- *Dorsal blocking splint* with the MP flexed is best for basal fractures;
- *Neighbour strap* for undisplaced condylar fractures, pulling towards the reduced direction
- *Derotation strapping* using tape to pull around a spiral fracture after reduction. This technique is difficult to use.
- *Gutter splint* for undisplaced or reduced fractures of the shaft or joint.

Surgical

Surgery has the advantage of allowing anatomical reduction of fracture fragments which can then be fixed rigidly. The handling of soft tissues is equally important to minimize postoperative swelling which impairs mobilization.

Surgical treatment is reserved for:
- Irreducible fractures
- Displaced intra-articular fractures
- Fractures with a tendency to rotate
- Multiple digit fractures
- Floating joint
- Percutaneous fixation
  - The least invasive form of fixation either with K-wires or screws. Surgical trauma and hence the ensuing stiffness is kept to a minimum.
  - The fracture is reduced with manipulation and held either manually or with reduction clamps. Very small (stab) incisions are used.
  - Due to the expansive extensor expansion at PP level, there may be difficulty starting early therapy due to transfixation of the extensor apparatus by the wires.
  - Most proximal phalanx fractures are amenable to percutaneous fixation unless the procedure is delayed.
  - Crossed K-wires should be inserted so that they do not cross through the fracture site as this will displace the fracture fragments.

- ORIF:
  - Open reduction and fixation with screws or plate and screws may be the only alternative if the fracture pattern is too complex or surgical intervention has been delayed. The handling of soft tissues is crucial to avoid tendon adhesion and to minimize unecessary swelling. The fixation must always be robust enough to allow early mobilization.
  - A midlateral approach is preferred if possible as it minimizes the risk of adhesions between extensor tendon and bone. The dorsal approach is preferred for condylar fractures. The interval between the central and lateral bands is preferred to the Chamay triangular tendon flap to avoid adhesions.
  - Current surgical techniques rely on availability of specialized low-profile plates and screws. These come in sizes between 1–2.4mm. The reduction can be held with special reduction forceps. The position should be checked with a fluoroscan before fixation. Occasionally, temporary fixation with a fine K-wire can facilitate insertion of screws or plates.
  - Screws may be used on their own as lag screws for long oblique or spiral shaft fractures as well as intra-articular fractures such as of condyles. The screw should be at least two widths from the fracture edge to avoid splitting the bone.
  - Plate fixation is carried out either in compression or bridging mode.
- External fixation is suitable for comminuted and open fractures.
- Interosseous wire loops using pre-stretched 28 or 30 gauge dental wire, supplemented by a single K-wire (the Lister method).

Postoperative course

It is crucial that therapy is started at the earliest opportunity (within 48–72h) to ensure the best outcome as stiffness is a major problem. Tenolysis is frequently required as tendon adhesions develop readily between tendons, bone and metal implant.

Fractures of the proximal phalanx

Mechanism

Commonly due to falls, ball games and direct trauma. May be open and comminuted.

Presentation

Painful and swollen digit sometimes with obvious deformity, i.e. dorsal angulation and/or rotation.

Anatomical considerations

The proximal phalanx can be divided into three areas:

- Base
- Shaft
- Condyles

Some basal fractures and all condylar fractures are intraarticular

Diagnosis

Clinical diagnosis, confirmed by X-ray. Rotational deformity NOT normally appreciated on X-ray. Check composite fist formation and direction of fingertip. All fingertips should converge towards the scaphoid tubercle.

Treatment

- Basal fractures
  - **Undisplaced:** splint in mid-flexion for 1 or 2 weeks then mobilize
  - **Dorsal angulation:** Usually in osteoporotic bone. Manipulate under LA into full flexion. Hold in dorsal blocking splint.
  - **Lateral angulation:** Reduce and neighbour strap. K-wire if unstable. In children, Salter–Harris Type III fracture.
  - **Collateral avulsion** Neighbour strap if undisplaced, fix from palmar approach if displaced. Salter–Harris III injury in children.
  - **Displaced intra-articular fracture** T or Y configuration. ORIF. May need graft if depressed ('pilon').
- Shaft fractures
  - Splint, wires, percutaneous screws or ORIF
- Condyles
  - **Type I** (unicondylar, undisplaced): splint 10 days the gentle mobilization with neighbour strap. Repeat X-rays to exclude displacement
  - **Type II** (unicondylar, displaced): closed reduction if possible, if not open approach between central slip and lateral band. Fix with mini-screws across both condyles.
  - **Type III** (bicondylar): unstable and challenging to fix. Oblique screws or, ideally, mini-fragment locking plate.
  - **Children** Similar principles.

Fractures of the middle phalanx

The middle phalanx has very little soft tissue cover dorsally. It is hence prone to direct trauma.

Mechanism

Commonly due to falls, ball games and direct trauma. Rotational mechanism such as dog pulling on lead or horse pulling on rein is also common. It may be open in relation to direct trauma. Fractures of the base of the middle phalanx are frequently intra-articular. These may cause a fracture dislocation of the PIP joint. Transverse fractures proximal to flexor digitorum superficialis (FDS) tend to tilt apex dorsal and fractures distal tend to tilt apex palmar.

Presentation

Painful digit frequently with obvious rotational deformity. Intra-articular fractures may present with subluxation or complete dislocation.

Diagnosis

Clinical diagnosis, confirmed by X-ray. Rotational deformity is not normally appreciated on X-rays, unless very significant (greater than 45°). Check composite fist formation and direction of fingertip. All fingers should converge to show towards scaphoid tubercle.

Treatment
- Shaft fractures
  - Splint, wires, percutaneous screws or ORIF
- Condyles
  - As for proximal phalanx
- Basal pilon fracture
  - *Dynamic external fixation:* impaction fractures or dislocations associated with comminution of the base of the proximal phalanx can be treated with dynamic external fixation with surprisingly good results. Many designs (Suzuki, Schenk, S Quatro etc.) available.
- Fracture dislocation
  - *Extension block splinting:* dorsal fracture dislocations involving more than 30% of the base of the middle phalanx can be treated with extension block splinting if the fracture can be reduced and joint congruency restored.
  - *Fragment fixation:* large palmar fragments can be fixed with screws from a palmar or dorsal approach.
  - *Small dorsal fragments* (avulsion of the central slip from a volar dislocation) can be reduced and held with a tension band suture.
  - *Small palmar fragments* do not generally require intensive treatment. Gentle mobilization is all that is needed as immobilization runs the risk of stiffness.
- Shaft fractures
  - Closed and undisplaced/minimally displaced fractures best treated with a gutter splint. Neighbour strapping not suitable to little finger due to discrepant length of adjacent ring finger.
  - Rotation difficult to control due to poor soft tissue envelope and unstable fractures require fixation. This is best achieved by K-wire fixation, rarely ORIF due to poor soft tissue cover and impingement of lateral bands.

Fractures of the distal phalanx
These are very common injuries. They appear in several contexts:
- As a closed injury to the tuft, shaft or the base
- As part of an open injury to the fingertip/nail bed or an amputation
- As a growth plate injury in children
- With traumatic avulsion of the FDP (rugby jersey finger)
- With avulsion of the terminal extensor tendon, i.e. a mallet injury

Mechanism
These injuries are the result of a crush injury in more than 80% of cases, commonly a workplace injury in adults; whereas in children crushing in a door or gate is more usual. In the case of FDP avulsion, although the initial description of this injury relates to rugby or American football, various mechanisms have since been reported and include:
- Sail rope or dog lead being pulled away from the patient's grasp
- Finger-pulling sport
- Rock and wall climbing
- Trying to stop bag being snatched away

In the case of a bony mallet injury, the mechanism is similar to the soft tissue mallet and involves forcible flexion of the digit whilst being held in extension by a taut terminal extensor tendon.

Presentation

The presentation depends on the nature of the injury as outlined in the list above. In closed injuries it is one of a painful and swollen terminal segment with varying degrees of limitation of DIP joint movement. The limitation is extreme in case of a rugger jersey finger. This injury presents with a very swollen and bruised digit with inability to flex the DIP joint. In case of a mallet injury, the typical droop can be observed. Both injuries may present with subluxation or dislocation of the DIP joint depending on the size of the fracture fragment. Open injuries and amputations present with varying amounts of bleeding.

Diagnosis

Clinical diagnosis is possible but the nature of the bony injuries and joint subluxation should be confirmed by X-ray. In children, there is usually a growth plate fracture.

Treatment

- **Closed tuft, shaft and extra-articular basal fractures** are treated with a foam-aluminium Zimmer splint.
- **Bone mallet** injuries are treated in splint for 6 weeks, Surgery avoided unless subluxation is present. (📖 see p. 143)
- **Subungual haematoma:** drain if painful with heated needle
- **Matrix injury:** if cosmesis an issue, remove the nail plate and repair under magification with fine dissolvable suture.
- **Nail plate dislocation** associated with a Salter–Harris Type I fracture in children (Seymour fracture). Clean and reduce, repair nail bed.
- **Displaced shaft fracture:** Closed fractures with sufficient displacement to cause nail bed embarrassment or dislocation of the nail plate should be treated with closed reduction. They may be percutaneously fixed with a K-wire in case of instability. This should preferably not transfix the DIP joint.
- **Open fingertip/nailbed injuries** are treated with washout, debridement and skin/nail bed repair with the appropriate suture materials. Stabilization of the fracture is performed with a minimal amount of metalwork to minimize risk of infection.
- **FDP avulsion:** 📖 see pp. 143–145

Soft tissue injuries of the hand

Wound care

Non-surgical

- Thorough cleaning
- Dressings
- Splints:
  - Position of safe immobilization (POSI), joints with the collateral ligaments in the longest position preventing contractures.
    - Wrist extended at 30°
    - MCPJs flexed at 60° (collateral ligaments longest here because of convex 'cam' shape of MC head)
    - PIPJs and DIPJs fully extended.
  - Splints should extend beyond the fingertips after tendon repairs in fingers. Finger movement may be permitted by using a splint to the level of MCPJs.
  - Dorsal blocking splints are used following flexor tendon repairs.
  - Volar splints are used following extensor tendon repairs.

Surgical

Debridement and wound excision

The term debridement originated during the Napoleonic Wars, meaning '*unbridling*' or decompression of missile wounds. It is often misinterpreted, and the term '*careful wound excision*' is probably clearer.

Careful wound excision is the cornerstone of the surgical management of soft tissue injuries.

- **Tidy** (fresh, less than 24h, sharp lacerations) can be sutured primarily.
- **Untidy** (delayed, crushed, devitalized, contaminated or infected wounds) should have necrotic tissue excised.
  - 1–2mm excision of the wound edges is adequate for simple wounds.
  - Substantial tissue excision required in grossly contaminated wounds, preserve nerves and vessels when possible.
  - Thorough wound lavage with several litres of warmed normal saline or Hartmann's solution.
  - **Adequate primary wound excision and early soft tissue reconstruction should be the aim for the majority of cases**.
  - High-energy transfer injuries should not be closed immediately.
  - Clear microbiological swabs must be obtained before delayed closure of infected wounds.

Cold sensitivity

- Cold sensitivity is common following injury or elective surgery. This has also been termed trauma-induced cold-associated symptoms (TICAS).
  - The symptoms are **pain and discomfort**, **stiffness**, **altered sensibility** and **colour change**.
  - Pain is the most troublesome symptom.
- Pre-existing symptoms of cold sensitivity are likely to be made worse by hand injury.
- It can be very disabling, and limit return to manual work outdoors, and sporting and recreational activities.
- Patients should be warned of its onset, and advised to have a lower threshold for wearing gloves, or preferably mitts (which are warmer than gloves).
- Duration:
  - Cold sensitivity is worse in the first 2–3 years following an injury, and then improves somewhat over the next few years.
  - It then usually reaches a plateau at a lower level, which is permanent.

Microvascular replantation

Digital replantation

Replantation is the microvascular restoration of the circulation of a completely amputated part.

Indication for microvascular digital replantation

- Thumb (always).
- Children (have to have a good reason not to).
- Multiple digits.
- Distal to FDS insertion for single digit.
- Single digit at patient request following informed consent discussion between patient and surgeon.

Contraindication for microvascular digital replantation

- Polytrauma precluding long replantation surgery
- Age, especially when nerve recovery unlikely
- Co-morbidity
- Single digit for patient who does not want long rehabilitation or wants early return to work (e.g. index finger of uninsured, self-employed manual worker).
  - Decision to replant or not should always be discussed with the patient.
  - Informed consent is often difficult at time of injury as emotions may run high, and long-term consequences of decisions are difficult to evaluate by some patients.

Transport of the amputated part to a replantation centre

- Wrap the amputated part in a saline-soaked swab.
- Put the swab and digit in a sealed plastic bag (it doesn't need to be sterile, just clean, e.g. blood sample bag, domestic freezer bag)
- Put the bag in a bowl of ice and water, which maintains a temperature of 2–4°C.
- ⚠ DO NOT PUT THE AMPUTATED DIGIT DIRECTLY ONTO ICE AS IT WILL FREEZE AND DIE FROM FROSTBITE EVEN IF REPLANTED.
- The part may be stored in a domestic refrigerator (not the freezer compartment).

Management at the replantation centre

- Speed is essential:
  - Book the operating theatre.
  - Start preparation of the amputated part under the microscope before the patient gets to theatre and while they are in the anaesthetic room.
- X-ray the hand **and** amputated part.
- Send blood for full blood count (FBC) and group and save (cumulative blood loss may be high in multiple replants).
- The use of brachial plexus blocks—axillary or supraclavicular—gives sympathetic block (producing useful vasodilatation), as well as good postoperative analgesia.
- Insert urinary catheter, and aim for urinary output of 1–2ml/kg of urine.
- Start intravenous infusion (IVI) and give crystalloid fluids.

- Give blood intraoperatively if there is excessive blood loss, keeping haemoglobin between 10–12 g/dl.

The sequence and techniques for replantation surgery

- Speed is essential:
  - Try to do as much as possible in a tourniquet time (2 hours). The work is much easier in a bloodless field, and it can be risky to reinflate the tourniquet once anastomoses are running, especially for multiple replants.
  - Do all the bone, tendon and nerve work before the vessels if you can, then you don't have to go back in and disturb your anastomoses.
- Surgeon factors:
  - These can be long procedures, and tiredness is a factor. Be as efficient as you can to speed it up, and take breaks every few hours to maintain concentration.
  - Remember to maintain your own hydration, and to eat if your energy and concentration is flagging.
- Preparation of the amputated part and recipient hand:
  - Preparation of amputated part may be concurrent with preparation of hand if enough experienced surgeons are present.
  - Wash away gross contamination in a bowl before skin preparation with surgical disinfection and draping.
  - Careful wound excision (skin, tendon, nerves and vessels as required).
  - ⚠ Protect neurovascular bundles (NVBs) carefully from saws and rotating K-wires, or use oscillating setting (if available) for K-wires.
- Bone fixation:
  - Bony shortening (with small oscillating saw) of untidy fracture site to clean edge. This may help to obtain end-to-end nerve repair.
  - No need to shorten bone in clean, guillotine-type amputation.
  - Bone fixation should be quick, simple and solid to allow early movement.
  - Crossed K-wires are quick, but can get in the way, and don't give much compression.
  - Lister technique (interosseous wire loop and oblique K-wire) quick, versatile, and gives compression.
  - 90°–90° interosseous wire loops are quick and unobtrusive; be careful to push the wire twist of the vertical loop flat against the bone so that it does not abrade extensor tendons
  - Low-profile titanium plates are secure, but sometimes require extensive periosteal/soft tissue stripping to apply, and may compromise vascularity when there has been extensive soft tissue damage from an untidy injury.
- Flexor tendon repair:
  - Repair should be strong enough for early movement (use 4-strand technique where possible)
  - Sometimes advisable to **only** repair the FDP to reduce the bulk in the flexor tendon sheath, and facilitate early movement.
  - Primary insertion of a silicone tendon-spacer may be the best option when there is an injury of the flexor tendons, tendon sheath and/or untidy fracture. Primary repair usually sticks in this situation.
- Extensor tendon repair:

- Continuous suture quick, easy, and glides well.
- Nerve repair:
  - ⚠ **Major determinent in the successful *functional* outcome of replant.**
  - Use interposition nerve grafts when segmental nerve loss.
  - Digital nerve graft— posterior interosseous nerve (PIN) from 4th compartment, just proximal to extensor retinaculum or lateral cutaneous nerve of forearm.
  - Common digital or mixed nerves at wrist and more proximally— use sural nerve or medial lateral cutaneous nerves of forearm as cable grafts.
- Vessel preparation:
  - ⚠ Vessels should be cut back to healthy intima. This is probably the most significant factor for achieving successful anastomosis in microvascular replantation.
  - Interposition reversed vein grafts may then be necessary.
  - End-to-end anastomosis is often possible in tidy amputations, and also after conservative shortening of untidy bone ends.
- Vein graft donor sites:
  - Vein grafts need to be a similar (small) calibre as the digital vessels.
  - Volar aspect of the distal forearm and wrist (although the donor scar is not good).
  - Lateral dorsum of the foot.
  - ⚠ Avoid 1st 2nd 3rd rays in the foot, as this may compromise the use of toe transfer as late reconstruction.
  - Put clip or tie on proximal end of vein, leaving distal end open ('the heart end', or 'blood flows into the open end') which then becomes the proximal end of the artery when the graft is reversed.
- Vein repair:
  - Do veins before artery if you can see the veins easily, then you can leave the digit to perfuse undisturbed after removing the clamps from the arterial anastomoses.
  - If veins cannot be seen easily, it may be necessary to repair the artery and let the digit perfuse to see where the draining veins are, and then repair them. This is more messy, with extra bleeding.
  - Vein grafts are not reversed when used to repair veins.
  - Can use the vein from an adjacent digit—one less anastomosis as proximal end is already attached.
- Artery repair:
  - Use reversed vein graft where segmental loss from injury or vessel preparation.
  - Y-shaped vein grafts for common digital arteries.
  - Can try distal end of artery to vein anastomosis in very distal replants (i.e. distal to DIPJ) if no recipient artery can be found. This works by reversed circulation through the capillaries.
- Thumb replant:
  - ⚠ Use a vein graft from the digital artery straight to the radial artery in the anatomical snuffbox for thumb replants if end-to-end digital arterial repair is unsuccessful.
  - This course is shorter to the ulnar digital vessel.

- Skin:
  - Skin should not be closed under tension.
  - Use split thickness skin graft for small skin defects. Can apply directly to vessels.
  - Larger areas with denuded tendon or open fractures need flap cover.

Proximal replantation (hand, forearm, arm)

- Replantations of the upper limb proximal to the MCPJs.
- Warm ischaemia time is the key determinant in the success of macrovascular replantation of parts containing muscle.
  - No muscle in digits, so can replant after many hours of cold ischemia (up to 94 hours published).
- These are dramatic injuries, so make sure you look after the **whole** patient.
- Always look for associated injuries.
  - These are usually very-high-energy transfer injuries (apart from sharp, guillotine-type amputations) and other injuries are common.

Pathophysiology

- Amputations are either **sharp, avulsion,** or **crush.**
- The amputated part contains muscle (unlike digital amputations).
- Reperfusion of ischaemic muscle allows toxic metabolites to enter circulation, leading to the systemic inflammatory response syndrome, and potentially multiple organ failure.
- The severity of reperfusion injury is proportional to muscle mass, duration of ischaemia, and the extent of direct mechanical damage to the muscle.
- Revascularized muscle swells, leading to compartment syndrome, and further muscle necrosis.
- Crush amputations lead to the worst reperfusion syndrome.
- Reperfusion syndrome:
  - Myoglobinuria
  - Hyperkalaemia
  - Metabolic acidosis
  - Renal failure
  - Coagulopathy
  - Acute respiratory distress syndrome (ARDS)

Transport of the amputated part to a replantation centre

- As above for digital part

Key points for proximal replantation
General

- Speed is more essential than digital replantation because of warm ischaemia.
- Muscle cannot tolerate more than 6–8 hours of warm ischaemia.
- Do not replant if more than 8 hours of warm ischaemia.
- Continue active cooling during the early part of replantation (i.e. on the operating table)
  - Avoid warm ischaemia whenever possible.

Bone
- Ideally, fix the bones rapidly, and then do the vascular repair, end-to-end, or with a graft with a stable bone platform.
  - Bone fixation after revascularization puts the vascular repair at risk.
  - If the bone fixation cannot be done quickly, consider temporary revascularization using a shunt.
- Rigid internal fixation is preferable.
  - Try to avoid difficult secondary bone surgery.
  - Consider a one-bone forearm or primary wrist arthrodesis in certain cases.

Vascular
- Perform fasciotomies and excise dead muscle **before** revascularization to avoid reperfusion syndrome.
- Allow venous bleeding after the arterial repair is flowing, to 'wash out' toxic metabolites before letting the clamps off the venous anastomosis.
- Repair venae comitans of radial and/or ulnar arteries to reduce bleeding (the deep venous drainage is more effective than superficial system).
- When the limb is not replantable, always keep 'spare parts' (e.g. radial or ulnar artery forearm flaps) for microvascular transfer to cover proximal stump, and maintain bony length for better function with a prosthesis.

Nerve
- Nerve repair is the major factor determining outcome.
- Bony shortening allows end-to-end nerve repair:
  - Reduces the distance of nerve recovery
  - Avoids the need for nerve grafts
- If secondary nerve grafting is anticipated, place both ends of the nerve in easily accessible positions.
- Good results in the upper arm and distal forearm and wrist:
  - The nerves are easy to repair.
  - The extrinsic muscles are already innervated in distal replants.
- Nerve repairs are difficult in the proximal and mid-forearm around the muscle branches.

Outcome of proximal replantation
- Outcome according to the Chen grading system:
  - Grade 1–IV
- Worse outcome in proximal forearm, where motor branches given off into long forearm muscles, as very there are multiple, small nerve branches which are difficult to orientate and repair.
- Better results in warmer countries where there is no problem with cold sensitivity.

Chen's outcome criteria for upper limb replantation[*]

Grade I
- Able to resume original work with the injured limb
- ROM >60%
- Complete sensory recovery
- M4–5 motor power

Grade II
- Able to resume suitable work
- ROM>40%
- Near complete sensibility
- M3–4

Grade III
- Able to carry on daily life
- ROM>30%
- Partial recovery of sensibilty
- M3

Grade IV
- Almost no useful function in the limb

[*] Chen ZW et al. (1981). *Orthopedic Clinics of North America.*

Revascularization

- Revascularization is the microvascular reperfusion of a part which is not completely amputated.
- This ranges from an injury to the flexor tendons and NVBs arising from a volar laceration, to almost complete amputation with a narrow remaining skin bridge. The sequence is the same as for microvascular replantation (as necessary).
- The difference between a revascularization and a replant is that there has been *warm* ischaemia (as the part is still attached) compared with *cold* ischaemia of a cooled, completely amputated part prior to replantation. This means that the delay to surgery following injury is more significant, and there will be more postoperative swelling after reperfusion.

Ring avulsion

- Ring is caught on an object (usually a protruding nail or wire fence), or in a machine, and the skin of the finger is pulled off as a sleeve, like the finger of a glove.
- Usually a bony fragment in the avulsed section, often amputated through the DIPJ or the proximal part of the P3, and the denuded skeleton and tendons are left intact.

Classification

See Classification of ring avulsion injury.

Treatment

- Class 1 ring avulsion can often be sutured following minimal wound edge excision. Often, there is a small dorsal skin defect requiring a skin graft. **The skin should not be sutured under tension as this is likely to promote venous congestion, leading to partial or complete loss of the digit.**
- Venous and arterial injuries require microsurgical reconstruction, frequently by the use of reversed interposition vein grafts, as there is significant intimal damage from the traction produced by the mechanism of the injury. The vessels must be cut back to a level where there is healthy intima to restore flow with no danger of subsequent thrombus formation.
- Complete ring avulsion amputations (Urbaniak class 3) can be replanted, and usually require vein grafts to the artery, and sometimes also the vein.

Classification of ring avulsion injury

Urbaniak[1]

I	Circulation adequate
II	Circulation inadequate
IIA	Circulation inadequate, only arterial damage
III	Complete degloving amputation

Kay[2]

I	Circulation adequate, with or without skeletal injury
II	Circulation inadequate, with or without skeletal injury
IIA	Arterial circulation inadequate only
IIB	Venous circulation inadequate only
III	Circulation inadequate, with fracture or joint injury
IIIA	Arterial circulation inadequate only
IIIB	Venous circulation inadequate only
IV	Complete amputation

1. Urbaniak JR, Evans JP and Bright DS (1981). Microvascular management of ring avulsion injuries. *J Hand Surg (Am)* **6**(1), 25–30.
2. Kay S, Werntz J and Wolff TW (1989). Ring avulsion injuries: classification and prognosis. *J Hand Surg (Am)* **4**(2), 204–13.

Amputations

General principles for elective amputation

Specific points for each level of amputation are discussed below.

- Involve the patient in the decision-making process regarding the indication for, and level of, amputation.
- Discuss the level with your local limb prosthesis service for more proximal amputations.
- Ensure amputated bone ends are smooth (no bony spicules, no sharp corners from saw cuts).
- Achieve good-quality soft tissue cover over bone. Proximal to the wrist, try to cover bones with muscle under skin flaps.
- Use fishmouth-type incisions with U-shaped curves, to avoid 'dogear' bulges.
- Ensure nerves are cut back under tension to ensure they are not placed in suture line (or painful neuroma results).
  - Consider intra-operative placement of an indwelling epidural-type catheter around major nerves for a few days following more proximal amputations.
- Apply compression to the amputation stump early, once the skin is healed. This reduces oedema, and speeds up fitting of a prosthesis when this is indicated.

Additional principles for emergency amputation

- Use reconstructive flaps to preserve length (rather than shortening limb or digits to get adequate soft tissue cover).
- Perform careful wound excision, ensuring skin flaps are viable.
- ⚠ If there is any doubt about the viability of any tissue, amputate distally, and wait to reassess vascularity, before completion of amputation at the 'definitive' level.
- Always consider the possibilities of 'spare part surgery', using amputated or mutilated parts for grafts, flaps, or immediate microsurgical reconstruction.
  - Remember that unreconstructable digits can be 'filleted' to provide flaps to cover more proximal losses.

Complications of amputation

- Bleeding from inadequate haemostasis.
- Infection.
- Neuropathic pain or phantom pain.
  - It may be worth starting drugs which modulate neuropathic pain (amitryptilline, gabapentin, pregabalin) peri-operatively to avoid or reduce this effect.
- Neuroma.
- Unstable soft tissue cover.
- Bony irregularity causing stump pain or difficulty with fitting of prosthesis.
- Lumbrical plus finger:
  - FDP causes paradoxical extension of PIPJ during attempted finger flexion, due to action of FDP on intact lumbrical
  - Occurs after amputation distal to PIPJ which divides FDP insertion, or FDP adhesions distal to lumbrical origin.

Digital amputation

General principles
- Can be at any level (see below).
- Try to preserve length, and think about the tendon anatomy.
- ⚠ DON'T SUTURE FLEXOR TENDONS TO EXTENSORS. This results in quadriga deformity.
  - The quadriga deformity is named after the steering arrangements on a Roman chariot, in which all four horses were controlled in unison by a shared set of reins.
  - The FDP tendons of the middle, ring and little fingers are usually conjoined. This means that if an FDP tendon from one of these fingers is held in an extended position (e.g. by suturing the flexors to the extensor), the others are unable to flex.

Indications for digital amputation
- Trauma:
  - Immediate (unsalvageable)
  - Late (stiff, painful, cold-sensitive, excluded from or interferes with normal hand use, insensate, failed reconstruction)
- Malignant tumour
- Ischemia:
  - Previous nerve damage
  - Berger's disease
  - Frostbite
- Infection (intractable osteomyelitis)
- Congenital polydactyly (📖 see p. 562)

Distal phalanx
- Following traumatic loss distal to eponychial fold, try to preserve length with volar advancement or cross finger flaps (📖 see p. 215)
- If length cannot be preserved, design fishmouth incision.
  - Try to keep the volar skin on the palmar aspect (rather than moving dorsal skin onto the volar aspect of the fingertip).
  - Excise germinal matrix (GM) of the nail completely (remember this extends more laterally than you think, 3–4mm lateral to nail fold—📖 see p. 170). The GM can be stained with methylene blue for easier identification.
- Shorten bone. Smooth off with bone nibblers.
- Preserve FDP attachment distal to DIPJ if possible. This maintains power grip with flexion of distal phalanx.

DIPJ
- Remove prominent condyles of the distal P2 with bone nibblers for smooth fingertip.

Middle phalanx
- Distal to FDS, preserve length to maintain FDS function.
- Proximal to FDS insertion, can shorten to level of tension-free skin closure.

Proximal phalanx
- Preserve length if distal to lumbrical/interossei insertion into extensor hood (if these are intact) as this maintains flexion of stump of P1 at MCPJ.

- If not, there is no benefit from preservation of P1 remnant; shorten through MCPJ.

MCPJ
- Usually fishmouth incision.
- If not, ensure design does not produce tight scar between webs of adjacent digits. This may require the use of Z-plasties.
- No need to remove articular surface of MC head in the same way as condyles of phalangeal bones, as it is not prominent, and does not interfere with grip.

Ray amputation
- The removal of a metacarpal and digit (i.e. whole digital ray):
  - Border digits—shortening of MC through base
  - Central digits—closure of the resultant cleft in the hand either directly or by transposition of an adjacent digital ray onto the base of the amputated metacarpal.
- This is a serious undertaking, and should not be performed by inexperienced surgeons. Poor technique can produce disastrous complications, compromising the function of the remaining digits.
- Patients (especially manual labourers) should be warned that grip strength is reduced.
- Avoid primary ray amputation during initial treatment of trauma on most occasions.
- Use zig-zag incisions in palm, and straight lines in a V-type excision on dorsum.
- Do not leave periosteal sleeve of MC in children as this will grow and ossify.

Indications for ray amputation
- Same indications for digital amputation.
- Incontinent hand following loss of middle or ring finger.
- Amputation of border digit, particularly index finger.
- To improve cosmesis following complete digital amputation.

Index finger ray amputation
- Incise around middle of proximal phalanx (P1) and down dorsum of 2nd MC. Use zig-zag incision in palm. Leave skin adjustment until the end of the procedure.
- Divide extensor digitorum communis (EDC) II and extensor indicis (EI).
- Incise periosteum of 2nd MC, and transect bone approximately 1–2cm above metacarpal base.
- Divide tendons of 1st dorsal interosseous (DI) and 1st lumbrical.
- Divide NVBs, flexor tendons (and allow to retract), and 1st palmar interosseous tendon.
- Divide volar plate and capsular structures, and remove index ray.
- Ensure digital nerves are transposed between interossei to protect them.
- Trim skin flaps at the end to ensure adequate cover.

Central digits (middle and ring) ray amputation
- Either close space by suture of adjacent deep transverse metacarpal ligaments, or transpose digital ray.
- Use a commisure flap to obtain a good webspace.

Transposition 2nd to 3rd MC
- Preferable to direct closure.
- The 2nd/3rd CMCJ complex is rigid, so following direct closure, the base of 2nd MC does not move ulnarwards, and II and IV are sutured together under tension, causing pain and loss of function.
- Divide 2nd MC though proximal third. Move ulnarwards, and fix onto base of 3rd MC with a strong plate.
- Check rotation of transposed index finger (by looking at alignment of nail plate), and ensure there is opposition to the thumb tip.

Transposition 4th to 5th MC
- Less important than 2nd to 3rd, as laxity of 4th/5th CMCJ allows 5th MC to move radially towards 3rd MC to close gap following direct closure.

Little finger ray amputation
- Incise around middle of P1 and down dorsum of 5th MC. Leave skin adjustment until the end of the procedure.
- Ensure base of 5th MC is preserved to protect insertion of FCU and ECU.
- Identify dorsal sensory branch of ulnar nerve.
- Divide EDC V and extensor digit minimi (EDM).
- Incise periosteum of 5th MC, and transect bone approximately 1–2cm above base.
- Divide tendon of abductor digiti minimi (ADM) and flexor digiti minimi (FDM), 3rd palmar interosseous and 4th lumbrical.
- Divide NVBs and flexor tendons (and allow to retract).
- Divide volar plate and capsular structures, and remove fifth ray.
- Ensure digital nerves are transposed between interossei to protect them.
- Allow hypothenar muscles to fall onto 4th MC to act as padding for ulnar border of hand (do not attempt to suture onto 4th DI muscle).
- Trim skin flaps at the end to ensure adequate cover.

Specific complications of ray amputation
- Decreased grip strength
- Non-union (of transposition)
- Neuroma of common digital nerves

Multiple digital amputations
- Preserve all viable tissue
- Always consider the use of 'spare parts' of unsalvageable digits for immediate reconstruction of others (as grafts, flaps, transposition or for microsurgical replantation, especially pollicization).

Trans-metacarpal amputation
- Not a common level for elective amputation
- In trauma, preserve bony length with flap (pedicled groin flap, free flap) as this may allow delayed reconstruction of digits using microvascular toe transfers, as long as there are 'enabling structures' (nerves, tendons, plus a suitable recipient vascular pedicle).

Trans-carpal amputation
- Don't shorten to this level in trauma for transmetacarpal loss. Functionally, the metacarpal hand is much more useful than a prosthesis on an elective trans-carpal amputation or wrist disarticulation.
- Preservation of the radiocarpal joint allows a greater ROM for a prosthesis.

Wrist disarticulation
- Preservation of DRUJ allows full pronation and supination of the forearm.
- Use fishmouth incision distal to the level of DRUJ to ensure good cover.
- Identify superficial branch of radial nerve (SBRN), median and ulnar nerves, and cut under tension to ensure that the (inevitable) consequent neuroma will not cause pain in the stump.
  - Alternatively, identify proximally through small exploratory incision and divide away from amputation site.
  - Remember each major nerve has a small vessel running axially along it, which must be cauterized using diathermy.
- Identify radial and ulnar arteries, and ligate securely before division.
- Ligate or cauterize the anterior and posterior interosseous arteries.
- Cut flexor and extensor tendons and allow to retract.
- Cut through wrist capsule to disarticulate either between carpal rows, or through radiocarpal joint.
  - Try to preserve TFCC and avoid damage to DRUJ.
- Close skin neatly in layers.
- Use a soft well-padded dressing and leave undisturbed for several days, ensuring limb is elevated.

Forearm
- Try and preserve as much length as possible, to maintain pronation and supination.
- For elective amputation, discuss length preoperatively with prosthetist
- Design a fishmouth-type incision, with the skin flaps distal to the level of bony transection.
- Leave the divided muscle ends longer than the bone to provide some padding.
- Ensure the major nerves are divided proximally to the skin flaps.
- Release the tourniquet to check haemostasis before wound closure.
- Use a vacuum drain.
- Leave the drain *in situ*, and the wound undisturbed for 5–7 days.
- Apply compression to the stump early, once the skin is healed.
- Arrange early review by the prosthetic team.

Through elbow (elbow disarticulation)
- The flare of the distal humerus affords better rotation of a prosthesis than a more proximal amputation.
- Use fishmouth anterior and posterior flaps to cover bone end adequately.
- Identify and ligate brachial vessels anteriorly.
- Identify and divide the median nerve and allow to retract under the biceps muscle.

- Identify and divide the ulnar nerve by medial epicondyle and cut under tension and allow to retract, or place under triceps muscle.
- Divide the attachments of the biceps tendon and brachialis muscle.
- Elevate the common flexor origin from the medial humeral condyle and enter the elbow joint anteriorly.
- Identify and divide the radial nerve under the brachioradialis, and allow to retract between the brachialis and brachioradialis muscles.
- Divide the extensor muscles.
- Divide the radiohumeral and ulnarhumeral joint capsules.
- Drape muscle over the humerus, but do not suture tight.
- Release the tourniquet to check haemostasis before wound closure.
- Use a vacuum drain.
- Leave the drain *in situ*, and the wound undisturbed for 5–7 days.
- Apply compression to the stump early, once the skin is healed.
- Arrange early review by the prosthetic team.

Above elbow

- Maintain all possible length.
  - All shoulder movement (especially abduction and adduction) is lost in a very proximal amputation which is functionally the same as a shoulder disarticulation.
  - Always use a flap and or skin grafts to avoid further shortening for direct closure.
- Use fishmouth anterior and posterior flaps to cover bone end adequately.
- Divide the brachial vessels.
  - Try to keep as much vessel length as possible if microvascular free-flap cover is anticipated, and 'park' the vessels here they will be easily accessible during the reconstructive procedure.
- Divide the median, ulnar and radial nerves and cover with proximal muscles.
- Divide the flexor and extensor muscle masses distal to the planned level of bony resection to allow good cover.
- Release the tourniquet to check haemostasis before wound closure.
- Use a vacuum drain.
- Leave the drain *in situ*, and the wound undisturbed for 5–7 days.
- Apply compression to the stump early, once the skin is healed.
- Arrange early review by the prosthetic team.

Nail injury

Anatomy

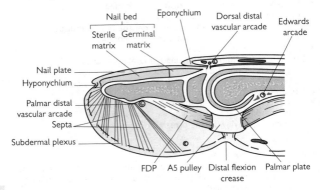

Fig. 6.1 Cross-section of the nail bed. FDP, flexor digitorum profundus.

The nail plate
- This is made up of tissue originating from the three areas of the nail bed (see below).
- Complete longitudinal growth (approximately 0.1mm/day) takes between 70 and 160 days.

The nail bed
- This consists of 3 parts; **the dorsal roof**, **the germinal matrix** (also known as the ventral floor) and **the sterile matrix** (also known as the ventral nail bed).
- The proximal end of the nail plate originates between the dorsal roof and the germinal matrix of the nail bed, enclosing it in a U-shaped fashion.

The nail fold (eponychial fold)
- The proximal nail plate sits under the **nail fold**.
- The skin over the dorsum of the nail fold is the **nail wall** (it lies dorsal to the dorsal roof of the nail bed).
- The thin membrane extending from the nail wall onto the dorsum of the nail plate is the **eponychium**.
- The **lunula** is the curved white opacity in the nail just distal to the eponychium, at the junction of the germinal and sterile matrices.

Hyponychium
- This is the mass of keratin between the distal nail plate and the nail bed. It is very adherent, and therefore resistant to infection.

Blood supply
Dorsal branch of the terminal trifurcation of the digital artery.

Function

- Support of the soft tissues at the very tip (hyponychium)
- Tool (scratching, picking, scraping, lifting etc.)

Nail bed injury

- Usually due to crush, which compresses and injures the (soft) nail bed between the (rigid) P3 and nail plate.
- AP and lateral X-rays should be obtained.

Subungual haematoma

The nail bed is highly vascular; closed trauma to the nail causes bleeding under the nail plate, with formation of a tight haematoma, causing the characteristic throbbing pain.

Treatment of subungual haematoma

Closed injuries (usually haematoma of less than 25% of visible nail bed) may be treated by trephine of the nail plate using a heated needle or paperclip. These should be explored if a significant laceration of the nail bed is suspected (see below).

Nail bed lacerations

These are either **simple**, **stellate** (from a burst-type injury) or **crush** (causing fragmentation of the nail bed). The nail plate may be dislocated from the nail fold.

Failure to explore these injuries acutely leads to late complications, such as distortion of the nail plate, or non-adherence of the nail plate to the nail bed.

Treatment of nail bed lacerations

- LA ring block
- Elevate the nail plate (keep it to use as splint)
- **Tip:** use small mucosal elevator or blunt dissecting scissor tips to get between the nail plate and the nail bed, then peel off the nail plate with a fine artery clip.
- Clean the sterile matrix.
- Repair the sterile matrix carefully (6/0 or 7/0 absorbable sutures), under loupe magnification.
- Loss of the sterile matrix can be reconstructed with SSG or split nail bed graft (either from adjacent injured digit, or from the great toe).
- If the nail bed is avulsed from the fold, it should be reduced and either sutured (if possible) or held in place by a splint.
- Use nail plate to splint nail fold.
- Replanted nail plate may 'take' and re-grow in young children.
- If nail plate lost or too damaged, use silicone sheet, or foil from a suture packet to splint nail fold.

Nail bed lacerations with fracture of distal phalanx

Approximately 50% of nail bed injuries have an associated underlying fracture of the distal phalanx (P3). The nail bed laceration communicates with the fracture, making it **an open fracture**.

Treatment of nail bed lacerations with a fracture of the distal phalanx

Follow principles for treatment of nail bed lacerations. In addition:

- Give IV antibiotics peri-operatively, and a course of oral antibiotics postoperatively.

- Copious irrigation before reduction of fracture.
- Undisplaced fractures may be treated conservatively after washout and nail bed repair. They are splinted by the soft tissues.
- Displaced fractures—use fine (0.8–1mm) K-wire for fracture, unless multiple small fragments, when it is better to let the soft tissues splint the fracture fragments without a wire.
- **Tip:** insert K-wire 2–3mm below hyponychium to get accurate placement into P3.
- Check lateral view with fluoroscan—easy to miss P3!
- Seymour fracture—dorsal dislocation of P3 from physis with overlying nail bed injury. Nail also dislocated from eponychial fold (📕 see p. 145).

Nail growth following injury

There is a delay in distal nail growth for 21 days following injury, when the nail thickens proximal to the injury site. This causes the bulge in an injured nail as it grows out. After this, the nail growth is faster than normal for 50 days, then it slows down for 30 days, after which time it becomes normal.

Reconstruction of nail complex

Reconstruction of the nail complex is difficult, and often imperfect, even in the most skilled hands. The categories below are guidelines; problems often overlap, and must be evaluated case by case.

Non-adherence of nail plate to nail bed

- Scarring of underlying nail bed, which is no longer adherent to nail plate.
- Keratin builds up under nail, and this may be mistaken for fungal infection.
- Treatment:
  - Excise the scar.
  - Close directly if possible
  - Replace defect with split nail bed graft, usually from a toe.

Split nail

- Caused by scar in dorsal floor/germinal matrix/sterile matrix complex.
- Treatment:
  - Excise and repair scar of sterile matrix.
  - Excise part of GM and replace with full thickness composite graft of GM from 2nd toe, with acceptable, but not perfect results.
  - Ablation of GM in severe cases

Nail spicule

- Usually remnant of GM complex following distal amputation
- Treatment:
  - Lift up flap of eponychium
  - Excise spicule and GM remnant

Hook nail (parrot-beak deformity)

- Caused by tight closure of a distal fingertip amputation, or loss of bony support for the nail bed.

- Treatment:
  - Release scarred tip
  - Elevate nail bed
  - Replace bony loss with bone graft (can absorb)
  - Local advancement flap
  - Microvascular partial toe transfer (complex solution)

Absence
- Congenital, or post injury
- Treatment:
  - Excise skin or scar in shape of nail and replace with full thickness skin grafts
  - Microvascular nail bed transfer

Technical tips
- Exploration of GM—ensure incisions are perpendicular to curve of eponychium to prevent deformity
- The GM stains with methylene blue. This is very useful to differentiate it from the rest of the nail bed, especially when performing nail ablation or removing nail spicules.

High-pressure injection injury

- Percutaneous injection of pressurized liquid or gas into the upper limb.
- This is a surgical emergency; the diagnosis should be made immediately, and surgical decompression performed urgently.

Pathophysiology

- Small entry wound
- Pressurized injectate spreads diffusely along fascial planes, flexor tendon sheaths, lumbrical canals, and NVBs.
- Rapid expansion within confined tissue compartments will lead to compartment syndrome.

Factors determining extent of injury

- Injected material:
  - Nature
  - Quantity
  - Temperature
- Kinetic energy transfer from injection

Epidemiology

- Incidence approximately 1 in 600 hand injuries
- Materials:
  - Grease
  - Paint
  - Paint thinner
  - Hydraulic fluid
  - Diesel fuel
  - Moulding plastic
  - Wax
- Distal non-dominant index finger most commonly affected.

Clinical features

- Often few early signs.
- Small puncture entry wound with minimal swelling masks severity of injury, especially to inexperienced physicians.
- Often overlooked, and present late to appropriate specialists, with massive inflammation, compartment syndrome and ischaemia.
- Radiograph useful to determine the extent of soft tissue involvement:
  - Shows soft tissue shadows, with gas and debris in the tissue.

Surgery

- These injuries should not be underestimated, and the primary surgical procedures should be performed by experienced senior surgeons.
- Exploration by junior surgical trainees is likely to undertreat this condition, and it is best to perform the necessary radical surgery during the first procedure.
- Wide decompression of finger and involved proximal compartments is required.
- Meticulous wound excision of all injectate and necrotic tissue, using loupe magnification.
- Delayed closure for non-organic injections.

- Open wound technique for organic injections.
- Secondary reconstruction of soft tissue defects often required using heterodigital flaps.
- Amputation may be the only option—do not shorten to the definitive level to close wound immediately, especially when there is extensive contamination.
- Oil granulomas may need to be excised late.

Outcome

- Variable
- Depends on nature of injection, and delay to treatment.
- Amputation rate 10–48%.
- Stiff digit in approximately 40%.

Extravasation injury

Leakage of drug or fluid from a vein into a surrounding tissue during intravenous administration.

Epidemiology
- Incidence low in specialist cancer treatment units.
- Incidence higher in general hospital environment.

Pathophysiology
- Damage to subcutaneous tissue and overlying skin.

Vesicant drugs
- Cause extensive necrosis.
- Inflammatory process continues for weeks after extravasation.

Irritant drugs
- Cause inflammation and pain.
- Usually acid or alkaline.
- High osmolality.

Vasoactive drugs
- Cause ischaemic necrosis.

Clinical features
Early
- Pain
- Erythema
- Swelling

Late
- Blistering
- Fixed staining of skin
- Skin necrosis

Delayed features
- Skin slough
- Ulceration
- Exposed tendons

Late complications
- Scars
- Joint contracture
- Tendon rupture
- Digital necrosis

Treatment
Early

Non-surgical
- Topical ice
- Topical steroid cream
- Hyaluronidase injection
- Steroid injection
- Saline injection to dilute toxins

- Specific antidotes:
  - Vasopressor agents—phentolamine
  - Cisplatinum—sodium thiosulphate
  - Doxorubicin—dimethylsulphoxide

Surgical
- Saline flush
- Multiple stab incisions
- Flush with saline and hyaluronidase
- Use liposuction for harmful vesicant substances

Late

Skin necrosis
- Dressings
- Splints
- Hand therapy
- May need SSG
- Occasionally wide excision and flap, when there is an extensive zone of injury with exposure of non-graftable structures, or across flexion creases.
- Occasionally amputation in unsalvageable part.

Outcome

- Early treatment with saline flush and liposuction prevents skin ulceration and preserves hand function.
- Only 15% healed without skin necrosis in delayed referrals.

Gunshot wounds

Pathophysiology

Energy transfer

- Gunshot wounds (GSW) and other missile injuries should be classified according to the amount of kinetic energy transfer imparted by the injury, rather than just the velocity of the projectile (i.e. high or low-energy transfer injury, rather than high- or low-velocity bullet).
  - This principle is demonstrated by the different injuries produced by the same shotgun at close or long range.
- Energy = Mass × Velocity^2

High-energy transfer

- Rifles
- Military projectiles (grenades, shrapnel from artillery, mines)
- Large calibre handguns
- Shotgun close range

Low-energy transfer

- Small calibre hand guns
- Shotgun long range

Entry wound

- Relatively small and proportional to the size of the missile.
- May be burns to the skin, and tattooing from propellant material in close range injury.

Cavitation

- As kinetic energy is transferred to tissues from the missile, the cavity around the wound track expands temporarily, creating a bigger wound with a vacuum. This phenomenon is known as **temporary cavitation**.
- Contaminants (clothing, propellant, soil) are then 'sucked' into the vacuum of the temporary cavity.
- Because of this, damage is always more extensive than it appears to be from the outside.

Secondary missiles

- Energy can be transferred to fragments of bone or contaminants, which then act as secondary missiles (usually high-energy transfer wounds), often opening up wound tracks in a different orientation from the original.

Exit wound

- Usually much bigger than the entry wound, due to energy transfer and secondary missiles.

Treatment of gun shot wounds

Resuscitation

- Remember to treat the whole patient, not just the GSW.
- ATLS primary and secondary survey.
- Resuscitate as necessary.
- Control haemorrhage, especially when there is a hole in a vessel (which spurts) rather than complete division (which usually goes into spasm).

Examination
- Vascularity and pulses
- Nerve function:
  - Motor
  - Sensory
- Muscle/tendon function

Investigations
- Plain X-ray
- Angiogram in vascular injury

Non-surgical
- Give tetanus toxoid if not covered
- Broad spectrum antibiotics, including penicillin if not allergic

Surgical
- Always use a tourniquet where possible
- ⚠ GSW should never be closed primarily

High-energy transfer
- Excise entry wound and exit wound.
- Extend wounds to explore wound track, including those caused by secondary missiles.
- Meticulous wound excision.
- Fix fractures.
- Immediate vascular reconstruction if required.
- Pack with gauze and leave all wounds open.
  - ⚠ Do not use 'tacking sutures' to close partially.
- Perform further wound inspection at 48–72 hours.
- Perform delayed closure, usually requiring SSG or flaps.
- Perform delayed nerve or tendon reconstruction, either at the time of the skin closure, or as a secondary 'late' procedure.

Low-energy transfer
- There is no consensus in the treatment of low-energy transfer GSW.
- There is now good evidence that in selected (mostly superficial) low-energy transfer GSW, the wound track can be managed by excision of the entry and exit wounds, and thorough washout of the wound track without opening it completely for exploration.
- The problem with this concept in the upper limb is the potential for injury to the complex functional anatomical structures along the track of the wound. Washout (rather than excision) of the wound track should **only** be done if there is no nerve or tendon injury on clinical examination, and the wound track is very superficial, and does not pass through the course of any major functional structures.
- Washout (rather than excision) of the wound track should not be performed for any military GSW, even if low-energy transfer.
- Wound tracks should be explored if there is any doubt about damage to underlying structures or compartment syndrome.

Burns

Body surface area

- Burn wounds are assessed according to percentage of body surface area (BSA) involved.
- The palm of the hand represents approximately 1% BSA.
- The whole upper limb is approximately 9% BSA.
- The percentage BSA involvement determines the requirement for fluid resuscitation.

Depth of burn

- Burns are classified by the depth of penetration through the skin).
- The depth of the burn wound determines the prognosis in terms of healing, scarring and requirement for surgical intervention.
  - Erythema
  - Partial thickness
    - Superficial
    - Deep
  - Full thickness
- It may be difficult to differentiate intermediate burns as superficial or deep partial thickness (which determines the treatment necessary). The burn wound often demarcates after several days and the depth may then be easier to assess.

Erythema

- Very superficial burn which has not penetrated the skin sufficiently to cause a wound.
- The skin becomes red and tender, but does not blister. This resolves after several days. It is easily mistaken for a deeper burn, which may then lead to overassessment of the % BSA.

Superficial partial thickness (1st degree)

The burn penetrates the superficial part of the dermis. They are sensate, and there is capillary refill.

They usually heal in 10–14 days with dressings and do not scar deeply.

Deep partial thickness (2nd degree)

The burn penetrates the deep part of the dermis. The sensibility varies, and there may be fixed staining of the tissue with no capillary refill.

They take weeks or months to heal with dressings. These are now mostly treated by early tangential excision and SSG.

Full thickness (3rd and 4th degree)

The burn penetrates the full thickness of the skin (3rd degree), and sometimes the deeper structures (fat, tendon, neurovascular structures, bone) (4th degree). These are insensate, and look and feel like leather.

Nature of injury

- Thermal:
  - The commonest cause.
  - Dorsal injury commoner than palmar.
  - Hand burns often from contact with heat source.
- Electrical
- Chemical

First aid
⚠ **Significant hand burns, and those patients requiring fluid resuscitation should be transferred to a specialist burns unit.**
⚠ **Remember your ATLS principles, as there may be other life-threatening injuries.**

Inhalational burns
- History of explosion, fire in enclosed space, or petrol burns.
- Hoarse voice, singed facial hair, perioral oedema, soot in airway in unconscious patient.
- Intubate if unconscious.
- Get urgent anaesthetic review, and consider paralysis and intubation if conscious and good history/examination for inhalational burns (always easier than emergency airway).
- Surgical airway (cricothyroidotomy) in emergency.

Systemic effect of burn injury
- Fluid resuscitation required if over 15% BSA in adults and 10% in children.
- Gain 2 good sites of IV access.
  - Venous cutdown preferred to central lines (which may lead to bacteraemia).
- Send blood for FBC, haematocrit, urea and electrolytes (U&E), creatine kinase (CK), group & save.
- Give crystalloid fluid, preferably Hartmann's solution (or normal saline if unavailable) according to the **Parkland** formula.
- Insert urinary catheter and monitor hourly urine output.
- The Parkand formula is merely a guideline. Fluids should be titrated according to the systemic condition of the patient, urine output and haematocrit.

Parkland formula for burn fluid resuscitation

1. Calculate the total fluid requirement (in mls) for 1st 24 hours:
   (4 × [weight in Kg] × [% BSA burn])
2. Divide this number in half.
3. Give first half over 1st 8 hours.
   (NB this 8 hours starts from the time of burning—may need to catch up if you treat several hours following injury).
4. Give second half over 2nd 16 hours.

Upper limb thermal burn wounds
- Remove from source of burn
- Cold water irrigation +++
- Hand bags—any clean plastic bag will do—secure around wrists LOOSELY with tape.
  - Good first aid
  - Easy to apply
  - Prevent dessication
  - Allow unrestricted swelling and some movement.

- Cling film—be careful not to apply circumferentially, which can cause constriction (and compartment syndrome) following swelling.
- Strict elevation
- Analgesia
- (Escharotomy—see below)
- Early splinting in functional position, ensuring 1st webspace abducted.
- Early K-wiring of PIPjs in extension may be indicated in severe burns.

Dressings
- Apply dressings to the hand after the first day or two, especially for superficial partial thickness burns, which do not require surgery.
  - These are tolerated better by the patients than hand bags
  - Allow better movement than hand bags.

Chemical burns
- Remove source of burn/contaminated clothing.
- Copious irrigation.

Surgical treatment

Immediate (escharotomy)
Circumferential deep partial thickness or full thickness burns may compromise the circulation of the upper limb. The treatment is immediate decompression by incision of the burn wound (the eschar, so escharotomy). There may also be a compartment syndrome, especially in electrical conduction burns.

- Escharotomy must be performed immediately, either in the emergency department or preferably in the operating theatre, as long as there is no delay transferring the patient.
- Although the burned tissue may be insensate, the surrounding tissue is sensate. Escharotomy is **not** pain free, and usually requires GA or at least some form of sedation (depending on the facilities available).
- Use cutting diathermy (on coagulation setting)—rather than scalpel to reduce bleeding. Cut veins are splinted open once the wound springs apart, and bleeding can be difficult to control.
- Go from distal to proximal to reduce bleeding. Intact proximal wound margin acts as a tourniquet while distal part is released.
- Incisions.
  - Use mid-axial incisions in the upper arm and forearm.
  - Extend onto dorsum of hand, and release intrinsics.
  - Extend over, and decompress carpal tunnel.
  - Use mid-lateral incisions in digits.
  - Fasciotomy mandatory in electrical burns.
- Ensure haemostasis following escharotomy **before** transfer to a specialist burns centre, as exsanguination is a possibility, especially in children.

Early

Tangential excision

Deep partial thickness burn wounds are shaved with a skin graft knife until bleeding dermis is reached. Can be done under a tourniquet to reduce blood loss, in which case the wound has a different appearance ('*If it's red it's dead, if it's white it's alright*'). SSG is then applied.

Deep excision

Full thickness burns can be excised completely (usually with diathermy) down to deep fascia, and then skin grafted. This can be done in the upper arm and forearm, but should be avoided in the hand where the surgeon should attempt to preserve the tendons and neurovascular structures where possible.

Split skin graft

The use of sheet, rather than meshed, SSG is desirable in the hand to minimize graft contracture. The junctions of grafts should be placed at joint creases where possible. Careful splinting and early mobilization after graft take is required, along with very intensive hand therapy, to achieve good results.

Late

The best treatment of burns scar contracture is prevention by early wound closure, splinting and early movement. The treatment of burns scars follows the general principles of reconstructive hand surgery (see Chapter 8).

Scar release/resurfacing

- SSG contracts, and should be avoided over joints.
- FTSG may be used to resurface small areas, but can still contract if placed in an area of deep scar, and will not revascularize ('take') on a bed of scar.
- Small local flaps can be used to reorientate scar bands. Traditional Z-plasty and other local scar revisions which require extensive undermining do not work well in burns scar or skin grafts, as the tips die, and further scar contracture results.
- The Y to V plasty is useful for burns scar revision as it does not require undermining of the skin flaps. It gains length at the expense of lateral laxity.
- Large areas of burns scar contracture or tight skin grafts usually require resurfacing with further full thickness skin grafts or by importing tissue in the form of pedicled or free flaps. The vascular pedicles of local flaps may have been affected by the burn wound or constricted by scar. Importing tissue by the use of a microvascular free flap, which is anastomosed onto deep vessels outside the zone of injury, is more reliable.

1st webspace

- 4- or 5-flap Z-plasty
- FTSG
- Free flap:
  - Free flaps more reliable than pedicled flaps

- Thin fasciocutaneous perforator flaps work well (anterolateral thigh flap, lateral arm flap) with long vascular pedicles and acceptable donor site morbidity.
- Pedicled flaps:
  - Radial forearm flap
  - Ulnar artery flaps
  - Becker (ulnar artery perforator) flap
  - Posterior interosseous flap
  - Pedicled groin flap

2nd to 4th webspace
- X to M plasty
- FTSG

Claw hand
- Procedures described for non-burned hands do not work well for burns scars.
- Flap cover may be required to allow useful release of MCPJs.
- Arthodesis may be more effective than attempts at release of the PIPJ and DIPJ.

Boutonnière deformity
- Often more complex pure subluxation of lateral bands of extensor mechanism, with absence of central slip and secondary contracture of PIPJ and volar skin.
- Tendon reefing procedures have limited benefit.
- Soft tissue cover is often difficult.
- Primary arthrodesis may be preferable.

Hand therapy for burns
- Early movement and correct splint application is the cornerstone of the management of the burned hand.
- Particular attention must be paid to the 1st webspace to prevent skin and/or adduction contractures.
- Fingers should be splinted in a functional position to prevent clawing and/or boutonnière deformities.

Electrical burns
- Flash burns commoner, and more superficial, than conduction burns (similar to normal thermal burn).
- Conduction burns deeper, and usually more extensive and serious.
- Conduction burns have entry and exit wound with burned tissue in between (similar to high-energy transfer gunshot wound).
- Usually extensive muscle damage (with high CK) and requirement for excision and fasciotomy.
- Check CK, C-reactive protein (CRP), U&E (beware high potassium), and consider early renal dialysis to prevent renal failure.
- May be devascularization of limb:
  - requires immediate vascular reconstruction (consider through-flow microvascular free flap).
  - fasciotomy and excision of dead muscle MANDATORY prior to revascularization.
- May be damage to major nerves.

Chemical burns

- Many possible agents.
- Alkali burns commonest.
- Alkali burns progress, as liquefaction allows deeper penetration of the chemical into tissues.
- Neutralizing agents discouraged because of exothermic reaction.
- Most treated by copious irrigation, followed by surgery if necessary.

Hydrofluoric acid burns

- Used in industrial glass etching and rust-removing compounds
- Fluoride ion penetrates tissue causing intense pain with local destruction
- Predelection for subungual region
- Intense vasospasm causes necrosis of fingertips
- May be lethal if untreated

Treatment

- Protect first aiders from injury by source
- Copious irrigation
- Calcium gluconate gel neutralizes HF
- Use topically or in glove
- May need systemic treatment with calcium gluconate

Frostbite

Cold injury can be classified as **freezing** (frostbite) or **non-freezing** (usually affecting feet, after prolonged immersion in near freezing water—trench foot).

Pathophysiology

- Cooling of body temperature (hypothermia) with peripheral shutdown as part of normal physiological response to cold.
- Exhaustion leads to hypoglycaemia with inability to generate sufficient heat to keep peripheries (hands, feet, nose, ears) warm.
- Dehydration with increased blood viscosity contributes to poor perfusion of small digital vessels, eventually 'clumping' of erythrocytes block end capillaries.
- High altitude:
  - Hypoxia from lower atmospheric pO_2 at altitude.
  - Hyperventilation from hypoxia causes dehydration from increased insensible fluid losses in exhaled breath.
  - Secondary thrombocythaemia (usually ↑ 1–2g/dl haemoglobin (Hb) as normal consequence of physiological acclimatization to altitude) contributes to increased blood viscosity with poor peripheral perfusion.
  - Cold temperature.
- Eventually tissues freeze progressively.
- Secondary injury on rewarming due to swelling and formation of microemboli.
  - Possibility of compartment syndrome.

Predisposing factors

- Cold still air temperature
- Windchill effect
  - 13 mph wind at +5°C gives effective temperature of −6°C
- Altitude
- Alcohol/drug abuse
- Exhaustion, with hypoglycaemia
- Relevant systemic conditions:
  - Peripheral vascular disease
  - Raynaud's disease
  - Diabetes
  - Hypothyroidism
- Previous cold injury (impairs normal physiological response to cold)
- Tobacco smoking

Classification

Frostbite is freezing of the tissues resulting in necrosis. It is a 'cold burn'.

Frostnip

Transient cold injury which returns to normal within 30 minutes of rewarming. This is analogous to superficial burn erythema.

Superficial frostbite

Permanent freezing cold injury affecting the epidermis and superficial layers of the dermis. This is analogous to a partial thickness burn. There is usually complete recovery following demarcation and peeling off of necrotic skin—known as the 'carapace' or 'eshcar'—(like the icing on a cake) leaving new pink tissue underneath. This explains the rationale of delaying surgical excision of frostbitten tissue, which often leads to unnecessary loss. There will be cold sensitivity proportionate to the depth of the frostbite.

Deep frostbite

Permanent freezing cold injury affecting (progressively) the full thickness of the skin, fat, tendon, muscle and bone. This is analogous to a full thickness burn. It leads to significant tissue loss and permanent cold sensitivity.

Affects

- Inhabitants of cold climates
- Mountaineers, especially high altitude
- Homeless sleeping rough
- Alcohol/drug abusers
- Industrial cold processing workers

Clinical features

Superficial frostbite

- Initially, white frozen skin (looks/feels like candle wax)
- On rewarming, swollen, mottled, purple skin. Pain+++.
- 24–48 hours, blister formation (clear or serosanguinous fluid)
- 2–7 days, blister fluid absorbs, tissue may turn black
- Days/months, black areas harden (carapace), and peel off revealing new, pink skin.

Deep frostbite

- Initially, white or purple-grey numb tissue
- On rewarming, tissue remains waxy and discoloured. Pain+++.
- Days/weeks, blister formation (dark fluid)
- Months, carapace formation, separation and eventual auto amputation of distal part.

Management

Immediate

- Treat systemic hypothermia and evacuate patient to a safe environment.
- Rehydrate patient
- Rapid rewarming at 40°C. This is very painful and requires strong analgesia.
  - Field conditions—warm water (hot bath temperature).
  - Hospital—use whirlpool bath with disinfectant solution.
- Keep patient and limb warm.
- Elevate limb.
- Deroof blisters (unless still in field conditions where clean dressings are not available).
- Clean non-adherent dressings.

- Consider aspirin or other anti-platelet aggregation drugs (dextran, prostaglandin infusion)
- Observe for compartment syndrome in severe deep frostbite injury— fasciotomy may be required.

❶ This is the only situation in which early surgical debridement may be indicated, especially if muscle is involved.

Late
- Manage frostbite wounds with clean dressings until desiccation of necrotic tissue has occurred (2–3 weeks)
- Wait for demarcation and separation of carapace (may take several months)
- Perform definitive surgical excision/amputation when frostbite is fully demarcated

Factitious injury (Secretans's)

General principles

- These are usually unexpected
- Suspect in wounds which you would expect to heal, and don't have a reason not to heal.
- The patient will often have seen other specialists with the same problem.
- Seek the motivation for doing it.
- Involve clinical psychologists if you are suspicious of factitious injury.
- Confront the patient about it with caution, as this can occasionally precipitate episodes of further self-harm, or even suicide.
- It is sometimes necessary to admit the patient to hospital to make the diagnosis.
- You will not cure this problem by surgery alone. You have identify and treat the underlying psychological reason(s), or they will keep doing it.

Factitious wounds

- Factitious wounds may heal after immobilization in a cast or occlusive dressing, only to recur when this is removed.
- Determined patients can still interfere with wounds despite POP, or seemingly impregnable dressings.

Factitious lymphoedema

- Usually caused by the self-application of a tourniquet.
- Less commonly by repeated blows (also causes bruising) or self injection (resulting in low-grade infection).

Munchausen by proxy

- Very occasionally factitious injury by proxy (children, elderly relatives or carers for elderly).
- The patient must be protected.
  - Hospital admission may be necessary to make the diagnosis and protect the victim.
- The assailants need psychiatric help.

Reconstruction

Principles of reconstruction of upper limb injuries

Principles of reconstruction of the upper limb
- Adequate, careful wound excision
- Stable skeletal fixation
- Reconstruction of vessel, nerve, tendon, bone:
  - immediate/delayed
- Primary healing:
  - direct tension-free closure
  - skin grafts to graftable areas—not across flexor creases, or to areas where secondary bone, nerve or tendon surgery is required
  - flap (replace 'like with like')
- Early movement
- → Good result

Restoration of a functional hand

Requirements
- Sensibility
- A flexible digit
- Another flexible (or rigid) digit
- Power and active movement
- Aesthetics

Sensibility
- Nerve repair
- Nerve transport
- Import sensate skin

Power
- Stability to allow power transduction
- Tendon transfer
- Functional muscle transfer

Bone reconstruction
- Maintain/restore skeletal length by external fixator, internal bridging plate or bone graft.
- When skeletal length has been lost, and there is scar contracture, interposition graft or distraction lengthening may be required.
- Can use approximately 5cm of non-vascularized bone graft in the hand if there is well-vascularized soft tissue cover.
- Immediate reconstruction of bone with non-vascularized bone graft is acceptable in a clean wound with good soft tissue cover.
- Longer defects may require the use of vascularized bone, especially in a previously infected, poorly vascularized, or extensively scarred wound bed.
- Vascularized bone may import the potential for growth in children.

Nerve reconstruction

- Successful nerve repair is the main determinant of good outcome in complex upper limb trauma.
- Tension-free end-to-end nerve repair is desirable.
- Where there is loss of nerve tissue and direct repair is not possible, immediate nerve reconstruction using cable grafts is acceptable in a clean wound with good soft tissue cover.
- Synthetic nerve guides are an alternative (but future evaluation needed).
- Following unreconstructable nerve injury or loss, consider:
  - the potential requirement for delayed tendon transfers when planning the immediate reconstruction.
  - nerve transfer
  - importing sensate skin using a flap from a different nerve territory.

Tendon reconstruction

- Immediate tendon reconstruction within the flexor tendon sheath will stick.
- Flexor tendons usually require 2-stage reconstruction:
  - Exception—rheumatoid arthritis
  - Exception—short segment of tendon graft in zone 3 , 4 or 5 repaired with a strong weave at either end, and followed by immediate mobilization.
- Immediate flexor tendon repair is unlikely to work in certain situations (e.g. flexor tendon injury over a burst-type phalangeal fracture with loss of the flexor tendon sheath).
  - Insert a silastic tendon rod primarily and reconstruct the pulleys if necessary.
- Do not reconstruct tendons acutely unless you know that the hand can be moved immediately.
- Delayed tendon reconstruction when passive range has been restored usually gives a better outcome.
- Consider reasonably early tenolysis (+/– scar resurfacing with a flap) after immediate tendon reconstruction in adults.
- Children may grow out of tendon adhesions.

Soft tissue

Issues to consider

The patient's needs
- Occupation
- Psychological issues
- Quick simple operation *versus* multi-stage, complex procedures.

The nature of the defect
- Site
- Size of defect
- Does it all need to be covered by a flap, or can it be skin-grafted?
- What is missing? E.g. skin, tendon, nerve, bone

The nature of the wound bed
- Clean—can cover now

- Dirty—needs further wound excision
- Infected—needs further wound excision/antibiotics
- Don't use SSG on infected bed until clear microbiology swabs (especially β-haemolytic Group A or G *Streptococcus*)
- Can use combination of wound excision and vascularized flap for chronically infected wounds

The timing of soft tissue cover

Donor site considerations, e.g. toe transfers for thumb reconstruction

- A great toe transfer looks more natural than second toe
- A second toe transfer provides a functional thumb
- BUT, the great toe gives terrible, disabling donor site when taken through or proximal to 1st MTP joint.

Spare part surgery

- Always consider how damaged digits or amputated parts can be used to reconstruct other digits.
- Even using discarded skin can save a skin graft donor site.

Tips for decision-making

Think about the long-term strategy

- Think about the whole, staged (if necessary) reconstruction.
- There is always a choice of available flaps.
- Think about use of available vascular pedicles, especially if required for later reconstruction with another flap, such as toe transfer.
  - Consider the use of through-flow flaps
  - It may be better to use a pedicled groin flap for immediate soft tissue cover, saving the available vessel for a later flap

Adequate wound excision is the key to success

- Wound excision and meticulous preparation of the wound bed is essential
- Inadequate wound excision is the commonest cause of infection under a flap, especially important when treating wounds which present several weeks after injury.

Assess tissue viability during wound excision

- Examine the base of skin flaps for perforator attachments
- Excise damaged skin up to healthy bleeding edges

Composite defects don't necessarily need composite flap reconstruction

- The geometry of bone, tendon, skin and vascular pedicle length may make it difficult to design a flap to meet all requirements in one stage.
- Staged reconstructions work well, and allow oedema to settle with return of passive ROM before tendon reconstruction.

Make provision for future access

- Think about cover for the next stage of reconstruction. Secondary bone, tendon or nerve reconstruction is much easier under a fasciocutaneous flap than under scar, SSG or a skin-grafted muscle or adipofascial flap.

Divide the defect into critical and non-critical areas

- Don't always think 'one defect, one flap'

- Critical areas (e.g. flexor surfaces, exposed fractures or bare bone, tendon or nerve repairs) need to be covered using flaps
- Non-critical areas may be covered by SSG

Think about donor sites
- Although pedicled forearm flaps are useful, the donor sites are terribly disfiguring, and now mostly avoidable by the use of microvascular free flaps or pedicled groin flaps.
- If you have to use the forearm as a donor site, consider fascial flaps cutaneous scars, but no skin-grafted secondary defect).

Involve the patient in decision making when there are options—informed consent
- The patient's views (which vary between individuals) are as important as the surgeon's in planning reconstructions, especially:
  - numbers and complexity of multi-staged procedures required
  - time required for rehabilitation after surgery
  - flap donor site choice
  - the end-stage of reconstruction—it is often possible to continue with minor adjustments for many years, and patients will usually tell you when they have had enough and are happy with what they have

*Do what you are good at, and can make work in **your** hospital*
- A successful, simple reconstruction is better than a clever, complex reconstruction which fails.
- Know your limits.
- If you feel a complex reconstruction is required, and you cannot do it, refer the patient to someone who can **early**.
  - This is especially important in children.

Surgical incisions

- The hand is second only to the face in awareness of appearance by both patients and those with whom they interact. Surgeons should always consider this when designing incisions.
- The planning of surgical incisions requires understanding of the different options, as well as experience in their use.
- Surgical incisions should:
  - Be extensible
  - Provide access to deep structures
  - Provide vascularized skin flaps (avoid very long, narrow flaps)
  - Avoid formation of scar contractures. Straight incisions across flexor creases (digits, palm, wrist, elbow, axilla) lead to scar contracture.
  - Avoid unnecessary dissection (leading to oedema and scarring)
- Scars should be placed on the non-dependent sides of the digits (e.g. radial side of little finger) where possible.

Types of incision

Dorsal

- **Straight** incisions are used on the dorsum of the wrist, hand and digits. These preserve longitudinal veins, and provide well-vascularized skin flaps with good access.
- **Horizontal** incisions across the MCPJ heads may be used for access to the MCPJs or intrinsic insertions into the extensor hood.
- **Zig-zag** incisions on the dorsum of the hand are unsightly and may create ischaemic skin flaps if the base is too narrow.
- **Lazy S or tri-radiate** (wine glass) incisions to approach the DIPJ.

Mid-lateral

- This runs along the side of the digit, dorsal to the neurovascular bundle, and therefore safe.
- It is designed by flexing the fingertip into the palm, and marking dots at the apices of the DIPJ, PIPJ and MCPJ creases. The digit is then extended and a line drawn connecting the dots.

Palmar

- **Bruner.**[1] These zig-zag type incisions are used in the volar aspect of the palm and digits. In the digits, they run from the mid-lateral line across the span of a phalanx to the contralateral mid-lateral line. In the palm they should be 1–2cm long, zig-zagging between palmar creases
- **Half Bruner.** These are similar to Bruner incisions, but zig-zag across half of the width of the digit.
  - NB A zig-zag incision should NOT cross the full width of the digit and back within the span of a phalanx. This leads to tip necrosis with flap loss.

1. Bruner JM (1967). The zig-zag volar-digital incision for flexor tendon surgery. *Plastic and reconstructive surgery* **40**: 571–4.

Suturing

Technique

General points

- Loupe magnification (2.5 to 4 x) is useful for all hand surgery.
- Soft tissues should be handled gently using fine instruments (fine toothed Adson's forceps, skin hooks).
  - Don't use your fine forceps for heavy soft tissue or bony work—use something stronger, such as toothed Gillies' forceps.
- Evert the wound edges and close dead space.
- Handle tendons minimally.
- Nerves and vessels should be sutured with microsurgical instruments, with the aid of an operating microscope.

Skin suturing

- The needle should enter the skin perpendicularly. Skimming through the skin edge at an acute angle leads to inversion of the wound.
- An equal volume of tissue should be taken in the bite of the needle on either side of the wound. When suturing skin of unequal thickness, this means taking differential-sized bites to get an equal *volume* of tissue in each one.
- Do not pick up the needle by the point with the needle holder. This blunts the tip, which then tears (rather than cuts) the skin and damages it.
- Putting the knot to one side of the wound after tying the first double throw helps to evert the wound edges.

Types of suture

Simple interrupted

A simple suture passing through either side of the wound.

Corner sutures

This suture passes through the skin edge, takes a subdermal bite of the corner of a triangular flap, and then is passed out through the adjacent skin edge. This is less traumatic to the tips of triangular flaps, and neater than simple interrupted sutures.

Mattress sutures

Insert a simple suture. Instead of tying it normally, take a further bite on the side where your needle has exited, and bring it out on the opposite side (where you started). Mattress sutures can be vertical or horizontal. They have the advantage over simple sutures of everting wound edges, and so can be interspersed between simple sutures to do this. They are difficult to remove when non-absorbable suture material is used. This is not a problem with absorbable suture material.

Subdermal

Continuous subdermal sutures are useful to close straight incisions in the arm, forearm and dorsum of the hand and wrist. The initial knot is placed deeply, and then small, equal bites are taken from either side of the dermis. The suture can be finished with a buried knot (large buried knots led to 'suture abscesses'), or the end brought through the skin and either tied in a knot through the skin or taped down.

It is now commonplace to use absorbable suture material for subdermal sutures. Non-absorbable suture material can also be used, which should be removed at 10–14 days after surgery.

Deep dermal

Interrupted deep dermal sutures are used to appose skin edges prior to skin suturing in the arm, forearm and dorsum of the wrist and hand. If placed in an 'in to out, out to in' fashion, and tightened along the axis of the wound (rather than across it), the knot is buried on the deep surface, reducing the chance of extrusion of suture material later.

Suture material

Most suture materials are now synthetic. Biological materials such as catgut and silk are still available, but tend to cause more inflammatory reaction than synthetics.

Choice of suture material should be made according to strength, handling qualities, half-life (absorbable sutures) and tissue reactivity.

Strength

Use the lightest suture material which is adequate.
- 3/0 (proximal) or 4/0 (distal) deep dermal sutures.
- 4/0 skin sutures in the upper arm, forearm, wrist and dorsum of the hand.
- 5/0 skin sutures in the palm and digits in adults.
- 6/0 skin sutures in the palm and digits in children.

Interrupted skin sutures

Non-absorbable
- Nylon [Polyamide 6] (Ethilon®, Ethicon, Johnson & Johnson International)
- Polypropylene (Prolene®, Ethicon, Johnson & Johnson International)

Absorbable
- Polyglactin 910 (Vicryl rapide®, Ethicon, Johnson & Johnson International)
  - Rubs out by 10–14 days

Continuous subdermal suture
- Polyglactin 910 (Vicryl®, Ethicon, Johnson & Johnson International)
- Poliglecaprone 25 (Monocryl®, Ethicon, Johnson & Johnson International)

Deep dermal suture
- Polyglactin 910 (Vicryl®, Ethicon, Johnson & Johnson International)
- Poliglecaprone 25 (Monocryl®, Ethicon, Johnson & Johnson International)
- Polydioxanone (PDS®, Ethicon, Johnson & Johnson International)

Site of suture

Digits and palm
- Simple interrupted sutures are used in the digits.
- Corner sutures are useful for insetting the tips of triangular flaps created by Bruner incisions.
- Horizontal mattress sutures are useful to evert the wound edges.

Dorsum of hand and wrist, forearm, and upper arm

- Simple interrupted or mattress sutures may be used for untidy wounds.
- Elective straight incisions may be closed using continuous subdermal absorbable sutures for the best cosmesis.

Removal of sutures

- Non-absorbable sutures should be removed at 10 to 14 days (this may depend on clinic times). If left longer than 14 days, unsightly, permanent suture marks will form.
- Absorbable sutures have the advantage that they do not need to be removed. This avoids disturbing wounds by suture removal, discomfort to the patient, and saves nursing time.
  - Polyglactin 910 (Vicryl rapide®, Ethicon, Johnson & Johnson International) sutures rub out by 10 to 14 days.

Wound care

Non-surgical

Cleaning
- This often requires some form of anaesthesia (LA/regional block/GA).
- Small, simple wounds can be cleaned without anaesthetic.
- Wounds should be cleaned mechanically using clean water or saline solution, and disinfectant.
- Contaminated wounds should be scrubbed.
- Ingrained dirt and grit should be scrubbed out (usually requires regional block or GA) to avoid tattooing of skin.

Dressings
Wound dressings should be:
- Non-constrictive:
  - Skin dressings and gauze strips should be applied in longitudinal strips (not circumferentially, which can restrict circulation).
  - Wool and bandage layers should be applied carefully to avoid constriction, particularly in the unconscious patient who is unable to tell you that the bandage is too tight.
- Non-adherent
- Absorbent
- Provide protection
- Immobilize the hand to protect repairs
- Be unrestrictive and light to allow early mobilization when required
- In general dressings applied in the operating theatre are bulky for proection and immobilization, and those applied postoperatively should be much lighter to allow hand therapy to continue.

First layer
- Paraffin gauze (tulle gras) is non-adherent for several days, after which it can stick to wounds. It is fenestrated to allow wound exudate to extrude. It is easily available, and cheap.
- Silicone sheet is non-adherent, and fenestrated. It is expensive.
- Suture strips should be avoided on digits, and where there is likely to be postoperative swelling.
- Infected or contaminated wounds can be dressed using iodine impregnated paraffin gauze (Inadine®) next to the skin, or by paraffin gauze with a layer of iodine soaked gauze on top.

Second layer
- Dressing: gauze swabs absorb wound exudate.
  - Gauze soaked in saline and wrung out adheres to wounds less than dry gauze.

Third layer
- Circumferential orthopaedic wool (Velband®) or extra gauze provides padding and support.

Fourth layer
- Crepe or clingwrap bandage hold the previous layers in position.

Splints
- Splints are designed to prevent full excursion of injured or reconstructed tendons, or to rest the hand after injury or infection.
- They can be made from plaster of Paris, fibreglass or thermoplastic material.
- The hand may be splinted safely in the position of safe immobilisation (POSI). This positions the joints with the collateral ligaments in the longest position preventing contractures.
    - Wrist extended at 30°
    - MCPJs flexed at 60° (collateral ligaments longest here because of convex 'cam' shape of MC head)
    - PIPJs and DIPJs fully extended.
- Splints should extend beyond the fingertips after tendon repairs in fingers. Finger movement may be permitted by using a splint to the level of MCPJs.
- Dorsal blocking splints are used following flexor tendon repairs.
- Volar splints are used following extensor tendon repairs.

Surgical

Debridement and wound excision
- The term debridement originated during the Napoleonic Wars, meaning 'unbridling' or decompression of missile wounds. It is often misinterpreted, and the term *'careful wound excision'* is probably clearer.
- **Careful wound excision is the cornerstone of the surgical management of soft tissue injuries.**
- **Tidy wounds** (fresh, less than 24 hours, sharp lacerations) can be sutured primarily.
- **Untidy wounds** (delayed, crushed, devitalized, contaminated or infected wounds) should have necrotic tissue excised and should NOT be closed primarily.
    - 1–2mm excision of the wound edges is adequate for simple wounds.
    - Substantial tissue excision is required in grossly contaminated wounds.
- Wound excision should be followed by copious irrigation with clean water or saline solution.
- Wound irrigation should follow (not precede) careful wound excision.
    - An initial (pre-excision) scrub may sometimes be required where there is gross contamination.
    - The use of pressurized irrigation (*pulse lavage*) systems before wound excision can drive dirt into the wound, and is not a substitute for appropriate wound excision.
    - Use several litres of warmed normal saline or Hartmann's solution. (you can use normal bags of IV fluid with the port cut off. These are usually sterile within the outer wrapper, so can be used per-operatively).
- Wound excision should be **systematic** (have a system!), examining and excising skin, fat, fascia, tendon, muscle and bone as required.
    - Arteries and nerves should be preserved whenever possible, but if necrotic or traumatized may require excision and reconstruction.
    - You should aspire to perform a definitive wound excision at the first operation whenever possible.

- Serial wound excision may be required in cases with gross contamination or necrotizing infection.
- The practice of multiple trips to the operating theatre (2nd look, 3rd look, 4th look) should be discouraged.
- **Adequate primary wound excision and early soft tissue reconstruction should be the aim for the majority of cases**.
- After wound excision, some untidy wounds can be closed primarily or by the use of skin grafts or flaps.
  - High-energy transfer injuries should not be closed immediately.
  - Clear microbiological swabs must be obtained before delayed closure of infected wounds.

Soft tissue healing

Primary healing

- Primary healing following surgery should be the aspiration of all hand surgeons. This permits early mobilization to achieve good results.
- Delayed healing leads to delayed rehabilitation.
- Appropriate design of incisions to provide well-vascularized skin flaps, and careful skin handling with good technique should always result in primary healing.
- In trauma, early flap or skin graft cover after careful wound excision may be required to achieve primary healing.

Secondary healing

- Most wounds will heal eventually by 'secondary intention' unless there has been radiotherapy, chronic infection, excessive local scarring or significant systemic problems.
- Delayed or secondary healing should be avoided in hand surgery; it leads to inflammation, oedema, stiffness and poor results.

Local factors leading to delayed wound healing

- Poor surgical technique:
  - Inadequate excision of contaminated, devitalized or infected wounds
  - Rough tissue handling
  - Inversion of wound edges
- Haematoma
- Infection
- Scar tissue
- Radiotherapy
- Previous cold injury

Systemic factors leading to delayed wound healing

- Age
- Poor nutrition
- Tobacco smoking
- Drugs (steroids, and other immunosuppressive drugs)
- Cancer
- Autoimmune/inflammatory diseases
- Diabetes

Grafts

- A **graft** is a piece of non-vascularized tissue which is detached from its site (and most importantly **blood supply**) of origin, and transferred to a different site, where it relies on the local blood supply to survive.
- Although skin is the most commonly grafted tissue, a graft may consist of any type of tissue (fascia, fat, tendon, nerve, vessel, bone, or composite tissue).

Skin grafts

- Skin grafts may be **split** thickness (of the dermis) or **full** thickness.
- These are named after surgeons who described their use:
  - **Thierche** grafts (thin split skin) although the term 'Thierche graft' is no longer in common use.
  - **Wolfe** grafts (full thickness skin),
- The site from which the skin graft is taken or harvested is known as the **'donor site'**. There are various choices of donor sites (see below) and these should always be discussed with the patient before surgery.

Skin graft 'take'

The process of a graft acquiring a blood supply from its new recipient bed is known as '**take**'. This is a race between the formation of new blood vessels to the graft against necrosis of the graft before it is revascularized. The recipient bed must consist of healthy, well-vascularized tissue.

Traditionally, skin graft take is said to consist of 3 phases, but recent work has demonstrated that the process is much more complex than this simplistic model:

- **Plasmatic imbibition:**
  - the diffusion of nutrients into the graft from the recipient bed
  - 0–24 hours
- **Enosculation:**
  - the joining together of adjacent blood vessel lumens in the graft and recipient bed
  - 48–72 hours
- **Neovascularization:**
  - the formation of new blood vessels from the recipient bed to the graft
  - 48 hours onwards

Recipient bed factors which prevent skin graft take
- Poorly vascularity
- Dense scarring
- Tendon denuded of paratenon
- Bone denuded of periosteum
- Infected tissue
- Haematoma under graft
- Irradiated tissue

Surgical factors which prevent skin graft take
- 'Shear' of graft:
  - inadequate fixation of graft or splinting of hand interferes with the process of graft take
- Thickness of graft

Split skin graft (SSG)

A shaving of skin (epidermis and superficial part of dermis) using hand-held or mechanical dermatome.

There is no limit to the size of SSG which can be used in the upper limb as long as the recipient bed is suitable.

Sites suitable for SSG
- Upper arm
- Forearm
- Dorsum of wrist and hand
- Dorsum of digits

Sites unsuitable for SSG
- Flexural creases (axilla, cubital fossa, and wrist):
  - scar contractures will develop.
- Palm and volar aspects of digits:
  - SSG on the palm is tight, insensate, and is not glabrous.
  - SSG will cause tight scars over flexor creases.
- Tendon denuded of paratenon
- Bone denuded of periosteum
- Vascular or nerve repairs or grafts
- Open fractures
- Injuries requiring immediate mobilization (SSG must be immobilized for 5–7 days to allow graft to 'take')

SSG thickness

SSG can be harvested in different thicknesses. Thin SSG will 'take' quicker than thick grafts, but thick SSGs are more durable, look more natural, and will contract less, as they contain more dermal components.

SSG harvest
- Hand-held dermatome (Watson skin graft knife):
  - Useful for harvesting small areas of SSG.
  - A rough guide for the correct setting of a hand-held skin graft knife is the thickness of a number 15 scalpel blade.
  - Their use requires a considerable amount of practice.
  - Unskilled use of a hand-held dermatome can easily produce an unhealed donor site, as well as poor-quality, untidy SSG
- Mechanical dermatome:
  - Usually driven by compressed air or battery.
  - These are easier to use, and are better for taking large pieces of SSG, as well as creating a more even donor site with fewer healing problems.
  - The usual setting for Zimmer® air dermatome is 8–10/1000 inch

SSG application
- SSG may be used in sheets (unmeshed), fenestrated using a scalpel, or meshed using a mechanical mesher, up to 6 times the original area.
- The most commonly used mesh ratio is 1.5 or 2 times.
- Meshed grafts allow the wound exudate to pass through the gaps in the mesh (known as 'interstices'), and allow the graft to expand when it is stretched across a wound, but are unsightly, producing a 'string vest' appearance.

- Unmeshed sheet graft is more likely to collect haematoma underneath it if applied to a new wound, but has a better long-term appearance.
- SSG is applied to recipient bed using glue, sutures, or skin staples to hold it in place and prevent graft 'shear'.
- The dressing must absorb wound exudates.
- The hand and wrist must be rested in a POP volar slab in a functional position for 5–7 days until the SSG has taken.

SSG growth
- SSG contracts with time, especially over flexor surfaces.
- SSG, and to a lesser extent full thickness skin graft (FTSG) has less potential for growth than vascularized skin flaps.

Choice of SSG donor sites
- The site of SSG harvest should always be discussed with the patient prior to surgery.
- Thigh:
  - lateral skin thicker skin than medial
  - medial thigh unsightly in young women
  - avoid medial thigh or overgraft (see below) in elderly patients
- Forearm:
  - unsightly
  - convenient, as within operative field
- Upper arm:
  - avoid medial upper arm in elderly as this does not heal
- Buttock:
  - well hidden
- Hypothenar eminence:
  - for small grafts (1–2 cm^2) to provide glabrous (palm) skin
  - must either take thicker (due to keratin), or raise initial flap of thick keratin layer prior to SSG harvest

Re-use of donor sites
- SSG donor sites may be used more than once.
  - The number of times depends upon the thickness of the graft taken, as the dermis does not regenerate.
  - This is useful in burns surgery, especially when the body surface area of the burn is larger than that available from which to harvest SSG.
  - Careless graft harvest, especially by a surgeon unfamiliar with the use of a hand-held skin graft knife, may result in an unhealed donor site. This is mostly avoidable by the use of a mechanical dermatome, careful technique and appropriate donor site selection.

Overgrafting of the donor site
- Overgrafting of the donor site with widely meshed (1 to 6) SSG may be appropriate for elderly patients with thin skin (especially those on steroids).
- Avoid the medial upper arm as a SSG donor site in elderly patients, as it may take many months to heal (if ever).

Full thickness skin graft
- A FTSG is a complete piece of skin, usually with a very thin layer of adherent subcutaneous fat on the undersurface.
- FTSG up to approximately 10cm^2 may be used in the upper limb on appropriate beds.

Sites suitable for FTSG
- Upper arm
- Forearm
- Dorsum of wrist and hand
- Dorsum of digits

FTSG harvest
- An ellipse of skin is excised with a number 10 or 15 scalpel blade.
- If a template of the defect is used, FTSG of the exact size and shape can be raised primarily (easier than trimming later), and the ellipse removed later to close the donor site.
- The subdermal fat is then removed from the FTSG using scissors.
  - This is easier to do if the last few millimetres of the FTSG is left attached to the donor site to provide an anchor for countertraction.
  - With experience, the FTSG can be harvested with minimal subdermal fat.

FTSG application
- FTSG is usually fixed with a 'tieover' dressing, sutured through the graft around the edge of the defect and then tied over cotton wool soaked in proflavine ointment or liquid paraffin.
- The hand and wrist must also be rested in a POP volar slab in a functional position for 7–10 days until the FTSG has taken.

FTSG growth
- FTSG provides a durable, more natural-looking reconstruction than SSG, and is less likely to contract, although it may still do so across flexor joint creases and within previous scar tissue.

FTSG donor sites
- Medial upper arm:
  - Either take below tourniquet (in operative field but hypertrophic, conspicuous scar), or remove tourniquet and take from proximal upper arm (requires re-prepping of skin, but well concealed, neater scar).
- Elbow crease (better in children).
- Ulnar border of the proximal forearm.
- Groin:
  - least conspicuous donor site scar
  - can take large area of graft
  - can pigment (dark brown), which is unsightly
  - ⚠ **Care must be taken to avoid taking medial pubic hair-bearing skin in pre-pubescent children, which subsequently develops pubic hair on visible areas on the hand.**
- The flexor aspect of the wrist crease is described in many books, but should be avoided as patients may be stigmatized by scars across the wrist mimicking suicide attempts.

Composite graft (skin and fat)
- A graft containing more than one type of tissue is known as a composite graft.
- Distal fingertip amputations may be replaced successfully in children as composite grafts (i.e. without revascularization) if done within 5 hours from injury.

Flaps

A flap is a piece of tissue with an integral blood supply.

Use of flaps

- To cover flexor surfaces.
- To cover vascular and nerve repairs.
- To cover poor recipient beds (📖 p. 212).
- To resurface SSG and joint contractures.
- To cover open fractures or joints.
- To import blood supply in infected or irradiated wounds.

Classifications of flaps

Tissue composition
- Skin (cutaneous)
- Skin and fascia (fasciocutaneous)
- Skin and muscle (myocutaneous)
- Skin and bone (osseocutaneous)
- Combinations of tissues—skin, bone, nerve, or tendon—(composite)

Blood supply
- Random pattern
- Axial
- Perforator

Geometrical
- Advancement
- Transposition
- Rotation
- Island

Site
- Local
- Regional
- Distant
- Free flap (microvascular free tissue transfer)

Tissue composition

Skin (cutaneous) or fasciocutaneous flaps

- These are the most useful tissue for cover of the upper limb.
- They are soft, pliable, and grow with the patient (important in children).
- They may be elevated easily for secondary reconstruction of underlying structures (e.g. vascular, nerve, tendon, bone).
  - This is safer than re-raising a muscle flap; the fasciocutaneous flap develops additional vascularity from ingrowth of vessels across the skin 'inset' (where it abuts the native skin around the edge of the flap) at the recipient site.

Muscle flaps
- Muscle flaps covered by SSG may also be used to reconstruct the skin envelope, but these are stiffer than fasciocutaneous flaps and more difficult to elevate subsequently.
- The muscle flap is more at risk from secondary surgery, as it is still reliant on its vascular pedicle, and does not pick up much blood supply from the recipient site.

Functional muscle transfer
- Some muscles (gracilis, latissimus dorsi) may be transferred and re-innervated (either by an adjacent intact nerve, or a nerve graft anastomosed to a distant donor nerve) to reconstruct **functional** muscle.
  - An example is transfer of the gracilis muscle to reconstruct the biceps, innervated by a fasicle of the ulnar nerve (Oberlin transfer) or nerve grafts to an intercostal nerve.

Bone flaps
- Also known as 'vascularized bone graft' (VBG), although it is a flap.
- The fibula is used most commonly, and is versatile.
  - It can be divided by osteotomy and 'double-barrelled'.
- Iliac crest, scapula, rib or vascularized radius may also be used.
- Vascularized bone flaps may be used to reconstruct metacarpals, the carpus, or segments of the radius, ulna or humerus.
- It can reconstruct larger defects than non-vascularized bone graft.
- It can be used in poor recipient beds (previous scar, infection or irradiation), in which non-vascularized bone would not survive.

Composite flaps
- Composite flaps are described (combinations of skin, bone, nerve, or tendon), although, in general, 'the more things you ask a flap to do the less well it does any of them'.
- The exception to this maxim is the use of great or second toe transfers to reconstruct digits in hand surgery. This technique is unique in providing the closest 'like for like' digital substitute.

Local flaps
- These are areas of tissue transferred to an adjacent recipient defect.
- In the hand, local flaps provide a 'like with like' tissue match.
- Design of these flaps requires knowledge of the flap anatomy, blood supply and geometry, as well as operative experience.
- Local flaps can be either transposition, rotation, advancement or island in their geometrical design.
- When designing a transposition or rotation flap, the defect is 'triangulated' and the flap planned and raised.
- Advancement flaps produce small triangular bulges (known as 'Burow's triangles' or 'dog ears') at their base, which should be excised.
  - Dog ears don't 'settle', so excise them at the time of flap cover.
- An island flap is a piece of tissue which is circumscribed completely on a vascular pedicle, and then transferred to the defect, sometimes passing under an adjacent bridge of skin.
  - An example is a neurovascular island flap to reconstruct a fingertip.
- The flap donor site is known as 'the secondary defect'.

- In some areas (e.g. the dorsum of the hand) this can be closed directly, taking advantage of areas of redundant skin.
- When it cannot be closed primarily, it is covered with a skin graft.

Regional flaps

- A regional flap is one which is elevated from a site in the vicinity of the primary defect, but not in contact with it, eg;
  - A cross-finger flap to one finger from an adjacent digit
  - A flap from the forearm to the hand, such as a reverse radial forearm flap or distally based posterior interosseous artery flap.

Distant flaps

- A distant flap (e.g. the pedicled groin flap to the hand) is a piece of tissue taken from a donor site distant from the defect. It is raised and transferred to the defect in multiple stages.
- *Stage 1:* the flap is raised on a pedicle, and inset into the defect. The pedicle is left intact until the flap becomes perfused by the tissue surrounding the defect, usually at about 3 weeks.
- *Stage 2:* the pedicle is divided as the second stage.
- The flap may be contoured or revised as a third stage.
- This technique is still useful, although it is inconvenient for the patient, and means the hand cannot be elevated.

Free flaps and reconstructive microsurgery

- Reconstructive microsurgical techniques were developed in the 1960s, first by surgeons replanting limbs and then digits, and later with the development of the 'free flap' in the early 1970s.
- Microsurgery techniques allow a piece of tissue to be taken from a donor site, including the artery and vein (and sometimes nerve) which supply it.
  - This tissue is then transplanted to the defect
  - The flap artery and vein are sutured to the recipient artery and vein under a microscope.
  - This is known as 'a microsurgical free flap' or 'free tissue transfer'.
- Local, regional, or distant options may be limited, and can require sacrifice of important structures. These may be avoided by the use of a one-stage reconstruction using a free flap.

Trauma

- The use of a flap in open fractures allows radical wound excision and immediate closure, promoting more rapid fracture healing and reduced bony infection rates.
- Flaps can be used to close wounds which are unsuitable for a skin graft (such as bare or fractured bone or tendon), or if the wound extends across the flexor surface of a joint.
- They provide more durable reconstruction than a skin graft, and some flaps can be made sensate in younger patients.

Oncology

- The use of flaps in oncological surgery allows radical excision of the tumour with an adequate margin of normal tissue, and limb preservation.
- The defect is reconstructed with a flap, which can be irradiated if necessary.
- Although flaps tolerate irradiation better than skin grafts, they are still affected by the radiation.

Revascularization

- When there is vascular insufficiency of an area from arteriosclerosis or trauma, the flap vessels can be anastomosed to recipient vessels both proximally and distally as a 'through-flow flap'.
- Only free flaps with the appropriate pedicle anatomy are suitable for use as a through-flow flap:
  - radial forearm flap
  - lateral arm flap
  - anterolateral thigh flap.

Composite defects

- Multiple flaps may be used together for complex reconstructions; one on the outside to reconstruct the skin envelope, and the other on the inside for bone or musculotendinous units.
  - e.g. an innervated functional muscle transplant, using a free gracilis muscle flap under fasciocutaneous flap, following an ischaemic contracture of the forearm.
- Although the idea of including all the necessary components of the reconstruction in the flap is seductive, composite flaps (e.g. dorsalis pedis flap with skin and extensor digitorum brevis tendons for a dorsal hand composite loss) may be disappointing. Many surgeons prefer to use a flap for soft tissue cover and either immediate or delayed tendon reconstruction with non-vascularized tendon grafts.

Useful flaps for upper limb reconstruction

Free flaps
Anterolateral thigh flap

Components
- Fasciocutaneous, fascial, cutaneous (thinned)
- Can be innervated for sensibility

Surface marking
- Line between anterior superior iliac spine and superolateral aspect of patella.
- Main perforators at (approximately) halfway point along this line.

Vascular pedicle
- Descending branch of lateral femoral circumflex artery.
- Can get long pedicle, with good calibre vessels.

Size
- Largest possible dimension for direct closure approximately 28cm x 8cm.
- Can take wider than 8cm, but need to use SSG on donor site.

Lateral arm flap

Components
- Fasciocutaneous, fascial, cutaneous (thinned).
- Can be innervated for sensibility.

Surface marking
- Line between deltoid insertion on humerus to lateral epicondyle of humerus.
- Main perforators along distal half of this line.

Vascular pedicle
- Posterior radial collateral artery.
- Pedicle relatively short, with small veins.

Size
- Largest possible dimension for direct closure approximately 6cm wide.

Gracilis

Components
- Muscle, myocutaneous.
- Can use as functional muscle transfer when innervated.

Surface marking
- Line between pubic tubercle and medial femoral condyle.
- Main perforators at approximately 10cm below pubic tubercle.

Vascular pedicle
- Medial femoral circumflex artery.
- Pedicle relatively short with small vessels.

Size
- Can take whole muscle including tendon.

Latissimus dorsi

Components
- Muscle, myocutaneous, skin—thoracodorsal artery perforator (TAP) flap
- Can use as functional muscle transfer when innervated

Surface marking
- Lateral border of posterior axillary fold below teres major, down to posterior superior iliac spine (PSIS), and across to midline.
- Fan-shaped muscle running under inferior border of scapula.

Vascular pedicle
- Thoracodorsal artery (from subscapular axis).

Size
- Can take whole muscle, but the most distal few centimetres on the iliac crest are unreliable.
- Size of skin paddle overlying muscle depends on body habitus of patient.

Fibula

Components
- Bone, osseocutaneous.

Surface marking
- Line over fibula on lateral side of leg.
- Main perforators to skin paddle in inferior third.

Vascular pedicle
- Peroneal artery.
- Nutrient branch of pedicle enters bone approximately 17cm inferior to the styloid process of the fibula.

Size
- Can take most of fibula.
- Must leave 6–8cm distally, above ankle synostosis, especially in children, to avoid valgus deformity.
- Small skin paddles can be closed directly.

2nd toe transfer

Components
- Whole toe, wrap-around, or PIPJ.

Vascular pedicle
- Usually taken on tibial digital artery. Find the common vessel to the great and 2nd toes in the first web space, and dissect retrogradely.
- This is supplied by the dorsal system in approximately 70%.
- The plantar system is more difficult to dissect, and results in a shorter pedicle.

Distant flaps

Pedicled groin flap

Components
- Fasciocutaneous

Surface marking
- Draw a line over the inguinal ligament from the pubic tubercle to anterior superior iliac spine (ASIS).
- Palpate and draw the femoral artery.
- The SCIA runs from the femoral artery two of the patient's fingerbreadths below, and parallel to, the inguinal ligament.

Vascular pedicle
- Superficial circumflex iliac artery (SCIA).
- Easiest to raise flap from lateral to medial.
- Stay above Scarpa's fascia layer until you reach the lateral border of the sartorius muscle, when the pedicle usually penetrates, and runs deep to the fascia.
- Tube the base to reduce raw area.

Size
- Width according to dimensions of patient, usually 6–7cm.
- Design in tennis racquet-shape to increase area of skin inset.
- Close donor site with hip flexed to reduce tension.

Regional flaps

Reversed pedicled radial forearm flap

Although the distally based radial forearm flap is reliable, it requires extensive dissection, sacrifices an axial vessel of the hand, and leaves a terribly scarred donor site in a very visible part of the forearm.

Components
- Fasciocutaneous, fascial, osseocutaneous, bone.

Surface marking
- Axis over radial artery.
- Greatest perforator density in distal third of forearm.

Vascular pedicle
- Radial artery.
- Can use venae comitans or cephalic vein (both better) for venous drainage.
- Has disadvantage of sacrifice of major axial vessel of the hand.

Size
- Either direct closure or SSG or donor site.

Reversed pedicled ulnar forearm flap
- Similar to RFF (radial forearm flap) based on ulnar artery.

Ulnar artery perforator (Becker) pedicled flap
- Skin flap based on perforator of ulnar artery 3–5cm proximal to pisiform.

- Can take 20cm long, and either close directly or SSG, depending on width.
- Can transpose through 180° to reach the palm.

Posterior interosseous artery (PIA) flap

Components
- Fasciocutaneous, fascial.

Surface marking
- Line from lateral epicondyle to mid-point of extensor retinaculum.
- Major perforator to skin at approximately halfway along this line.
- Easiest to mark with arm resting over patient's chest.

Vascular pedicle
- Posterior interosseous artery
- Runs between EDC and EDM, with PIN
- Be careful not to damage muscular branches of PIN in proximal third of forearm.

Size
- Either direct closure or SSG or donor site.

Local flaps

- There are many different flap possibilities for digital reconstruction, with multiple eponyms.
  - These should not be attempted without proper training.
  - A relatively trivial injury can be turned into a more serious loss by a poorly executed local flap.
  - The technical details are beyond the scope of this book, and the reader should consult *Green's Operative Hand Surgery*[1] and the original papers in the hand, plastic and orthopaedic literature for more information.

Cross-finger flap (XFF)

- This is used to resurface the volar surface of the damaged digit.
- A 'trapdoor' of dorsal skin is raised from an adjacent finger.
  - Take the flap as an 'aesthetic unit', i.e. a rectangle between the IPJs, usually over the P1 or the middle phalanx (P2).
- A FTSG is used to reconstruct the donor site.
  - Apply the FTSG **before** you inset the flap onto the injured digit.

De-epithelialized cross-finger flap

- This is used to resurface the dorsum of the damaged digit.
- A 'trapdoor' of dorsal skin is raised from an adjacent finger leaving the adipofascial layer intact, with base on the opposite side from the defect.
- The adipofascial layer is raised, based on the same side as the injured digit.
- The adipofascial layer is turned over onto the defect, and the trapdoor of skin is replaced on the donor site.
- The adipofascial de-epithelialized XFF is covered using a SSG.

1. Green DP, Hotchkiss RN, Pederson WC *et al.* (2005). *Green's Operative Hand Surgery*, 5th edn, Churchill Livingstone.

Distal V-Y advancement flap (Tranquilli Leali, Atasoy)

- A V-shaped flap is raised on a subcutaneous pedicle (it is **not** islanded on the vessels), usually at, or just proximal to the DIPJ.
  - Design it the same width as the columns of the lateral nailfolds.
- Hold it under tension distally, and divide fibrous septae sequentially to gain advancement.
- Secure with an hypodermic needle through P3 so the flap is not inset under tension (which causes a tight fingertip).
- Suture loosely, and do not try and close the tail of the Y tight.
  - It is better to leave the tight areas open, as these heal well.

Neurovascular island (NVI) advancement flap

- These flaps are a little larger than the distal V-Y flaps, and are islanded on the NVB.
- They are designed as a **V-Y** (Venkataswami oblique triangular flap) or **step-advancement** (Evans modification).
- The dissection has to continue to the level of the A2 pulley (more proximal than you think) to get sufficient distal movement of the flap.

Reconstruction from axilla to hand

Axilla

Skin graft
- SSG can be used on a suitable bed in the axilla for immediate cover.
- Usually results in contractures, especially when crossing the anterior or posterior axillary folds.
- Contractures require delayed resurfacing with a flap.

Local flaps
- Fasciocutaneous perforator flaps

Regional flaps
- Pedicled latissimus dorsi flap
- Parascapular flap
  - Can be islanded and passed through the quadrangular space.
- Thoracodorsal perforator (TAP) flap.

Free flaps
- Thin, fasciocutaneous flaps better than skin-grafted muscle flaps

Elbow

Local flaps
- Fasciocutaneous perforator flaps
- Distally based lateral arm flap

Regional flaps
- Islanded pedicled latissimus dorsi flap (with or without skin)
- Proximally based radial forearm flap
- Proximally based ulnar forearm flap

Free flaps
- Thin, fasciocutaneous flaps
- Muscle flaps with SSG
- Through-flow flaps are useful to reconstruct brachial artery injuries

Dorsum of wrist and hand

SSG
Dorsum
- Can use SSG, but can limit flexion

Local flaps
- Small random pattern flaps, especially on dorsum (more lax skin)

Regional flaps
- Proximally based radial forearm flap
- Proximally based ulnar forearm flap
- Becker (ulnar artery perforator) flap
- Distally based posterior interosseous flap

Distant flaps
- Pedicled groin flap

Free flaps
- Thinned fasciocutaneous flaps
- Muscle flaps with SSG

Volar wrist and palm

SSG
- SSG tight and insensate
  - Causes contractures across volar wrist and palmar creases
  - Difficult to do secondary surgery under SSG

Flaps need to be thin, sensate, and adherent

Regional flaps
- Becker (ulnar artery perforator) flap
- Adipofascial turnover flaps from wrist or forearm

Free flaps

Fasciocutaneous flaps
- Thinned, sensate anterolateral thigh flap
- Thinned sensate lateral arm flap
- Free posterior interosseous artery flap

Fascial flaps
- Anterolateral thigh fascial flap
- Lateral arm fascial flap

Muscle flaps
- Thick muscle flaps are stiff and wobble during grip
- Thinned gracilis muscle flap with SSG
- Thinned latissimus dorsi flap with SSG
- Serratus anterior muscle flap with SSG

Reconstruction of digits

General principles

- Preserve length.
- Provide sensate, well-padded, glabrous skin without neuroma.
- Provide a trouble-free nail (otherwise consider ablation of GM)
- Use local tissue (especially sensate, glabrous skin on the fingertips) where possible.
- Use flaps from the same (damaged) digit—homodigital flaps—when these give a good reconstruction.
  - This avoids the use of other, uninjured digits—heterodigital flaps—as donor sites
- Always consider the use of spare parts in multiple injuries.
- Skin grafts on the volar aspect of digits are tight, insensate, and contract with growth in children.
- Raw areas of glabrous skin heal well
  - (McCash principle from surgery for Dupuytren's disease)
- When shortening through the P3, proximal to the nailfold, ensure that all of the GM is excised (📖 see p. 170).
  - If you leave the GM intact with lack of bony support, a hooknail deformity will result.
- Consider syndactylising fingers with one flap (usually regional or free flap) in multiple digital injuries, and divide later.

Classification of fingertip amputations

Dorsal oblique
- Distal V-Y advancement flap

Transverse
- Distal V-Y advancement flap
- Venkataswami or Evans neurovascular island flap

Volar oblique
- Venkataswami or Evans neurovascular island flap
- Cross-finger flap (for more oblique loss)
- Microvascular free toe pulp flap

Flaps for the volar aspect of finger and fingertips

Local flaps
- *Atasoy* distal V-Y advancement flap
- Venkataswami or Evans neurovascular island flap
- Homodigital reversed neurovascular island flaps
  - Sacrifice one digital artery
  - Potentially unreliable
  - Need careful design and experienced surgeon
- Cross-finger flap (for more oblique loss)

Distant flaps
- Pedicled groin flap (often for multiple digits)

Free flaps
- Free toe pulp (can be sensate)

Flaps for the dorsum of the fingers
Local flaps
- Random pattern transposition flaps
- Random pattern rotation advancement flaps
- De-epithelialized cross finger flap
- Dorsal metacarpal artery (flag) flaps (Lister)
- Dorsal metacarpal artery perforator (Quaba) flaps
- Reversed dorsal metacarpal artery (Maruyama) flaps

Regional and distant flaps
- Distally based posterior interosseous artery flap
- Pedicled groin flap

Free flaps
- Toe web
- Single slip of serratus anterior
- Free posterior interosseous artery flap

Partial toe transfers
- Various parts of the great and second toes can be used to reconstruct fingertips, pulp, nail complexes and joints.

Microvascular toe joint transfer
- This is a very technically demanding procedure.
- Results in adults are disappointing;
  - 27° active ROM for toe PIPJ to finger.
- Useful in children to import growth potential.
- May be useful in adults to reconstruct composite dorsal skin, extensor tendon and joint loss (with good flexor tendon and volar skin).

Thumb reconstruction

- Thumb reconstruction follows the principles outlined in the previous section, and many of the techniques for finger reconstruction are applicable.
- Reconstruct an opposable thumb whenever possible, with a stable skeleton, and painless, well-padded, sensate skin cover.
- Restore the 1st webspace.
- Microvascular toe transfer provides the best total thumb reconstruction:
  - This requires microvascular skills and facilities.
  - Not all patients want to lose a toe, in which case other methods are available.
- Non-vascularized bone graft must be intercalated (i.e. vascularized bone at each end) to prevent absorption.
- Pollicization of the index (or other) finger may be indicated when the CMCJ has been lost with the thumb.

Flaps for the dorsum of the thumb

Local flaps
- Random pattern transposition flaps
- Random pattern rotation advancement flaps
- De-epithelialized cross finger flap
- 1st dorsal metacarpal artery (Fouchet) flap

Regional flaps
- Distally based posterior interosseous artery flap

Distant flaps
- Pedicled groin flap

Free flaps
- Toe web
- Single slip of serratus anterior
- Free posterior interosseous artery flap
- Free lateral arm flap

Flaps for the volar aspect of thumb and thumb tip

Local flaps
Bipedicled neurovascular island flaps
- Moberg flap
- O'Brien neurovascular island flap
- V-Y neurovascular island flap (Elliot)

Single-pedicled neurovascular island flaps
- Venkataswami oblique triangular flap
- Evans step advancement

1st dorsal metacarpal artery (Fouchet) flap

Distant flaps
- Pedicled groin flap

Free flaps
- Free toe pulp (can be sensate)

Restoration of the 1st webspace

General principles
- This is one of the most useful procedures in hand reconstruction.
- The 1st webspace is a complex, U-shaped structure between the 2nd metacarpal and the proximal phalanx of the thumb.
- You have to release the contracture **AND** provide abduction force.
- It may require deepening and/or widening.

Structures to release
Skin
Soft tissue
- Dorsal fascia
- 1st dorsal interosseous
- Adductor pollicis

Joint
- 1st CMCJ release
- ? Osteotomy of 1st MC

Local flaps
- Single Z-plasty
- Four-flap Z-plasty
- Five-flap Z-plasty ('Jumping man')

Regional flaps
- Radial border index (usually no graft)
- Ulnar border thumb (? Graft and gives access to ulnar collateral ligament for congenital reconstruction)
- Dorsum index finger (e.g. cleft closure)
- Rotation flap from dorsum of hand
- Distally based posterior interosseous artery flap
- Reversed radial forearm flap

Free flaps
- Groin flap (best donor site, especially for children)
- Anterolateral flap
- Lateral arm flap
- Posterior interosseous artery flap

Partial and complete thumb reconstruction
Techniques
Microvascular
- 2nd toe:
  - Smaller than normal thumb, but good function
  - Acceptable donor site
- Great toe:
  - Donor site poor
  - Don't take proximal to MTPJ, as interferes with gait

- Wrap-around great toe (Morrison):
  - Minimizes donor site morbidity
  - Can use with intercalated bone graft
  - Do not use in children as no epiphyses with transfer
- Trimmed toe (Wei):
  - Allows functional IPJ with FPL
  - Great toe narrowed for better size match.
  - Do not use in children, as epiphyses damaged by narrowing procedure.

Pollicization
- Use of the index (or other) finger to make a thumb.
- Use other fingers if damaged and index intact.
- Use in the absence of 1st CMCJ or for congenital absence or some types of hypoplasia.
- Modified Buck–Gramcko technique.
- The MCPJ of the shortened index acts as a 1st CMCJ.
  - It must be rotated to prevent hyperextension.
- Pollicize damaged index for CMCJ prior to toe transfer.

Two-stage osteoplastic technique
- *Stage 1:* pedicled flap (groin, RFF, PIA) with non-vascularized pe.g. of bone graft.
- *Stage 2:* neurovascular island (Littler) flap, usually from radial side of ring finger provides island of sensate skin for opposable surface.
- Advantage: does not require microvascular skills/facilities
- Disadvantage: bone graft absorbs.

One-stage osteoplastic technique
- Reversed pedicled radial forearm flap, including vascularized radius in the flap.

Options for each level (in order of ascending complexity)
Distal to IPJ
- Functional loss not great, and many patients manage well.
- Restore 1st web (see above)
- 1st metacarpal distraction lengthening
- Microvascular wrap-around or trimmed toe gives length, sensibility and a near normal appearance.

Through proximal phalanx with intact MCPJ
- Deepen 1st webspace to use thumb metacarpal (*phalangization*)
- 1st metacarpal distraction lengthening
- Osteoplastic techniques.
- Pollicization of inured digit.
- Toe transfer:
  - Great toe a little wide
  - Wrap-around toe does not provide IPJ
  - Trimmed toe restores movement at IPJ

Proximal to MCPJ
- Pollicization of injured digit +/− toe transfer
- 2nd toe transfer

Proximal to 1st CMCJ
- Pollicization of injured digit +/− toe transfer
- Pollicization of normal digit.

Skin conditions

Surgical incisions

The hand is second only to the face in awareness of appearance by both patients and those with whom they interact. Surgeons should always consider this when designing incisions.

The planning of surgical incisions requires understanding of the different options and experience in their use. They should:

- Be extensible
- Provide access to deep structures
- Provide vascularized skin flaps (avoid long, narrow flaps)
- Avoid formation of scar contractures
  - Straight incisions across flexor creases (digits, palm, wrist, elbow, axilla) lead to scar contracture
- Avoid unnecessary dissection (leading to oedema, scarring)

Types of incision

Dorsal

- **Straight** incisions are used on the dorsum of the wrist, hand and digits. These preserve longitudinal veins, and provide well-vascularized skin flaps with good access.
- **Horizontal** incisions across the MCPJ heads may be used for access to the MCPJs or intrinsic insertion into the extensor hood.
- **Zig-zag** incisions on the dorsum of the hand are unsightly and may create ischaemic skin flaps if the base is too narrow.
- **Lazy S or tri-radiate** (wine glass) incisions are used to approach the DIPJ.

Mid-lateral

- This runs along the side of the digit, dorsal to the neurovascular bundle, and therefore safe.
- It is designed by flexing the fingertip into the palm, and marking dots at the apices of the DIPJ, PIPJ and MCPJ creases. The digit is then extended and a line drawn connecting the dots.

Palmar

- **Bruner**. These zig-zag type incisions are used in the volar aspect of the palm and digits. In the digits, they run from the mid-lateral line across the span of a phalanx to the contralateral mid-lateral line. In the palm they should be 1–2cm long, zig-zagging between palmar creases.
- **Half Bruner.** These are similar to Bruner incisions, but zig-zag across half of the width of the digit.
  - NB: A zig-zag incision should NOT cross the full width of the digit and back within the span of a phalanx. This leads to tip necrosis with flap loss.

Nail

Anatomy
📖 See Chapter 6.

Injuries
📖 See Chapter 6.

Nail distortion
Although trauma is the commonest cause of nail distortion, patients often present with a chronic problem; secondary causes should not be overlooked.

Nail pits
Associated with psoriasis

Nail ridge
A transverse ridge (Beau's line) can be precipitated by an episode of severe illness. The line progresses along the nail plate.

Infection
- Fungal
- Bacterial
- Viral

Nail bed tumours

Benign
Glomus cell tumour

Exquisitely tender. May erode terminal phalanx. Treat by removal of nail plate, careful elevation of matrix, complete excision of tumour and then repair of matrix with 8.0 absorbable suture.

Nail bed cyst

Some cysts are rather more distal, causing a blemish on the nailfold. These can be excised by elevating the nailfold, removing the cyst and then and then carefully repairing the fold again.

Mucous cyst

A ganglion cyst from the DIPJ emerges from the weak area between the extensor insertion and the collateral ligament. Usually provoked by a small osteophyte. Pressure from the cyst onto the germinal matrix can cause unsightly grooving of the nail. This usually recovers with excision of the cyst.

Malignant
Malignant melanoma (MM) and squamous cell cancer (SCC) can both present under the nail. May be overlooked. Treated by amputation. Lymphadenopathy also treated.

Benign skin tumours

Epidermoid cyst

Clinical features
- Derived from cells buried under the skin, which then form a spherical, subdermal, transilluminable cyst, sometimes with a visible punctum.
- Usually occur on the palmar skin of the digits.
- May be a history of a previous laceration or amputation.
- In the fingertips, may compress the bone of P3, producing a lytic lesion on X-ray.

Treatment
Excision: Excise around the capsule, also excising the punctum with an overlying ellipse of skin.

Actinic keratosis (AK)
Precursor of skin malignancy—10% transform to squamous cell carcinoma. Cumulative exposure to sun damage, less commonly occupational or medicinal exposure to radiation. or to some chemical agents.

Treatment
- *Superficial areas* of keratosis: treated effectively by topical agents such a 5-fluorouracil, or liquid nitrogen spray.
- *Persistent areas*, or those which ulcerate, should be biopsied (at the junction between the lesion and normal skin, sometimes from multiple sites in bigger lesions) to obtain a tissue diagnosis to exclude malignancy.
- *Wide excision* with direct closure, flap or graft.

Keratin horn
This is a keratotic mass, longer than it is wide. There is an underlying SCC in approximately 10% of keratin horns.

Calcinosis (systemic sclerosis)
- This is a manifestation of systemic sclerosis or scleroderma, either as an isolated condition, or as part of the CREST syndrome:
  - Calcinosis
  - Reynaud's syndrome
  - Eosophageal stricture
  - Scleroderma
  - Telangectasia
- Small nodules of calcium are laid down in the fingertips. This can extrude, causing painful ulcers and loss of function.
- The skin is tight and sclerotic, attempts at surgical removal usually result in a non-healing wound.
- Infection should be treated urgently to avoid ulceration.
- The vascularity (and therefore wound healing) of the digits in scleroderma can be improved by sympathectomy of the common digital arteries in the palm.

Malignant skin tumours

Malignant skin and soft tumours present in many ways in the hand. Although many are obvious, some may present in a subtle, insidious fashion, and clinicians should always be wary of unusual or chronic presentations, and sometimes question the previous diagnosis.

The rest of the upper limb, and axillary and supraclavicular lymph nodes, should always be examined in patients with suspicion of a malignant tumour.

Terminology

Primary or local lesion
The original primary tumour.

Satellite lesion
Small lesions developing around the primary lesion from microscopic local tissue invasion.

In-transit metastasis
A recurrent lesion developing in the line between the primary lesion and the regional lymph node basin.

Distant metastasis
Haematogenous spread of tumour to distant sites (e.g. lung or bone).

Skin cancers

Risk factors
- Genetic tendency:
  - Some phenotypes, e.g. light skin type
  - Autosomal dominant e.g. Ferguson–Smith syndrome
  - Autosomal recessive e.g. xeroderma pigmentosum
- Chronic sun exposure (SCC, MM, BCC)
- Ionising radiation
- Immunosuppresive drugs e.g. post-transplant
- Old age (a form of immunosuppression)
- Carcinogenic chemicals, e.g. arsenic
- Viral infection, e.g. human papilloma virus
- Chronic wounds, e.g. Marjolin's ulcer in chronic burn wound

Principles of surgery for skin cancer of the upper limb
- Do not treat these cases unless you are experienced and trained in their management.
- Obtain an histological tissue diagnosis before definitive treatment.
  - Exception: for small lesions, can excise with adequate margin and close primarily before histology .
- The specimen should be clearly marked (for histology) to orientate it for planning of further surgery.
- **If defect can be closed primarily**; perform excision biopsy with margin of 2–3mm.
- **If defect cannot be closed primarily,** perform (dependent on the level of suspicion):
  - **Either** an excision biopsy with 2–3mm margin (and leave wound open until pathology result available).
  - **Or** an incision biopsy.

- Appropriate wider excision and reconstruction can be performed when the pathology result is available.
- During definitive surgery, consider frozen section histology to check clearance for very aggressive tumours, or when visible margins are indistinct.
- Excision margins in the hand must be considered individually for each case:
  - The effect on function and reconstructive options must be considered carefully when planning excision margins in the hand.
  - It is often difficult to get adequate deep clearance of aggressive tumours without destroying hand function by excision of important dynamic structures.
  - Partial or complete digital amputation is usually necessary when the tumour has penetrated bone.

Staging of skin cancer of the upper limb
Investigations

- Histology
- Clinical examination of lymph nodes
- MRI scan of local disease
- CT scan of the axilla, neck and chest in the presence of lymphadenopathy.

Clinical stages

Stage I   Local disease
Stage II   Lymph node involvement
Stage III   Distant metastasis

Squamous cell carcinoma

- SCC is the commonest skin cancer seen in the upper limb.
- A locally invasive malignant skin tumour which can metastasize to other organs of the body.
- SCC in the hand more likely to metastasise to the lymph nodes than SCC elsewhere.
- It arises from the keratinizing cells of the epidermis or its appendages.

Presentation of SCC

- Indurated nodular or keratinizing or crusted tumour that may ulcerate.
- May present as an ulcer with no keratinization.
- There is a wide spectrum of presentation, from small well-differentiated lesions to large, poorly differentiated lesions which metastasize.
- Mostly seen on sun-exposed areas (dorsum of hand, forearm, upper arm).
- Regional lymphadenopathy may be present.
- Subungual lesions.

Bowen's disease

This is a precursor, *carcinoma in situ* SCC, and is still known by this eponym. Once a histological diagnosis has been made, it is usually treated as a well-differentiated SCC. A more conservative approach may be necessary in elderly patients with multiple lesions who are unfit for extensive surgery.

Marjolin's ulcer

This is development of an SCC in a chronic wound (originally described in unhealed burn wounds).

Prognosis

The most important determinant of outcome is the presence of lymph node metastasis. The degree of differentiation (well-, moderately, poorly differentiated), size, and depth of the tumour all affect prognosis, and this information should be included in the histopathology report for accurate staging.

Treatment

Local disease

- Surgical excision is the treatment of choice, 1–2cm margin according to degree of differentiation and site.
- Radiotherapy can be used for lesions where surgical morbidity would be high (e.g. amputation), or in patients not fit for surgery.
- Cryotherapy and curettage are also described.
    - These methods do not provide an accurate histological staging, and have no advantage over surgery in local control or long-term survival.
    - Complete excision is difficult to achieve, and to assess pathologically.
- Moh's surgery (sequential excision under histological control) has a high success rate but is time consuming and unpleasant for patients.

Treatment of lymphadenopathy

- Fine-needle aspiration cytology (FNAC) to get histological diagnosis.

- Open biopsy if result equivocal.
- Lymph node dissection in the presence of histologically proven lymph node metastasis.
- There is no survival benefit from prophylactic lymph node dissection in node-negative disease.

Keratoacanthoma (KA)

- KA is a difficult entity to classify in the spectrum of benign and malignant epidermal tumours.
- Difficult to differentiate between KA and well-differentiated SCC.
- Rapidly growing, exophytic, keratin-filled tumour, often with central crater.
- Tends to regress spontaneously (approx 10% recur).
- KA should be treated as potentially malignant (at the benign end of the spectrum of SCC).
- Lesion should be excised with 1cm margin.

Malignant melanoma

- Incidence 10/10000 in UK
- Female:male = 2:1
- Increased incidence with increasing proximity to Equator (and sun)
- Incidence rises with age to 50 and then slows (especially females)
- Some racial variation. Commoner in lighter-skinned races
- Potential for distant metastases

Clinical diagnosis of MM

Major features
- Change in size
- Irregular border of lesion
- Irregular pigmentation

Minor features
- Largest diameter ≥ 7mm
- Inflammation
- Bleeding (rare in early MM)
- Change in sensation

Types of MM

Lentigo maligna melanoma (LMM)
- MM with radial growth phase, usually arising from large pigmented lentigo. These can progress into invasive vertical growth phase.
- There is no potential for metastatic spread of isolated LMM.
- They should be treated by initial biopsy for diagnosis, followed by complete excision.

Superficial spreading MM
- Commonest form of MM

Nodular
- No radial growth phase
- Locally invasive, with high potential for distant metastases

Acral lentiginous
- Palms, soles, digits, on glabrous skin
- Higher incidence in dark-skinned races

Desmoplastic
- Usually amelanotic
- Deeply invasive

Histopathology

The following information must be included in a pathology report of a MM:
- Thickness of tumour (Breslow thickness)
- Depth of penetration of the dermis (Clarke's level I to IV)
- Growth pattern:
  - Radial growth precedes development of vertical growth phase (dermal invasion)

Malignant melanoma Thickness, Nodal, Metastasis (TNM) classification: American Joint Committee on Cancer (AJCC)

Thickness (T) Thickness

T1	<1.0mm
T2	1.01–2.0mm
T3	2.01–4mm
T4	>4mm

Nodal (N) Number of metastatic nodes

N1	1 node
N2	2–3 nodes
N3	4 or more nodes
	In-transit metastasis

Metastasis (M) · Site

M1	Distant skin, subcutaneous or nodal
M2	Lung
M3	Any other distant or visceral metastases

Staging

Stage I	T2 tumour without ulceration, N0, M0
Stage II	Up to T4 tumour with ulceration, N0, M0
Stage III	Any T, any N, M0
Stage IV	Any T, any N, any M

Investigations for malignant melanoma

- Stage I Histology
- Stage II Chest X-ray, CT scan chest, abdomen, pelvis, serum lactate dehydrogenase
- Stage III Should be assessed by multidisciplinary team including surgeon, oncologist, pathologist, radiologist, palliative care specialist

Treatment of malignant melanoma

Local disease

The mainstay is surgery. The margin of excision is calculated according to the tumour (Breslow) thickness.

Excision margins for malignant melanoma

Lesions <1mm	1cm margin
Lesions 1–2mm	1–2cm
Lesions 2.1–4mm	2cm
>4mm	2–3mm

Treatment of lymphadeopathy (MM)
This is the same as for SCC, with the exception of SNB.

Sentinel node biopsy (SNB)
- The sentinel node is the first node in the dominant draining lymph node basin (axilla for upper limb) to be invaded by tumour.
- The sentinel node is identified by lymphoscintigraphy (injection of radioactive dye and location using a gamma probe), and injection of methylene blue dye into the biopsy scar at the time of wider excision (the SN turns blue).
- This should only be done in the context of a clinical trial until the survival advantage has been evaluated.

Adjuvant therapy
- No survival benefit for any adjuvant therapies so far.
- Radiotherapy occasionally used for palliation to control unresectable local disease—not very effective.
- Several trials in progress.

Information required for histopathology report of malignant melanoma

Thickness of tumour (Breslow thickness)
The Breslow thickness is measured (in millimetres) from the top of the granular layer of the epidermis to the deepest melanoma cells in the dermis.

Depth of penetration of the dermis (Clarke's level I to V)

I	Intra-epidermal or *in situ*
II	Into papillary dermis
III	Fills and expands papillary dermis
IV	Into reticular dermis
V	Into subcutaneous fat

Clarke's level tumour thickness for malignant melanoma (1965)[1]
Growth pattern
- Radial growth precedes development of vertical growth phase (dermal invasion)

1. Clarke WH (1965). The histogerens and biological behaviour of primary human malignant melanoma of the skin. *Cancer Research.* **29:** 705–727.

Other malignant skin tumours

Merckel cell tumour
- Rare, aggressive tumour derived from neuroendocrine cells.
- Lymphadeopathy common at presentation
- Treatment similar to MM depending on stage of disease.

Basal cell carcinoma (BCC)
- Rare in the hand.
- A slow-growing, locally invasive malignant skin tumour which originates from the pleuripotential epidermal cell of the epidermis.
- Mainly affects Caucasians.
- Almost never metastasizes (few cases in world literature).

Presentation of BCC
- Presents as ulcerated lesions with heaped-up edge, and surrounding telangectasia.
- Mostly seen on sun-exposed areas (dorsum of hand, forearm and upper arm).
- Spectrum of morphological types, which vary in degree of differentiation and invasiveness:
  • Nodular BCC has discrete, pearly edge, and can be treated safely by excision with 3mm margin.
  • Multifocal BCC has indiscrete margin, with microscopic spread beyond visible margins. Local invasion is very aggressive. Requires wide excision to obtain clear margins.

Prognosis of BCC
- Depends on the morphological subtype.
- Usually cured following complete excision of nodular BCC.
- Multifocal aggressive tumours may recur despite wide excision.
- Most recurrences in first 5 years after treatment.
- Patents who have had one BCC at higher risk of developing further tumours.

Treatment of local disease
- Excision, with predetermined margins according to morphology.
  • Further surgery may be indicated if histology shows incomplete excision, depending on tumour type, and fitness of patient.
- Moh's surgery:
  • Favoured by some dermatologists.
  • This involves serial excision of the tumour (with narrow margins), and serial histopathological examination of the tumour and excision margins, until adequate clearance is achieved.
  • It is time-consuming and resource-intensive, and may lead to delay in reconstruction of significant defects when the patient has to be referred to another surgeon for this.
  • Some studies have shown higher complete excision rates and less uneccesary removal of marginal tissue from Moh's compared with comventional surgery.
- Destructive:
  • Curettage

- • Cautery
  - • Cryotherapy
  - • CO_2 laser.
- • Radiotherapy:
  - • For lesions where surgical morbidity is high.
  - • Patients unfit for surgery.

Dupuytren's disease

Dupuytren's disease (DD) is a fibromatosis which occurs in the palm and/
or digits.

The DD tissue either appears as **nodules** in the palm, or **cords** of disease, usually starting in the palm, and progressing distally into the fingers,
in the line of the fibres of the normal palmar fascia.

Epidemiology

- No proven cause.
- Prevalence varies geographically, suggesting a genetic influence:
  - Highest prevalence in Scandinavia (up to 30% men over 60 years in
    Norway)
  - Rare in African and Asian people.
- Variable level of penetrance and gene expression.
- Prevalence lower in women, with later age of onset.
- Approximately 15% of men over 60 years affected in UK.
- It is usually less severe in women.
- The incidence is the same in men and women in 8th and 9th decades.
- Bilateral in 50%.
- Most often right hand in unilateral cases.

Risk factors

Family history

- Suggests genetic cause.
- No gene yet isolated.

Diathesis

- Hueston used the term *diathesis* to describe DD in certain patients:
  - early onset of aggressive disease
  - involvement of multiple digits and the radial side of the hand
  - knuckle (Garrod's) pads
  - bilateral disease
  - ectopic disease (outside the hand—sole of the foot, Peyronie's,
    other forms of fibromatosis)

Diabetes

- Strong association in type 1 and type 2 diabetes.

Alcohol

- Higher incidence associated with high alcohol intake
- Higher incidence in alcoholics (probably combination of smoking **and**
  drinking)

Trauma

- Suggested association with sharp injury to palmar fascia.

Smoking

Smoking appears to be associated with the formation and progression
of DD, as well as producing microcirculatory ischaemia, which is likely to
complicate surgery.

Epilepsy
- Probably due to anti-epileptic drugs
- Previous studies suggest association between DD and epilepsy.
- Recent study of 800 patients found no association between DD and epilepsy.

Cell biology of DD

Three phases of DD
The development of DD has been shown to be mediated by proliferation of fibroblasts, which subsequently develop into myofibroblast cells, which produce abnormal Dupuytren's tissue. The myofibroblast has morphological characteristics of both fibroblasts and smooth muscle cells. It can contract actively, and is modulated by TGFβ.

Luck described 3 histological phases of DD in 1959:
- **Proliferative** phase leading to nodules.
  - There is more genetic modulation activity in nodules compared with cords.
- **Involutional** phase in which cells align themselves to lines of stress.
- **Residual** phase leaving scar-like cords.

Cytokines
Various cytokines are associated with the development of DD, including:
- Transforming growth factor alpha
- Platelet-derived growth factor
- Fibroblast growth factors
- Epidermal growth factor
- Nerve growth factor

Matrix metalloproteinase (MMP) inhibitors
- Examination of DD tissue and serum from affected patients has shown altered levels or upregulation of certain MMPs.
- These changes are also reported in patients with frozen shoulder.

Normal anatomy
- The palmar fascia is a system of retinacular fibres which provide a fibrous skeleton for the hand, providing reinforced channels, and anchoring the palmar skin to the underlying structures during normal movements to provide grip.
- Contrast this with the dorsal skin of the hand, which is easily wrinkled
- **Bands:** normal palmar fascial structures
- **Cords:** diseased fibres
- A three-dimensional understanding of the normal anatomy of the palmar fascia (and how it changes when infiltrated by DD) is essential to be able to plan and perform surgery for the condition.
- The fibres of the palmaris longus (if present), or the longitudinal fibres of the palmar fascia, merge with the deep fascia of the forearm or the anterior surface of the flexor retinaculum, and pass distally into the palm.

- These longitudinal fibres then pass distally as a pre-tendinous band over each digital ray, splitting distally to pass on each side of the flexor tendon, and inserting in 3 layers.
- The transverse fibres (of Skoog) pass horizontally underneath the longitudinal fibres, and extend distally, to the level of the distal palmar crease. The NVBs are deep to these fibres (and therefore safe from dissection) proximal to this level.

Layers of insertion of the longitudinal palmar fascia
- **Layer 1 (superficial)**
- The most superficial fibres insert into the skin of the distal palm, midway between the proximal and distal palmar creases.
- **Layer 2 (intermediate)**
- The spiral fibres pass on either side of the flexor tendon (deep to the NVB) to reach the lateral digital sheet. They are made up from a combination of (from proximal to distal) the **longitudinal fibres** of the palmar fascia, the **spiral fibres of Gosset**, and the **lateral fascia of the digit** (lateral digital sheet, or retrovascular band).
  - The **lateral digital sheet** receives fibres from the **natatory** ligament (in the webspace), and contributes fibres to **Cleland's** (posterior to NVB) and **Grayson's** (anterior to NVB) ligaments.
- **Layer 3 (deep)**
- The deepest longitudinal fibres pass deeply on either side of the flexor tendons and MCPJs.

Vertical fibres
- Superficial fibres connect the palmar fascia to the skin
- There are 3 types of deep fibres:
  - The septa of Legueu and Juvara
  - The fibres of the deep layer of the pre-tendinous band
  - Vertical bands which run from the palmar fascia to separate the flexor tendon sheath and lumbrical canal.

Digital fascia
- The various layers are defined by their position and relationship to the digital NVBs.
- **Grayson's ligament** arises from the side of the flexor tendon sheath to insert into the mid-axial skin, passing volar to the NVB.
- **Cleland's ligament** arises from the side of the phalangeal bones to insert into the mid-axial skin, passing dorsal (deep) to the NVB.
- **The lateral digital sheet** runs lateral to the NVBs, receiving fibres from the spiral fibres of Gosset, and the natatory ligament more proximally.
- **The retrovascular band** is longitudinal fibres running deep to the NVBs.

Diseased anatomy

The cords of DD contract and displace the NVBs, as well as infiltrating intsjo.

Pre-tendinous cord (palmar)
Runs in the palm above the transverse fibres of Skoog to the layer of the distal palmar crease, where it diverges into the digital cords.

Central cord (digital)
This follows layer 1 and passes further distally into the digit, often with skin involvement. It attaches to the base of the P2 on either side, as well as to the tendon sheath.

Lateral cord (digital)
This runs from the natatory ligament (anterior to the NVB) to the lateral digital sheet. In the little finger, it attaches to the ADM cord, if present, causing PIPJ flexion.

Spiral cord (digital)
This arises from the longitudinal pretendinous fibres and follows layer 2 as the spiral cord to the lateral digital sheet, where it is attached to the P2 by Grayson's ligaments.

As the spiral cord contracts, the NVB can be displaced at any level between 2 fixed points, from the mid-palm (under the transverse fibres of Skoog) to the base of the P2, even crossing the midline.

1st web space
The natatory ligament in the free edge of the web is usually involved.

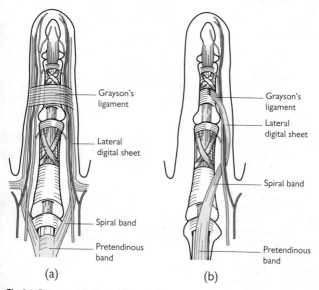

Fig. 8.1 Formation of spiral cord. (a) The parts of the normal fascia that compose the spiral cord; (b) with contraction, the spiral cord straightens and the neurovascular bundles spirals around it and is displaced towards the midline.

Presentation
- May start as palmar nodule(s), which are often painful.
- Nodules may progress to cords.
- Bilateral in 50% of patients.
- The right hand is affected more commonly than the left, irrespective of hand dominance.
- The ulnar (ring, then little) fingers are most commonly affected, then middle, thumb and index fingers.
- Often involvement of ADM, with ADM cord forming in the tendon going into the ulnar side of the little finger.
- Garrod's knuckle pads.
- Isolated trigger finger with involved fibres wrapping around the A1 pulley.
- Ectopic sites:
  - Plantar fibromatosis (Leddehosen disease) in 5–20%
  - Peyronies' disease in 2–4%.

Examination
- Chart the extent of the disease in the notes.
- Arrange clinical photographs.
- Function. Ask about compromised function, and get patient to tell you what they *can't* do, and *want* to be able to do after surgery.
- Range of movement and angles:
  - Measure the active and passive ROM of all digits.
  - Make a fist (MCPJ/PIPJ flexion).
  - Full finger extension (MCPJ/PIPJ/DIPJ extension).
  - Hook grip (MCPJ extension, PIPJ/DIPJ flexion).
  - Measure the angles across joints in full flexion and full extension.
- Flexion deformity (cord causing loss of extension) and/or joint contracture (joint infiltration by DD)?
- Extensor mechanism:
  - Look for boutonnière deformity.
  - Test for central slip attenuation using Bouvier manoeuvre (bend MPJ passively and look for automatic extension of the PIPJ as far as the contracture allows).
- Vascular status of the digit:
  - Colour
  - Capillary refill
  - Digital Allen's test
- Document distal sensibility in all of the digits.
  - If it is already absent or reduced from previous surgery, it is important to note this, or you may get the blame for reduced sensibility after your surgery.

Informed consent points
- Explain condition of DD.
- Explain operation, and realistic expectation (i.e. extent of improvement which can be achieved in that patient's hand).
  - Discuss donor site choice in dermofasciectomy.
- DD cannot be cured by surgery, and is likely to recur, even after the most careful and expert surgery.

- You will need to have some help at home for the first few weeks after surgery (especially patients living alone).
- Patients are advised to stop smoking, especially before dermofasciectomy.
  - Smoking increases chances of delayed wound healing, infection, graft loss and poor result.
- Small risk of nerve damage, especially if extensive or recurrent disease.
- Small risk of haematoma.
- Small risk of infection.
- You will have your hand in a dressing following surgery.
- You must keep the hand elevated following surgery.
- You will need to have hand therapy following surgery.
  - This is equally as important as the surgery to achieve a good result.
  - You may need to wear a splint.
- The skin will take 2–3 weeks to heal completely.
- Risk of stiffness, especially after extensive surgery.
- You will experience cold intolerance, which can initially be alarming, as the digit turns blue. Wear gloves in the cold weather.
- Small risk of CRPS (explain).
- Driving after 3–4 weeks.
- Heavy manual work at least 6–8 weeks (depends on extent of surgery).
- 3 months to full recovery.

Surgical procedures

Indications for surgery

- Loss of function:
  - Inability to rest palm flat due to flexion at MCPJ (usually >20°)
  - Supination of digit caused by spiral cord.
- PIPJ involvement causing functional difficulty (usually >30° Little and ring, >20° middle and index).
- Rapid progression of disease.
- There is no real role for early preventative surgery as recurrence is inevitable. This should be delayed until symptomatic, even in young patients with a strong diathesis.

General principles

- No consensus about surgery for DD, and the decision-making can be difficult.
- Avoid unnecessary dissection and undermining of skin.
- Change scalpel blades frequently.
- Do as much sharp dissection using a scalpel (rather than scissors).
- Find the digital NVBs in an easy, safe place which is uninvolved by DD, such as the base of the P1 proximal to the MCPJ crease (just distal to the edge of the Skoog fibres), and follow distally into the digit.
- Dissect around NVBs gently with tenotomy scissors.
- Close straight line incisions with Z-plasties, so that the transverse limbs of the Z are placed across joint creases.
- Leave thin or involved skin flaps open, or replace with FTSG.

Skin incisions

- Each surgeon develops personal preferences for skin incisions based on their own experience.

- The normal rules for skin incisions in the hand apply, but with some additional principles.
- Excessive skin undermining and dissection should be avoided:
  - This is more likely to allow dead space for haematoma (and subsequent infection).
  - Promotes recurrence.
  - Increases risk of skin necrosis.
- Care must be taken raising thin, narrow-based skin flaps over DD with skin involvement.
  - It may be better to excise the skin, and use a FTSG to avoid the complications of delayed healing.
- Tip necrosis of skin flaps leads to infection with delayed healing (and therefore postoperative mobilization), which is likely to cause stiffness.

Straight line (Skoog) incisions
- Can be used over longitudinal cords of disease, as long as they are closed with Z-plasties, placing scars in the line of PIPJ and DIPJ creases.
- Minimize undermining of the skin.
- Z-plasties lengthen the scar to allow straightening of the finger.

C-shaped incisions
- C-shaped incisions, with approximately 1cm limbs, can be used for segmental fasciectomy (Moerman's technique).

Transverse incisions
- Can be used in the palm, either alone, or in combination with longitudinal incisions.
- Avoid the creation of distally based flaps of skin in the webspaces (by a combination of multiple longitudinal and transverse incisions. These are poorly perfused (their blood supply is proximally based), and may die. If you have done this inadvertently, use a FTSG.

The open palm technique
- Described by McCash.
- Leaves transverse palmar incisions open to allow drainage of haematoma, and can compensate for some degree of skin shortage following correction of a contracted digit.
- These heal in 2–6 weeks, and allow good mobilization with minimal pain.
- Isolated transverse incisions make access to longitudinally orientated NVBs difficult, and require extensive undermining of the palmar skin to resect cords of DD.

Fasciotomy
- Division of a diseased cord (fasciotomy) can be performed open or closed, usually under LA, with a hypodermic needle or the tip of a number 11 scalpel blade.
- It is usually reserved for isolated cords in the palm above the transverse fibres of Skoog.
- Although there are some enthusiastic proponents of percutaneous fasciotomy, the main indication is for elderly patients with a discrete palmar cord, who want a simple procedure to straighten the MCPJ for function or hygiene.

- There is a risk of digital nerve injury with the closed percutaneous technique. It is dangerous in the digits.
- If done as an open procedure, it is as easy to perform a Moerman's-type segmental fasciectomy, which may give a longer-lasting improvement.
- When performed as part of a fasciectomy, division of the cord allows the finger to be extended for surgical access to the digital DD.
  - Dissect as much as you can safely before dividing the cord; this provides useful countertraction, and makes the dissection a little easier.

Fasciectomy

This is excision of involved fascia. There are several degrees of fasciectomy (according to the amount of disease and the surgeon's preference) and the terminology is a little arbitrary, and therefore confusing.

Segmental fasciectomy (Moerman's technique)

Short (1–2cm) segments of the diseased cords are excised through small C-shaped incisions. The 'C' can alternately be reversed, as multiple incisions, progressing distally in the palm. This breaks up the cords, allowing return of extension, with minimal post operative effects, as the surgery is relatively non-invasive. It also makes a 'firebreak' between the ends of the cord, which cannot then join up and continue to contract. It has the advantage of being possible under LA infiltration for small areas.

Limited or regional fasciectomy

Variable excision, usually of longitudinally orientated cords of disease, in the palm and/or digits. This is the most commonly performed procedure for uncomplicated primary DD.

The transverse fibres of Skoog in the palm should be preserved where possible (these are usually not involved in primary disease). This means that they act as a 'waterproofing layer' for further surgery, and the surgeon can be sure the NVBs are deep to these fibres, proximal to the level of the distal palmar crease.

Radical fasciectomy

The concept of radical fasciectomy is to treat the disease like a 'cancer', and perform an extensive resection of all visible fibres, longitudinal and vertical.

Published operative series have not shown reduced recurrence rates. The rate of postoperative haematoma and delayed wound healing is high, and the hand becomes much stiffer than after more conservative surgery.

This operation has become less popular, as it does not seem to confer any advantage over more limited fasciectomy, and has higher complication rates.

Dermofasciectomy

This is a technique in which normal or diseased skin, fat, and fascia is excised, usually down to the mid-lateral lines in an 'aesthetic unit', and replaced by FTSG. This removes much of the tissue which can potentially become involved by extension of, or recurrent disease.

Grafts take better in the digits than in the palm in isolation. Grafts crossing the MCPJ into the palm from the finger appear to take better than isolated grafts in the palm.

Indications for dermofaciectomy
- Extensive skin involvement,
- Secondary skin shortage from contracture,
- Insertion of a 'firebreak' of FTSG in early, aggressive or recurrent disease.

PIP contractures
- With practice, during examination of the hand, you can usually tell if the loss of extension of the PIPJ is due to a tight cord across the joint, or from infiltration by DD into the joint itself, or a combination.
- In general, the more surgery you do to the PIPJ, the more stiff and swollen it will be postoperatively, and the longer the patient will take to recover (if at all).
- The main danger is loss of pre-operative ROM in flexion, or a painful joint, both of which are very disabling.
- Release of PIPJ structures should be performed serially, and with great caution. It is probably better not to gain full extension of the digit, and retain pre-operative flexion, than to get full extension and a very stiff and painful PIPJ.
- When there is infiltration of the flexor tendon sheath by DD, transverse incisions in between the pulleys (usually between A2 and A3, and A3 and A4) can produce surprising improvement in extension. A FTSG can still be used to resurface this area, despite gaps in the tendon sheath.
- Splints are more important following PIPJ release, as the extensor mechanism over a joint, which has been flexed for a long time, is unlikely to be strong enough to maintain the extension gained by the surgery.

PIPJ structures to be released
- Flexor tendon sheath
- Accessory collateral ligaments
- Check rein ligaments
- Proximal edge of volar plate

Recurrent disease
- Surgery for recurrent disease is usually more challenging than for primary Dupuytren's.
- Various causes:
  - **extension** of previous disease in an adjacent (unoperated) field,
  - **recurrent** disease at the site of previous surgery. In either case, it should be approached with a different mindset.
- Frequent involvement of the PIPJ and DIPJ and skin. There will be skin shortage from established contracture, and often extensive infiltration by the Dupuytren's tissue.
- Have a low threshold to perform dermofasciectomy.
- Assume one or both digital vessels may have been divided in the primary surgery.

Postoperative therapy

- **Elevation** of the hand postoperatively is vital to prevent unnecessary swelling, and to allow any wound exudate to follow gravity proximally and not to accumulate under the skin flaps or graft.
- **Rest.** A period of (4–7 days) rest and elevation allows the immediate postoperative swelling to subside and the wounds to settle. This varies according to individual preference, and logistical factors such as availability of clinics and therapists.
  - Immediate movement on the first day after surgery tends to cause pain and stiffness.
- **Dermofasciectomy.** Immobilization for 7 to 10 days in a volar POP cast or firm wool-and-crepe dressing is required to allow complete take of FTSG in dermofasciectomy, after which time the soft tissues will stand up to intensive hand therapy.
- **Week 1.** The patient should work on flexion; this is functionally the most important movement to regain, and also prevents splitting of wounds by forced extension (which causes delayed wound healing with its adverse sequelae).
- **Week 2.**
  - Push extension.
  - Hook grip. Extension of MCPJs with flexion of PIPJ and DIPJ. This exercises palmar flexion, and stretches the extensor mechanism over the PIPJ.
- **Splints**
  - The use of splints should be decided on an individual basis.
  - Early splinting should be used with caution as it can stretch the skin flaps and lead to delayed healing and delayed progression with hand therapy.
  - Postoperative splinting is unlikely to improve what gain in extension has been made by surgery, but can be important to maintain it.
  - Splinting is important following PIPJ release, when the extensor mechanism may be attenuated, and may not be strong enough to keep the finger extended.

Per-operative complications

- Buttonholing of skin during dissection of skin flaps
- Nerve injury:
  - Should be rare in primary disease.
  - Commoner in revision surgery for recurrent disease.
- Vascular injury:
  - Should be avoided.
  - Commoner than nerve injury.
  - Can lead to vascular compromise during secondary surgery, especially if you do not know what happened during the first procedure.
- Vascular compromise:
  - Revision surgery with vascular injury during primary procedure.
  - Extension of chronically flexed digit (with fibrosis around NVB) stretching the digital artery.

Postoperative complications
- Haematoma
- Infection
- Wound breakdown/graft loss
- Swelling
- Stiffness
- Loss of flexion
- Cold sensitivity
- CRPS
- Recurrent disease

Other treatment

Enzymatic fasciotomy with collagenase is being developed and is in the early clinical trial stage. It may have a role for cords in the palm which cause MP contracture.

Osteoarthritis of the hand

Introduction

Osteoarthritis

Common disease of diarthrodial joints. Primary aetiology is characterized by progressive degeneration of articular cartilage: a manifestation of an abnormal state of chondrocyte metabolism, loss of certain tissue components, alterations in microstructure and changes in biomechanical properties.

Normal cartilage comprises a large highly organized extracellular matrix that is synthesized and maintained by a sparse population of highly specialized cells called chondrocytes. The normal function of articular cartilage is dependent on its composition and its microstructure. In addition the chondrocytes responsible for its maintenance are sensitive to applied load, therefore its structure is also determined by its function.

Biochemical changes include increased hydration, decreased proteoglycan content, altered structure and variation in collagen predication, fibril size and arrangement.

Biomechanical changes include a decrease in the tensile, compressive and shear moduli (stiffness) and an increase in the permeability.

The thumb

The thumb is the key to function in the hand. It should be long, strong, stable and pain-free. There are 4 joints:

- Scaphoid–trapezium–trapezoid (STT)
- Trapezium-metacarpal (carpometacarpal)
- Metacarpophalangeal (MCPJ)
- Interphalangeal (IPJ)

The thumb carpometacarpal joint is most commonly affected by idiosyncratic arthritis, whereas the MCPJ is most commonly affected after injury. Painful degeneration of any of these joints will significantly compromise hand function: treatment, and thus restoration of function, is usually reliable.

Digits

Whilst spontaneous arthritis is not at all uncommon in the proximal and distal interphalangeal joints, pain is unusual. The joints become swollen and stiff. They may become unstable and deviate laterally.

- Bouchard's nodes—proximal interphalangeal joints
- Heberdon's nodes—distal interphalangeal joints

Function may be inhibited particularly by stiffness or pain in the little and ring fingers (spoiling power grip), or by pain and instability in the index and middle fingers (spoiling apposition against the thumb).

Aetiology

Osteoarthritis in the hand has many causes.

Primary idiopathic

This is the most common cause. Especially seen in females after the menopause, there is often a clear family history. The thumb base is most frequently affected, the interphalangeal joints occasionally and the metacarpophalangeal joints very rarely. The arthritis is characterized by a discrepancy between the physical or radiological signs and the symptoms of which the patient complains. Some patients have advanced radiological changes yet minor symptoms and *vice-versa*.

Post-traumatic

The thumb and finger joints are prone to injury, exposed to compressive, shearing and distractive forces at work and leisure. Subsequent articular cartilage incongruity or instability may lead to degenerative change within months or even many decades later. However, even marked incongruity or instability may never lead to symptoms or functional problems.

Post-infective

Most commonly seen after an infected DIPJ ganglion cyst or tooth-injury to the MCPJ ('fight-bite'), a joint can be rapidly destroyed.

Metabolic

Occasionally, spontaneous osteoarthritis is associated with metabolic disorders, for example haemochromatosis with 2nd or 3rd MCP arthritis.

Digital joint replacement

Whereas the biomechanics, biomaterials and surgical techniques for hip and knee replacement has been refined such that reliable long-term outcomes are almost assured, arthroplasty of the small joints of the hand is still uncertain.

Biomechanics

The soft tissue envelope around the MCPJ and PIPJ is complex. The joint movement and posture is affected by the tension of the collateral ligaments and by the relative length and tone of the tendons (FDS, FDP, intrinsics, EDC) that traverse the joint ('kinetic chain').

The finger MCPJ is not a simple ball-and-socket. It is wider at the palmar surface than the dorsal surface, allowing collateral stability for power grip and thumb pinch in flexion yet allowing collateral laxity for span in extension. MCPJ replacement should maintain both the length of the joint and the collateral ligament insertion. Also, the joint is not a hinge; the head is offset anterior to the alignment of the metacarpal shaft so that on flexion the proximal phalangeal base glides as well as hinges. The design should reproduce this anterior offset.

The PIPJ is a bicondylar joint which acts almost as a hinge, but with a few degrees of rotation on flexion to allow convergence of the fingers into the palm. The collateral ligaments attach very close to the surface so that minimal bone resection is essential to maintain stability and proper axis of rotation.

Implant for the MCPJ and PIPJ must allow for these complex movements, so a constrained hinge is not suitable.

Biomaterials

Silastic

Used for more than 30 years. Acts as a spacer which is particularly helpful when the inadequate soft tissues have been reconstructed in rheumatoid. However, the implants do not reproduce the normal kinematics of the joint, they do not provide stability and they do not resist soft tissue tension well. The implants impart most of their movement by pistoning rather than flexion–extension. Range of movement is limited (usually about 15 to 50°) and they tend to break eventually. In the osteoarthritic hand, the ligaments are usually stable and bone stock is preserved; this gives the opportunity for anatomical replacement which requires different biomaterials.

Metal on polyethylene

These materials have been proven in replacement of the hip and knee; anatomical surface replacement implants are available for the MPCJ and PIPJ.

Pyrolytic carbon

This material is produced by chemical vapour deposition, when hydrocarbon gas injected into chamber and heated to 1300°C. The breaks carbon–hydrogen bond and pure carbon remains. This material can be fashioned into an anatomical shape. The modulus of elasticity is similar to bone; there is negligible wear (it is used as a bearing in some mechanical heart valves).

Fixation

The ideal fixation method has not been established for digital replacement.

- Press-fit: pyrolytic carbon is held by appositional bone growth rather than true bone ingrowth. A thin layer appears around the implant on radiographs which does not represent failure.
- Ingrowth: plasma spraying, hydroxyapatite coating, sintered finish and porous polyethtlene are all options but none are established in small joints
- Cement: advantages—immediate fixation; grouting the discrepancy between the implant shape and medullary canal; accurate placement. Disadvantages: heat damage, brittle due to thin layer and stiffness.

Scaphoid–trapezium–trapezoid joint

Otherwise known as the STT or triscaphe joint.

Aetiology

Spontaneous (commonly seen in cadavers). Possibly associated with rotatory instability of the scaphoid—a flexed scaphoid will alter joint forces across the STT joint. Assocated with scapholunate incompetence. Occasionally follows trauma.

Symptoms and signs

Radiological change not always symptomatic. Pain in the radial side of the wrist. Patient characteristically points to the scaphoid tubercle (at the front of the radial side of the wrist) whereas in carpo-metacarpal (CMC) arthritis the patient points to the dorsal aspect of the thumb base.

Tender over the scaphoid tubercle. Pain reproduced by the examiner moving the wrist radial-wards and ulnarwards under compressive load. There may be a volar wrist ganglion associated with STT arthritis.

X-rays show sclerosis and reduced joint space at the STT joint. On the lateral view there may be a dorsal intercalated segment instability (DISI) deformity. Look for associated thumb trapezium–metacarpal arthritis (which alters treatment options).

Non-operative treatment

Non-operative

- Adapt
- Splint
- Cortisone injection. Fine bore needle, passed into the front of the joint. If in doubt can be done under fluoroscopic guidance.

Operative treatment

There is no ideal treatment for this condition. Each of the surgical options carries significant drawbacks. No RCT data to guide choice. STT fusion most widely studied.

STT fusion

Fusion deletes pain from the arthritic joint. Transverse incision over dorso-radial aspect of wrist, fluoroscopy helps to localize level (can be performed through a palmar approach). Extensor pollicis longus (EPL) and ECRL retracted. Capsulotomy. Wrist moved into radial deviation and extension, scaphoid tubercle pushed backwards to achieve a scaphoid angle of 55–60° relative to long axis of radius (these manoeuvres improve radial deviation after surgery). STT joint held with percutaneous wires passed under fluoroscopic control. Confluence of STT joint removed with osteotomes or a circular core-reamer. Separate incision over radial styloid. Tip excised subperiosteally (to improve radial tilt; do not remove too much otherwise the palmar ligaments are destabilized) and periosteum closed. Cancellous bone harvested through radial styloid base. Packed into STT joint. Wounds closed with dissolvable subcutaneous suture, Plaster splint 6 weeks then X-ray and wire removal. A circular plate or memory staples are elegant alternatives to K-wire fixation.

Complications

This operation has a reputation for a fairly high complication rate. Non-union, pin-site problems. Loss of radial tilt and flexion due to impingement of the STT block on the radius, without the usual flexion of the scaphoid (minimized by pre-positioning the scaphoid and excising the tip of the radial styloid).

Outcome

Flexion–extension 70%; grip 70%. Good pain relief in most.

Trapeziectomy and undercut trapezoid

For patients with trapezium–metacarpal arthritis as well as STT arthritis, the trapezium is removed and then the distal edge of the trapezoid is undercut by 4–5mm. This procedure could be performed in isolated STT OA, hoping to reproduce the generally reliable results of trapeziectomy, although sacrificing a normal trapezium–metacarpal joint is debatable.

Outcome

No robust outcome studies.

Excision of distal pole of scaphoid

Dorsal or anterior approach. Joint identified under fluoroscopy. Distal quarter excised with saw or osteotome. Check for impingement. Careful closure of capsule-periosteum.

Complications

Concerns raised about destabilizing the scaphoid which extends as unconstrained distally and controlled by lunate through intact scapholunate ligament. Must be avoided in those with a pre-existing DISI. Do not excise too much distal pole. Capsular reconstruction to avoid this complication has been described.

Outcome

Very few data in the literature.

Other procedures

Interposition of a pyrocarbon disc. No published long-term results.
Arthroscopic assessment and debridement. Technically difficult, small-bore scope required.

Thumb CMCJ arthritis

Othersise known as basal joint or trapezium–metacarpal joint.

The thumb plays a pivotal role in hand function, often represented as the pillar of the hand, providing oppositional strength for prehension. Functionally the most important joint is the carpometacarpal joint which slides (whereas all the other joints in the hand are essentially hinges). Arthritis in this joint can, therefore, be debilitating. Commonly affects women in their fifth to sixth decade (about 15% affected). Postmenopausal women are affected 5 to 10 times more commonly than men.

Aetiology

- Ligament laxity due to hormonal changes
- Weakness of the palmar oblique ligament causing lateral subluxation of the metacarpal base, altering joint load and precipitating arthritis
- Hypoplasia and increased radial slope of the trapezium joint
- Chronic stress to an incongruous joint
- Abnormality of the abductor pollicis longus
- Biomechanical associated with synovial inflammatory mediators
- Imbalance of the two main forces, both of adductor pollicis and the abductor pollicis longus acting on the first metacarpal
- Acute trauma or previous fracture (Bennett's)
- Cumulative trauma. No good evidence that the pathology is caused by overuse in an occupation; rather, symptoms may be exposed by the demands of work.

Clinical features

Symptoms

Pain in the thumb base, precipitated by activity. Patient tends to point to the dorsoradial side of the thumb base (whereas in STT arthritis patient points to the scaphoid tubercle). Forceful pinching and grasping large objects exacerbate the pain. In earlier stages stiffness is not normally present; in fact the converse tends to be true, joints in the early stage tend to be lax. As the joint becomes inflamed and osteoarthritic there is an increasing tendency toward subjective and objective stiffness. With increased stiffness pain normally subsides.

Signs

Prominent metacarpal base. In early stages the joint may be lax; the metacarpal base can be passively subluxated into and out of the saddle joint. The strong pull of the APL during pinch allows the base of the 1st MC to subluxate dorsally. Adductor pollicis however tends to pull the distal part of the metacarpal palmarwards, leading to narrowing of the 1st webspace and eventually to fixed contractures. As the adduction deformity becomes fixed, the MCP joint hyperextends (attenuation of the palmar plate) to provide an adequate thumb-index span. Tender over the joint, painful coarse crepitus on passive movement.

Differential diagnosis

- STT arthritis
- De Quervain's tenosynovitis
- Radioscaphoid arthritis

X-rays

There is poor correlation between radiographic severity and clinical symptoms.

Posteroanterior (PA) and oblique views and most usefully the Robert's view are requested to assess stages of the disease. The **Robert's view** is acquired with the hand hyperpronated and the X-ray beam directed anteroposterior (AP), creating a clear image of all three articulations of the trapezium.

Radiographic staging is commonly performed using a classification system proposed by Eaton.[1]

Table 9.1 Eaton classification

Eaton classification	Description
Stage I	Articular contours are normal. Possible widening of the joint space because of laxity of the ligamentous support.
Stage II	Slight narrowing of the trapeziometacarpal joint. Minimal sclerotic changes of the subchondral bone. Presence of osteophytes less than 2mm in diameter. Scaphotrapezial (ST) joint appears normal
Stage III	Joint space markedly narrowed or obliterated with cystic changes, sclerotic bone and varying degrees of dorsal subluxation. Subchondral sclerosis and osteophytes measuring more than 2mm in diameter may be present. The ST joint appears normal
Stage IV	Complete deterioration of the TM joint as in stage III and ST joint is narrowed by sclerotic and cystic changes

CMC stress views

PA view of both thumbs taken simultaneously while patient pushes the radial aspect of each thumb tip against the other forcefully. This tends to cause the MC to sublux laterally if the joint is lax.

1. Eaton RG and Glickel SZ (1987). Trapeziometacarpal arthritis: staging as a rationale for treatment. *Hand Clinics* **3**: 455–469.

Non-operative treatment for thumb CMC OA

Hand therapy

Aims

- Decrease pain in the thumb
- Maintain 1st webspace
- Maintain functional strength for pinch and grasp and thus independence in functional tasks
- Educate the patient in joint protection
- Increase stability

Splinting

Static splinting maintains optimal joint alignment and reduces the forces that may lead to further joint deterioration or deformity.

Helpful for the CMC joint that is becoming progressively hypermobile or unstable.

Provides rest and support, however once removed it will no longer have a therapeutic effect.

The most effective splint in immobilizing and resting the basal joint is the long opponens or thumb spica. This typically positions the base of the thumb in relative palmar abduction, incorporating slight flexion and medial rotation, thus helping to maintain the 1st webspace and increasing the natural stability of the joint by increasing the congruity of the joint surfaces.

Little has been published on the efficacy of non-operative splinting in the management of basal joint disease. Further debate concerning whether to immobilize the wrist or not. Fluoroscopically it has been shown that the short opponens splint (thumb spica extending to the level of the wrist but not immobilizing the wrist) does indeed stabilize the basal joint on trapeziometacarpal radiography.

Exercise

Only prescribed in the early stages of instability in the absence of inflammation or marked pain. Where a joint is inflamed, rest and support is more appropriate. Flexibility exercises are designed to maintain the pliability of the surrounding soft tissues. Particular attention should be given to preventing adduction contractures of the 1st webspace.

An important deforming force of the CMC joint is the strong pull of the adductor pollicis muscle. The pull of the adductor combined with weakness of the opposing thenar intrinsic muscles may result in a significant adduction deformity of the thumb. Therefore strengthening the thenar musculature as well as the APL extrinsic abductor and long extensor may be beneficial in maintaining dynamic stability of the CMC joint. However, isolation of the EPL for exercise is not desirable since it encourages retropulsion of the thumb and subluxation of the arthritic basal joint.

As a rule exercise should not cause pain that lasts for more than two hours.

The goals of resistive exercises are to promote muscular-based stability about the base of the thumb and maintain the strength required for the performance of functional activities, however it is important to have an understanding of individual patient's needs and their clinical presentation to tailor a conservative programme to their specific requirements.

Education
- Avoiding stressful activities such as lateral pinching and gripping
- Maintaining pain-free functional strength and flexibility
- Energy conservation (optimal activity versus rest cycles) by dividing stress among multiple joints or extremities
- Using assistive devices or splints

Oral medication
- Paracetamol-based
- Non-steroidal anti-inflammatories

Steroid injection

Transient pain relief by reducing inflammation. The duration of response is unpredictable; unlikely to last long in stage III and IV. Can be repeated on two or three occasions. Combining injections with splinting may be effective in decreasing inflammation and thus pain.

Operative treatment for thumb CMCJ OA

Indications

Failure of non-operative measures to relieve pain and maintain function. The recommendation for surgery tends largely to be based on the clinical picture. Surgery becomes an option when symptoms are refractory to the aforementioned modalities and the patient's ability to perform activities of daily living is severely impaired or pain is not satisfactorily relieved.

Surgical options

- Osteotomy
- Volar ligament reconstruction
- Excision arthroplasty:
  - Partial
  - Total
  - Ligament suspension
- Replacement:
  - Hemiarthroplasty
  - Silicon interposition
  - Anatomic joint replacement
  - Non-anatomic joint replacement
- Fusion
- Denuruation

Volar ligament reconstruction

Indications

For stage I or early stage II disease.

Incompetence and degeneration of the volar beak ligament (anterior oblique ligament) provokes cartilage failure at the front of the joint. Reconstruction of volar ligament reduces metacarpal into trapezium socket and may give symptomatic relief. Does not compromise alternative surgical procedures if it fails.

Procedure

Palmar approach. Thenar muscles reflected. FCR identified just proximal to trapezium ridge. FCR is used because its insertion on the base of the 2nd MC, simulates the vector of the palmar oblique ligament (also known as the AOL—anterior oblique ligament) and it is conveniently located in the groove of the trapezium. FCR traced distally, removing trapezoid ridge with rongeur. Mid-forearm incision. FCR split in two. Drill hole across base of 1st metacarpal. Half of FCR passed through hole palmar-to-dorsal, re-turned across front of joint imbricating in loose capsule, reattached to residual FCR. Plaster resting splint until sutures removed. Thermoplastic splint supporting thumb metacarpal in abduction, MP joint in slight flexion for 3 to 4 weeks.

Outcome

About 70% have good clinical outcome. Few long-term data. Persisting symptoms can be treated with alternative surgical methods.

Osteotomy

Indications

For stage I or early stage II of the disease: joint-preserving procedure, does not preclude further surgery.

OA tends to start in the volar half of the CMCJ; extension osteotomy shifts contact stresses dorsally away from the compromised volar joint surface and may give symptomatic relief.

Procedure

Dorsal incision over thumb metacarpal. Extensor pollicis brevis reflected. APL insertion carefully preserved. Osteotomy across proximal 1/5th of metacarpal using cooled saw blade and no periosteal stripping. Distal second cut at 25 degrees, aimed to emerge at palmar exit of first cut. Palmar cortex broken manually. Wedge of bone removed. Osteotomy closed and held with kwires or low-profile plate. Plaster 5 weeks holding thumb base abducted and MPJ flexed 10–20°.

Outcome

About 70% good results (in short to medium term). Small risk of non-union.

Excision arthoplasty

First described by Gervis (1949). Arthritic joint deleted by removal of the entire trapezium. Some surgeons have modified this to removal of the distal half of the trapezium.

Procedure

Dorsal or palmar approach. Capsulotomy, trapezium removed piecemeal. Check STT joint by distracting 2nd metacarpal and inserting Macdonald's dissector to display joint. If STT OA significant, excise 3–4mm of distal surface of trapezoid. Careful and robust capsular repair holding thumb base in abduction and pronation.

Rehabilitation

Splintage: studies range from no immobilization to up to 6 weeks of immobilization. Splints should support the thumb CMCJ in abduction and slight pronation; the MP joint should be slightly flexed.
Mobilization: Dependent largely on pain. Recent studies have recommended mobilization at 2 weeks with good results. Graded activity is recommended at 4 weeks with adduction, pinch grip and strengthening activities deferred until week 6 after surgery. Aim is to encourage proper functional posture (thumb base abducted and pronated, then MP joint flexed). Otherwise there is a tendency for the opposite to occur.

Outcome

About 85% are pleased with result. Pinch grip about 70% of normal. Good results are durable at 10-year follow-up. Takes 4–9 months to finally settle. Small risk of dystrophy, scar pain.

Resection and interposition

A rolled-up segment of palmaris longus or FCR ('anchovy') can be placed into the space. The volume of tendon available, and its viability, unlikely to alter the load through the new joint.

Resection and ligament suspension

A tendon can be redirected across the metacarpal base to reduce the tendency of the metacarpal base to impinge on the distal pole of the scaphoid and to encourage an abducted posture.
- FCR
- FCR (split or whole), with anchovy of residual FCR
- APL
- Many others described

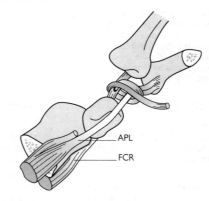

Fig. 9.1 Ligament reconstruction with APL.

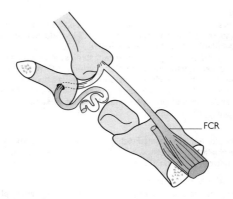

Fig. 9.2 Ligament reconstruction with split FER.

Joint replacement

Aim

- Preservation of thumb length
- Stable yet mobile joint surface
- Durable material
- Durable fixation into bone

Contraindicated in poor bone stock (e.g. rheumatoid arthritis, unstable joints, malaligned joints, patients likely to place high functional demands)

Silicone interposition

Good results reported in the past. Poor mechanical tolerance of compression. Popularity waned because of **dislocation**, **cold flow** wear of the silicone, **silicone synovitis** in the wrist joint, fracture.

Non-anatomic joint replacement

Various ball-and-socket designs (e.g. de la Caffiniere, ARPE, Cardan, GUEPAR) have been used.

Pyrocarbon metacarpal base hemiarthroplasty with convex surface placed into a reciprocal concavity reamed into the trapezium. No long-term results.

Anatomic joint replacement

Hemiarthroplasty (e.g. pyrocarbon) for those stable joints with a well-preserved trapezium surface. No long-term results

Cobalt chrome-polythene. Materials have a good pedigree from knee and hip arthroplasty. However, secure fixation into trapezium is difficult. Risk of dislocation and early loosening.

Fusion

Indications

Grade III and IV OA joint destruction. Instability secondary to ligamentous laxity (e.g. Ehlers–Danlos). Offers a secure, stable and often pain free base for the thumb.

Contraindications: OA of the STT joint or thumb MCP joint. The functional price for losing retroposition and opposition is high for those needing dexterous movement of the thumb.

Procedure

Dorsal approach over CMCJ, carefully preserving the radial artery and superficial radial nerve. Capsulotomy and minimal periosteal reflection. Joint denuded of cartilage (various techniques—burr, osteotome, peg and socket reamers). Bone graft if needed from beneath Lister's tubercle. Fixation (wires, plate, compression screw). Angle about 35° palmar abduction, 30° radial extension and 15° pronation. Plaster cast 6 weeks then X-ray.

Outcome

High complication rate (especially non-union and unacceptable stiffness). Theoretical risk of secondary degenerative changes at the MP joint or the scaphotrapezial joints due to compensatory techniques. Patients do not like the substantial loss of thumb movement.

MP joint hyperextension

This is a common deformity which develops as the thumb base adducts. It can also occur after trapeziectomy if the metacarpal falls into adduction.

Options

- *Leave alone:* the deformity will correct, helped by careful active exercises and splintage—if there is only minimal hyperextension
- *Temporary K-wire:* hold the joint into 30° flexion for 6 weeks after trapeziectomy
- *Sesamoid arthrodesis:* the most suitable procedure for marked hyperextension with good passive flexion. Through a small radial–palmar incision over the sesamoid, the sesamoid and metacarpal neck cartilage is denuded with burr, Bone surfaces apposed and held with a screw, suture or K-wire. The joint is transfixed at 30° for 4 weeks.
- *Fusion:* MP joint at 25–30° allows excellent function. Techniques include compression plate, tension band or single compression screw. Indicated in particular when simultaneous OA in MCP. Contra-indicated if thumb CMCJ fused.
- *Volar tenodesis:* Re-routed APL.

Which surgical technique for CMC arthritis?

Fusion vs excision

No evidence that pinch grip or patient satisfaction is superior in fusion. Lesser risk of complications with excision. Fusion not generally recommended except in exceptional circumstances.

Excision alone vs excision with ligament suspension

Three recent randomized studies have shown no significant differences with respect to pain, stiffness/weakness, functional disability, ROM, hand/pinch strength or height of the pseudoarthrosis.

The only difference is the length of surgery and a higher complication rate with ligament suspension. A role exists for ligament suspension in those with an unstable joint after capsule repair.

Joint replacement vs excision

RCT evidence is not available; anecdotally, recovery from replacement arthroplasty is usually quicker than after trapeziectomy. Pinch strength and function seem to recover more quickly. Patients who have had a replacement on one side and trapeziectomy on the other tend to prefer the replacement. However, issues of durability and complications with replacement should be considered.

Finger carpometacarpal joint

Aetiology

Idiopathic osteoarthritis is extremely unusual in the finger CMCJ (whereas it is common in the thumb CMCJ and finger IPJs). Most commonly seen after a fracture-dislocation of the little finger CMCJ. The ring CMCJ is sometimes involved in the injury; rarely the middle and index (which are very stable joints, needing extreme violence for dislocation).

Non-operative treatment

Many displaced 5th CMCJ injuries ('reversed Bennett's') or comminuted basal 5th MC fractures settle with time despite radiological OA. Cortisone injections may settle the pain for a while.

Surgery

5th CMCJ OA

If the 4th CMC is preserved (check on CT) then excise base of 5th MC and fuse 5th to 4th metacarpal. This preserves flexion-supination ('metacarpal descent') at the base of the ulnar side of the hand, contributing to power grip.

4th, 3rd 2nd CMCJ OA

Fusion (K-wires, screws, plates).

Metacarpophalangeal joint

The metacarpophalangeal joint rarely develops osteoarthritis in the absence of an underlying cause. The loss of function in a painful, stiff joint is significant, reducing power grip and especially in the index, pinch grip against the thumb.

Aetiology

Infected tooth bite

A punch to an opponent's tooth readily breaches the five layers over the MCPJ (skin, fat, tendon, capsule, synovium), introducing virulent oral flora into a closed space. Severe infection develops within 24–48 hours; failure to recognize and promptly treat the injury (thorough lavage, antibiotics) leads to destruction of the articular cartilage.

Haemochromatosis

Rare haematological condition. Genetic disorder causing the body to absorb an excessive amount of iron from the diet: the iron is then deposited in various organs, mainly the liver, but also the pancreas, heart, endocrine glands, and joints. Iron studies (serum ferritin, transferrin saturation) are recommended if MCPJ arthritis is found in the absence of any predisposing cause.

Injury

- Comminuted fracture of metacarpal head (most common).
- Instablity after dislocation or collateral ligament injury.
- Comminuted fracture of base of proximal phalanx.

Non-operative treatment

Cortisone injection

Valuable, can last for a long time. Repeat as required.

Splintage

Cumbersome. No ideal position.

Surgery

Fusion

- Indication: not an ideal operation in the fingers, usually salvage for failed joint replacement or intractable instability. However, very suitable for thumb MP joint where function is minimally affected by MP fusion because pain-free stability much more important than movement (no role for thumb MP replacement except after CMC fusion).
- Procedure: Dorsal approach, split extensor, excise joint with cooled saw. Angle of fusion −45° for all fingers, slight supination of index and middle for apposition against the thumb. For the thumb MP, about 25° flexion. Techniques: compression plate (recommended), tension band wire, K-wires.

Replacement

- Implant choice: if soft tissues stable (usually they are in osteoarthritis), use anatomical surface replacement (pyrolytic carbon, metal–metal, metal–polythene). Occasionally use silastic implant (unstable soft tissues, salvage of failed surface replacement).
- Procedure: dorsal approach, split extensor, minimal bone resection, preserving collateral ligaments.
- Rehabilitation: depends on implant (manufacturer's recommendations) stability of fixation, stability of soft tissues. Early movement when possible.
- Complications: dislocation, stiffness, infection, loosening.
- Outcome: very few data in literature. More reliable than PIPJ replacement (because surrounding soft tissue envelope less complex and proper centre of rotation easier to achieve). Early study and different design: pyrocarbon MP joint 80% survivorship at 10 years. Recent study >90% satisfaction and 99% survivorship at one year.

Proximal interphalangeal joint

The PIP joint is the most important joint within the finger. It needs to be painless and either stable (index and middle for thumb apposition) or flexible (ring and little for power grip).

Aetiology
- Idiopathic osteoarthritis (Bouchard's nodes)
- Trauma (intra-articular fracture, instability after ligament injury)
- Infection

Non-operative treatment
- Adapt
- Analgesics
- Cortisone injections
- Splint

Surgery
Fusion
- Indications: preferred for index and middle to regain stable pinch against thumb (unless movement is crucial and insecurity of PIP replacement understood). Unstable collateral ligaments or unbalanced tendons (swan neck, boutonnière)
- Approach: dorsal tendon splitting; excise bone with cooled saw or cup-and-cone reamer
- Angle: **index and middle** 20–30° flexion and slight supination, (tailored to allow pulp apposition with thumb), **ring and middle** 40–50° (to contribute to power grip yet allow reasonable opening of grasp)
- Fixation: compression plate recommended, K-wires, tension band.

Replacement
- Indications: preferred for little and ring finger where flexion for powergrip more important than stability. Avoid if collaterals unstable or tendons unbalanced (swan-neck, boutonnière)
- Approach:
  - Dorsal: central tendon split, avoid detachment of central slip
  - Chamay: dorsal incision fold-back of extensor, central slip insertion preserved
  - mid-lateral: z-shaped exposure through ulnar collateral (index, middle, radial collateral (ring, little). Palmar plate divided, joint opened. Extensor preserved. Collateral closed with non-dissolvable sutures. Careful rehabilitation to avoid stressing
  - Anterior: A3 pulley elevated on one side, tendons retracted, palmar plate detached proximally. Advantage: preservation of extensor gliding surface
- Technique: minimal bone resection, preserve collateral ligaments and central slip, centre of rotation perfect to maintain tendon balance
- Implant: unconstrained pyrocarbon, metal–metal or metal–polyethylene, occasionally silastic. Do not use a constrained implant (there are torque and collateral stresses through the PIP joint on flexion–extension which will predispose to loosening)

- Rehabilitation: hand therapy essential. Depends on integrity of central slip and implant fixation
- Results: few data available. No long-term outcome studies. Perhaps 1/3 do well (i.e. useful range of painfree motion), 1/3 equivocal (pain relief even if stiff). 1/3 unsatisfactory (stiff, unstable, dislocation. loosening, swan neck, boutonnière).

Rehabilitation after PIP replacement
- Early mobilization but avoid lateral forces
- Active flexion and extension
- Night splintage for protection
- Gradually increase passive extension with splint
- Passive flexion at 3 weeks if permitted by surgeon (immediately if anterior or lateral approach)
- 6 weeks after surgery:
  - Maximize extension of PIP joint
  - Increase resistance to exercises
  - Increase function
  - Avoid heavy twisting activities until 12 weeks after surgery

Distal interphalangeal joint

Aetiology
- Idiopathic (Heberdon's nodes)
- Infection (most commonly after ganglion cyst rupture by patient)
- Injury (fracture, dislocation. Unusual, even with a displaced mallet fracture)

Non-operative treatment
- Adapt (often will spontaneously stiffen and pain resolves)
- Analgesia
- Thimble splint (awkward in index and middle as spoils pinch)
- Cortisone injection (30 gauge needle)

Surgical treatment

Fusion
- Angle is controversial. Some prefer flexion in little and ring to contribute to grip, others prefer straight in little and ring to avoid catching on gloves and pockets. Index and middle fused straight or nearly straight with very slight supination for apposition against the thumb.
- Approach: dorsal incision H- or Y-shaped. Preserve blood supply to nail bed. Avoid damage to germinal matrix. Excise joint with cooled saw or cup-and-cone reamer.
- Fixation: intramedullary screw (recommended if straight fusion needed. Larger screw usually need in thumb as wider medulla). K-wires an alternative (but may get infected before fusion achieved). Buried intra-osseous loop and oblique wire (not recommended).

Replacement
- Not presently indicated for fingers. Technically possible in the thumb with digital implants but indications unclear.

Pulmonary hypertophic osteoarthropathy
Seen in up to 10% of thoracic malignancy. Periosteal thickening and new bone formation in digits, clubbing of nails. Joint pains, especially early morning.

Infection

General principles

History

Presenting complaint
- Take a careful history. The patient may associate the infection with an unrelated event, or have forgotten something which is relevant.
- Ask specifically about foreign body injury.
- If an explanation for the infection is not immediately forthcoming, ask about occupation and hobbies.

Past medical history
- Ask about diabetes (more prone to infection, more severe and more resistant to treatment).
- IV drug abuse (infection from injection, immunosuppression, poor compliance with treatment).
- Inflammatory arthritis, organ transplant, or other systemic conditions leading to immunosuppression.
- Ask about previous exposure to infection (such as *Herpes simplex*).

Drugs
- Check tetanus status.
- Steroids and other immunosuppressives.

Occupation and hobbies
- Gardening and thorn injuries.
- Pets and animal bites.
- DIY and sharp injury.

Examination
- Record temperature, pulse, blood pressure.
- Compare with unaffected hand.
- Examine nails and nail folds.
- Examine joints (pain, ROM).
- Look at flexor tendon sheath and palmar spaces to exclude involvement.
- Look for axillary lymphadenopathy.
- Mark the edge of rapid onset cellulitis with permanent marker pen for subsequent comparison.

Investigations
- Microbiology:
  - Send pus or tissue (fresh, *not* in formalin) for culture and sensitivity.
  - Get urgent gram stain in severe infections.
- X-ray:
  - Fracture or radio-opaque foreign body.
- Ultrasound scan (USS):
  - To detect radiolucent foreign body (wood splinter, thorn).
- Blood tests:
  - ↑ White cll count (WCC)
  - ↑ CRP
  - ↑ CK in muscle necrosis following severe necrotizing infection.

Monitor both daily in severe infections, especially those requiring surgery.
↓ CRP indicative of recovery.

Treatment

General measures
- Hydration
- Analgesia
- Manage blood sugar very carefully in diabetes
- Elevation

Antibiotics
- Start empirical antibiotics until microbiology culture results available.
- Give IV for severe or rapidly progressive infections.
- Prescribe sensitive antibiotics when culture results available.
- Discuss severe cases with microbiologist.

Surgery
- Use high arm tourniquet. Do not exsanguinate limb; elevate the limb for several minutes before the tourniquet is inflated.
- Incise and drain, with incision over central prominent part of abscess.
- Use mid-lateral, rather than Bruner (zig-zag) in digits if possible (less exposure of tendon sheath and NVB).
- Excise wound when extensive necrosis or necrotizing progression of infection.
- Send wound swabs and tissue for culture.
  - Phone lab to ensure immediate gram stain result obtained.
  - Perform further wound excision if required.
- Allow to heal by secondary intention or delayed closure only after clear microbiology culture results.
- ⚠ Do not close infected wounds primarily—leave them open. Pack lightly with antiseptic-soaked dressing gauze.

Microbiology

Cellulitis

Acute
- *Staphylococcus aureus* is commonest infecting organism.
- *Streptococcus.*

Chronic
- *Candida*

Soil or faeces
Anaerobic organisms, yeasts and *clostridium tetani.*

Necrotizing infections
Combined, synergistic, *staphylococcus aureus, streptococcus* (often β haemolytic Group A or G), and mixed anaerobes.

Bites
- *Dog bites:*
  - *Streptococcus viridans*
  - *Pasteurella multocida*
  - *Bacteroides*
- *Cat bites*
  - *Pasteurella multocida*
- *Human bites*
  - *Staphylococcus aureus*
  - *Eikenella corrodens*
  - *Alpha-haemolytic streptococci*
  - *Bacteroides*

Antibiotic policy

Antibiotic practice varies geographically. These guidelines are empirical for practice in the UK, based on the latest evidence. Severe cases must be discussed with your local microbiologists. You should always check the tetanus immunization status of the patient. Doses should be checked in the Formulary and adjusted accordingly for weight, age, severity of infection, interactions and allergy.

Cellulitis

- Flucloxacillin:
  - Erythromycin if penicillin-allergic
- Penicillin
- Plus clindamycin for Group A haemolytic *Strep.*

Soil contamination

- Flucloxacillin
- Penicillin
- Metronidazole

Animal bites

- Co-amoxiclav (ampicillin with claevulinic acid):
  - Ciprofloxacin plus clindamycin if penicillin allergic

Methicillin-resistant *Staphylococcus aureus* (MRSA)

Topical

- Iodine dressings
- Mupirocin cream

Systemic

- Teicoplanin or vancomycin

Necrotizing fasciitis

- Flucloxacillin
- Penicillin
- Clindamycin
- Metronidazole
- Gentamycin (check renal function)

Cellulitis

Cellulitis is infection of the skin and soft tissues. It is most commonly bacterial (usually *Group A beta-haemolytic streptocoocus*, sometimes *Staphylococcus aureus*), but may be caused by other agents. The infection usually originates from a cut, puncture wound or crack in the skin, but it is sometimes difficult to find out how it started.

The skin is hot, red and tender. The infection may spread, sometimes rapidly, and can progress to abscess formation, especially in palmar spaces or the flexor tendon sheath (these should be sought when examining patients). Regional lymph nodes may be enlarged and tender.

Severe cellulitis, especially in the immunocompromised, may lead to systemic sepsis and progress to a necrotizing soft tissue infection (see p. 284).

Treatment
- In early stage, oral penicillin and flucloxacillin until microbiology results available.
- If more severe with systemic signs (raised temperature, spreading cellulitis, lymphadenopathy, malaise) intravenous penicillin and flucloxacillin, plus clindamycin.
- If penicillin allergic, clarithromycin or erythromycin for early cellulitis, and teicoplanin plus clindamycin for severe infections.
- Elevation and splintage.
- If not resolving, reconsider possibility of deeper infection.
- Once resolving, continue oral antibiotics for 10–14 days.

Abscess

An abscess is a collection of pus in a confined space.

Fingertip (nail, nail fold, pulp)

(☐ see p. 170)

Paronychia

- A collection of pus in the lateral nail fold (paronychium) is known as paronychia.
- Follows ingrowing nail, manicure, nail-biting.
- Early cases—oral antibiotics and trim ingrowing nail.
- Established cases: elevate and remove outer ¼ of nail plate from the matrix.
- Chronic infection is associated with fungal infection (see below).

Felon

- A collection of pus in the pulp of the digit is known as a **felon**. Remember that the multiple vertical fibrous septa in the fingertip divide it into multiple spaces.
- It usually presents after inoculation from a puncture wound.
- *Staph. aureus* most likely pathogen.
- Drainage is via a unilateral midaxial incision or midline palmar incision. 'Fishmouth' incision over the distal pulp 2–3mm below the hyponychium (under nail plate) is effective but risks necrosis.
- In more severe infections affecting the nailfold *and* pulp, it is sometimes necessary to remove the nail plate to drain the pus. This can lead to loss of adherence of the nail plate to the underlying sterile matrix (oncholysis), which allows build up of keratin under the nail plate, and may predispose to fungal infection.

Whitlow

- *Herpes simplex* infection of the nail fold or finger tip pulp is known as a Whitlow.
- Seen in dental and medical personnel, and sometimes in children.
- Diagnosis by characteristic history of episodic infection and examination finding of itchy vesicles.
- Primary treatment by systemic antivirals (acyclovir).
- Surgery should be avoided unless severe secondary bacterial infection.

Subdermal

- Can be anywhere in the hand.
- Suspect flexor tendon sheath or deep space involvement if overlying.
- Drainage by appropriately orientated incision over prominence of abscess.
- A foreign body must be considered (history, X-ray, ultrasound). Thorns such as blackthorn can be particularly virulent.

Deep spaces

These spaces can become infected by penetrating injury or by spread from a flexor synovial sheath infection. The anatomy is crucial to successful diagnosis and treatment.

Webspace (collar stud)

Infection in the webspace may present as two abscesses, one on the palmar and one on the dorsal side of the hand (giving the 'collar stud' or 'hourglass' appearance). The two are separated by the fascial connections around the webspace and the superficial transverse metacarpal ligaments.

The incision to drain them should NOT be placed across the webspace, or a tight scar results.

They should be regarded as two separate abscesses, with palmar and dorsal approaches.

Palmar spaces

Anatomy

There are three deep spaces in the palm which can become infected: the thenar and mid-palmar spaces are separated by a vertical septum running from the 3rd MC to the palmar aponeurosis. The mid-palmar and hypothenar spaces are separated by a septum attached to the 5th MC. The thenar (index) and mid-palmar (middle, ring, little) spaces extend distally into the lumbrical canals.

Thenar space

Contains 1st lumbrical. FDS and FDP to index pass over this space. Lies over 2nd MC.

Mid-palmar

Contains 2nd, 3rd, 4th lumbricals. Lies over 3rd and 4th MC.

Hypothenar

Contains hypothenar muscles over 5th MC. Less important, as not continuous with long flexors or lumbricals.

Parona's space

Space bound by pronator quadratus, FPL, FCU and long finger flexors. Infection derives from ulnar or radial bursa. Median nerve compression common.

Necrotizing fasciitis

This is a severe, progressive infection caused by a *synergistic* (i.e. one potentiates the effect of the others) combination of virulent organisms (aggressive beta haemolytic Group A or G *streptococcus*, other Gram-positive, Gram-negative and anaerobic organisms). Infection spreads along fascial planes. Severe systemic illness eventually overwhelms the patient (coagulopathy, shock). Muscle necrosis (rhabdomyolysis) leads to increased creatine kinase (CK) which may contribute to renal failure.

Usually presents late by nature of its evolution.

Unusual in fit young people. It is seen mainly in neglected severe infections, diabetes, alcoholism, drug-abusers and other conditions leading to immunosuppression, elderly and infirm patients, or those with intellectual or psychiatric problems which lead to delayed recognition and subsequent treatment.

Investigation

- Raised white cell count, raised CRP.
- Blood cultures.
- X-rays—may show gas formation.

Treatment

Patients are septic, and must be treated **immediately** by radical surgical excision of infected tissue, beyond visible margins, as infection may progress at the subdermal level along fascial planes. Amputation may be necessary.

- Repeat debridement as required.
- Antibiotics to cover broad spectrum.
- Likely to need intensive care support when systemic inflammatory response leads to failure of respiratory, cardiac and renal systems.

Flexor tendon sheath infection

Anatomy

The flexor tendon sheath encloses the flexor tendons in the digits and extends into the palm. The tendon is reinforced in the digits and over the MCPJs by a series of annular (A1 to A5) and cruciate (C1 to C3) pulleys, with normal tendon sheath in between them (📖 see Chapter 13, p. 391).

The sheath around FPL extends from the insertion of FPL distally to the wrist proximal to the flexor retinaculum (radial bursa).

All of the FDS and FDP tendons are surrounded by a common sheath (ulnar bursa) from a short distance above the wrist to a level just distal to the flexor retinaculum in the index, middle and ring fingers. It continues distally around the little finger, becoming its tendon sheath.

Clinical features

Kanavel's signs

- Digit held in flexed posture
- Pain on passive extension of the affected digit
- Tender along line of flexor tendon sheath
- Fusiform swelling of digit

In the thumb and little finger, the infection can spread within the sheath into the distal forearm because of the continuation of the sheath (radial bursa around FPL, ulnar bursa around little finger tendons).

Investigations

- Blood tests:
  - ↑ WCC
  - ↑ CRP
- Microbiology:
  - Pus and tissue should be sent for microscopic examination and culture

Treatment

Antibiotics

In mild cases, the infection may settle following IV antibiotics, prescribed empirically. Sensitivities may become available if pus has been sent from surgery.

Clinicians should err towards surgical exploration if there is any doubt about the severity of the infection, or if significant improvement is not seen after 24 hours of IV antibiotics.

Surgery

Surgery is indicated for more severe cases, or those which progress.

Surgical technique

Distally, the flexor tendon sheath is approached by a transverse incision across the volar DIPJ crease, exposing the A5 pulley, and incising the tendon sheath at the proximal edge of the A5 pulley.

Proximally, a 1–2cm transverse incision is made over the A1 pulley in the palm (at the level of the proximal palmar crease on radial side of hand, distal palmar crease on ulnar side of hand), and the tendon sheath is incised at the distal edge of the A1 pulley.

Pus can be seen within the flexor tendon sheath, causing it to bulge outwards. When the sheath is incised and pus extrudes, a pus swab should be taken and sent for microbiology, requesting immediate gram stain with culture and sensitivities. (The laboratory technician should be contacted to do this straight away, rather than leaving the specimen overnight.)

After 'milking' the pus out, the tendon sheath is irrigated with copious amounts of saline, from proximal to distal (to prevent the infection tracking more proximally in the hand and wrist). This can be done using a 16 or 18G IV cannula, or a paediatric umbilical catheter.

In severe infections, it may be necessary to explore the whole digit, and excise necrotic tissue. Extension of the initial exploratory incisions is best achieved by mid-lateral rather then Bruner zig-zag incisions (these leave the tendon sheath exposed if left open in a swollen digit).

Dressings

Vaseline gauze, iodine-soaked dressing gauze, padding, plaster splint in the position of function.

Postoperative

- High elevation.
- Inspect the hand daily, and return to the operating theatre for further irrigation until the digit improves clinically. (The cannula may be left *in situ* to continue irrigation on the ward. This is difficult for the nursing staff, and painful for the patient, and is not recommended.)
- Bath hand in iodine/water solution daily.
- Start exercises to move in flexion and extension immediately by Hand Therapists.
- Ensure the hand is splinted in functional position when resting.

Bites

General principles

Bites cause infection from inoculation, and injury from mechanical trauma to soft tissue and bone.

Fragments of teeth may be embedded in wounds. Bites can cause fractures, especially if the injured part is held between both jaws as a 'hammer and anvil effect'. There may be skin loss requiring reconstruction.

Bite wounds of the upper limb should never be closed primarily.

History

Take a careful history about mechanism of injury (single versus multiple bites, jaws closed around hand, etc.) and type of animal.

Check tetanus status.

Examination

Examine wounds, check tendon and nerve function.

Investigations

- X-ray:
  - Fractures
  - Fragments of teeth
- Blood tests:
  - ↑ WCC
  - ↑ CRP

Monitor daily in severe infections, especially those requiring surgery. Falling CRP indicative of recovery.

- Microbiology:
  - Pus swabs
  - Tissue for culture

Microbiology

- *Dog bites*
  - *Streptococcus viridans*
  - *Pasteurella multocida*
  - *Bacteroides*
- *Cat bites*
  - *Pasteurella multocida*
- *Human bites*
  - *Staphylococcus aureus*
  - *Eikenella corrodens*
  - *Alpha-haemolytic streptococci*
  - *Bacteroides*

Treatment

Antibiotics

- Give tetanus toxoid booster if required.
- Start IV empirical antibiotics (take advice from local microbiologist):
  - Penicillin
  - Clindamycin
  - Metronidazole
  - Gentamycin
- Change to sensitive antibiotics when culture results available.

Surgery

- Excise wound edges.
- Explore wounds, and extend for access if necessary.
- Excise crushed or devascularized tissue.
- Send microbiology swabs/tissue for culture.
- Thorough wash with saline solution.
- Leave wounds open.
- Antiseptic dressings.
- Volar POP splint in functional position.
- Inspect wound 24–48 hours. Return to theatre if necessary. Send further microbiology swabs.
- Delayed closure/reconstruction when wounds clean/cultures negative.
- Closure only after clear microbiology culture results.

Intra-articular

General principles

- Any joint can be infected, Usually from penetrating injury but very occasionally haematogenous.
- Bacterial enzymes rapidly destroy articular cartilage, aggravated by raised intra-articular pressure.
- Intra-articular infections may be caused by any of the infective agents discussed previously.
- Gout, pseudogout can mimic infection (examine X-rays for crystal deposition; microscopy of aspirate for crystals).
- Thorns, teeth and other foreign bodies may puncture the joint capsule, inoculating the joint with infection, and the joint may then appear uninvolved.
- Prophylactic exploration may avoid subsequent joint infection, and permanent damage.

Joints should be explored when there is a penetrating injury over the joint, even if there does not appear to be a puncture wound through the extensor tendon.

Thorough lavage (arthroscopic in wrist), cannula or preferably open lavage in smaller joints.

Antibiotics, (initially best-guess then according to microbiological evidence). Splintage until symptoms settle then therapy to avoid stiffness.

Punch injury ('fight bite')

Injury from an opponent's tooth penetrates the MCP joint. Frequently missed. Develop a destructive septic arethritis within 48 hours. With the fist clenched, the 5 layers of tissue (skin, fascia, tendon, capsule, synovium) are very thin and easily breeched. When examined with MCPJ extended, the penetrating nature may be overlooked as each layer overlaps the next.

Investigation: X-rays to demonstrate tooth, fractures and bone defects.

Treatment: early recognition, thorough washout, antibiotics (augmentin) and delayed repair of the capsule and tendon.

Thorn/foreign body injury

Infection following a clear history of thorn injury should always be explored surgically. Have a low index of suspicion to do this. There is usually a tiny fragment of thorn in the wound (and sometimes joint). Progression to severe infection is usually rapid, leading to destruction of the joint surfaces.

Septic boutonnière

Delayed treatment of an infection of the PIPJ may lead to a septic boutonnière deformity. The path of least resistance for the pus is the thin dorsal capsule between the lateral bands and the central slip of the extensor mechanism. This can lead to attrition of the central slip.

After the infection has been drained, isolated attrition of the central slip can be reconstructed (📖 see p. 436). Arthroplasty or arthrodesis may be necessary following destruction of the joint surfaces, along with a Fowler's-type tenotomy of the lateral bands to correct the extension deformity of the DIPJ (📖 see p. 365).

Myxoid cyst

A degenerative myxoid cyst from the DIPJ ruptures and becomes infected, causing joint destruction. An acute infection may need surgical lavage, followed by splintage and antibiotics. Persisting pain, once sepsis has resolved, may justify surgical arthrodesis. Many will spontaneously fuse.

Gonoccoccal arthritis

Neisseria gonorrhoeae. Low-grade temperature, migrating joint pains, sometimes acute isolated purulent arthritis of one joint. Treatment: joint aspiration. Intravenous ceftriaxone until resolving then oral antibiotics for 10 days.

Osteomyelitis

- Osteomyelitis of the upper limb usually originates from an open fracture or infection of the adjacent soft tissues.
- Haematogenous spread is rare.
- Acute infections are usually bacterial, most commonly *Staphylococcus aureus*.
- There may be vascular compromise following trauma.
- Underlying peripheral vascular disease increases the risk.

Symptoms
- Pain
- Swelling
- Occasionally leakage

Investigation
- X-ray shows areas of sclerosis and periosteal reaction (may not appear for 2 or 3 weeks)
- CRP (useful in monitoring response to treatment)
- Isotope bone scan
- CT scan to show sequestrum
- MRI scan to show sequestrum and local invasion

Treatment
- Treat causative infection if still present
- Stabilize skeleton (usually external fixation)
- Usually requires 6–8 weeks of antibiotics. May need long-term central line (discuss with microbiologists).
- Excision of infected bone with reconstruction of bone (+/– soft tissues) as necessary
- Amputation may be only option in digits

Chronic infections

Bacterial

Actinomycosis

- *Actinomycosis israelii* normal flora of oral cavity.
- Usually from punch injury.
- May occur in dentists.
- Starts as abscess.
- Soft tissues become hard and indurated.
- Infection may invade bone.
- 'Yellow sulphur granules' (*Actinomycosis* organisms) from draining sinus characteristic late stage finding.
- Treatment by penicillin (erythromycin or tetracycline if allergic).

Syphyllis

- Ulcers (chancre) occur on fingertips.
- Acquired by orogenital contact.
- Often lymphadenopathy.
- Test by swab and serology.

Viral

Viral warts

- Caused by Human papilloma viruses (HPV)
- 95% common warts (*Verruca vulgaris*)
- 5% flat warts (*Verruca plana*)
- Commoner in children
- Spontaneous resolution in 50% at 1 year, 90% in 5 years.

Treatment

- Topical, usually 16% salicylic acid
- Cryotherapy
- Cauterization
- Surgical wide excision

Fungal

- Often treated by family doctors or dermatologists, so may not be familiar to hand surgeons.
- Diagnosis by cultures:
  - Nail clipping or skin scraping in cutaneous infection
  - Biopsy in subcutaneous or deep infection
- Treatment by topical or systemic antifungal drugs

Cutaneous

- Skin
  - Commonest cutaneous fungal infection is trichophytosis (*Trichophyton*) known as *tinea* or *ringworm*
  - *Candida albicans* in clenched fist syndrome
- Paronychial
  - *Candida albicans* in over 70%
- Common in those who immerse hands in water frequently
- Treatment by:
  - Keeping nails dry

- Topical antifungal agent
- (Eponychial marsupialization)

Nail (Onychomycosis)
- Known as *tinea unguium*
- *Trichophyton rubrum* commonest agent
- *Candida albicans* affects whole nail plate
- Can get secondary bacterial infection with *Pseudomonas*
- Treatment by:
  - Topical antifungal agent
  - Removal of nail plate in extensive infection
  - Oral anti-fungal drug

Subcutaneous

Spirotrichosis
- *Sporothrix schenckii*
- Seen in farmers and gardeners, but rare overall
- Ulcers with lymphadenopathy
- Need fluorescent antibody staining or special culture for diagnosis

Deep
- These are rare, and affect synovium, joints and bone.
- Infective agents:
  - *Aspergillus*
  - *Blastomyces*
  - *Coccidioides*
  - *Cryptococcus*
- Treatment by surgical excision and systemic antifungal agents

Leprosy (Hansen's disease)
- *Mycobacterium leprae*
- 224,717 cases worldwide (WHO 2007), with numbers falling due to drug treatment programmes.
- Primarily infection of nerves (plus skin lesions).
- Early recognition and treatment can provide cure.

Signs
- Anaesthesia:
  - Skin patches
  - Cutaneous nerves
  - Peripheral nerve trunks, causing regional blocks
- Thickened nerves:
  - Ulnar nerve first (and most commonly affected) nerve trunk involved in upper limb, usually at elbow
  - Median nerve, usually at wrist
  - SBRN (sensory branch) of radial nerve as it comes out from under brachioradialis in forearm
- Skin lesions:
  - Painless, poorly defined, hypopigmented patch
  - Sensibility may be reduced or normal

- Nerve compression and palsies

Diagnosis
- Mainly clinical
- Confirmed by detection of acid-fast bacilli:
  - Skin slit smears
  - Skin biopsy
  - Nerve biopsy
  - Nasal scrapings (determine whether patient infectious)

Treatment
- Elimination of *Mycobacterium leprae* by multidrug therapy
- Relief of pain
- Preservation of sensibility:
  - Steroids
  - Nerve decompression
- Prevention and correction of deformity:
  - Hand therapy
  - Reconstructive surgery
- Rehabilitation

Mycobacterium
Slow onset, so often delayed diagnosis.

Swabs often negative so tissue samples if possible. False-negative results not uncommon.

Prolonged culture necessary on Lowenstein–Jensen medium (37° for *M. tuberculosis*, 32° for *M. Marinum*).

Ziehl–Neelson staining—positive for acid-fast bacilli.

Treatment includes surgical debridement and prolonged combination chemotherapy.

Modes of presentation (in decreasing frequency)
- Cutaneous:
  - *Myobacterium marinum* in West
  - *Mycobacterium tuberculosis* in East
- Tenosynovitis:
  - *Myobacterium marinum* (50% cases)
  - *Mycobacterium kansasii*
  - *Mycobacterium avium-intracellulare*
- Arthritis:
  - Mainly *Mycobacterium tuberculosis* in wrist joint
- Osteomyelitis:
  - Approximately 0.1% of cases of TB

Tuberculosis (TB)
- Mostly *Mycobacterium tuberculosis* (rarely *Mycobacterium bovis*)
- TB is the commonest chronic infection of the hand.
- Affects synovium, so imitates rheumatoid arthritis.
- May need repeat biopsies to get diagnosis (organisms sparse)
- Treatment by chemotherapy

Atypical Mycobacteria
- *Myobacterium marinum*:

- From trauma to hand in water inhabited by fish (fishermen, fish tanks, swimming pools, sewage plant workers)
- Commonest cause of cutaneous TB in West
- 50% cases of tuberculous tenosynovitis
- Need special cold culture (32°C)
- Prolonged chemotherapy (according to microbiological advice)
- *Mycobacterium kansasii*:
  - Waterborne
  - Usually causes tenosynovitis (50% cases) or cutaneous lesions

Herpes simplex

📖 see p. 282.

Protozoa

Cutaneous Leishmaniasis

- Seen in inter-tropical and temperate regions
- Transmitted by phlebotomine sandflies (20 species)
- Bites ulcerate, and leave multiple permanent raised scars
- Treatment by topical antimony, or amphoteracin B.

AIDS

Immunodeficient patients infected by the Human Immunodeficiency Virus (HIV) may present with unusual or atypical infections (mycobacteria, fungi, viruses and parasites). The *Kaposi's sarcoma* is pathognomic, and may present in the upper limb.

Conditions mimicking infection

Occult malignancy

- ⚠ Beware of malignancy in long-standing or unusual infections (most commonly malignant melanoma).
- If there is any doubt, perform a small incisional biopsy of the nail bed for histopathology (if you send tissue scrapings, this may merely show necrosis).

Gout

Chronic gout may present as a caseating lesion in the hand. This can be confused with infection or rheumatoid arthritis. Serum urate should be checked when the diagnosis is in doubt.

Gout or pseudogout of the wrist can present like an acute septic arthritis. X-rays may show crystal deposition. Treat with arthroscopic lavage with microscopy and culture of fluid. Splintage, and analgesia.

Barber's interdigital pilonidal sinus

Pilonidal sinus is an occupational condition, usually seen in barbers cutting men's hair (women's hair is usually longer and softer!). The sharp, cut hairs pierce the webspace skin and form a sinus. Usually only one webspace is affected (most commonly the 3rd). Treatment is by excision and primary closure or secondary healing, depending on the presence of infection.

Nerves

Neuroanatomy

Innervation of the arm

Sensory

The arm has a characteristic sensory innervation.
- Dermatomes according to cervical nerve root level
- Territory of individual peripheral cutaneous nerves

Motor

The motor supply to the arm can be considered from various perspectives:
- Myotomes according to cervical nerve root level
- Muscle groups supplied by each peripheral nerve
- Cervical nerve root supply of each joint movement
- Peripheral nerve supply of each joint movement

Microanatomy of a nerve

A peripheral nerve has a typical architecture.
- **Neuron**: cell body.
  - Motor cell body in the anterior horn cell,
  - Sensory in the dorsal root ganglion.
- **Peripheral nerve**: bundles of axons with efferent and afferent fibres.
  - Convey pseudomotor and vasomotor fibres from ganglion cells in the sympathetic chain.
  - Some nerves are predominantly motor, some predominantly sensory.
  - The larger trunks are mixed, with motor and sensory axons running in separate bundles.
- **Axon**: extension of the nerve cell body.
  - Microtubular axonal transport systems both antegrade and retrograde.
  - May be myelinated or, more commonly, unmyelinated.
  - Small-diameter fibres carrying crude sensation and efferent sympathetic fibres are unmyelinated but wrapped in Schwann cell cytoplasm.
- **Action potential**: electrochemical signal.
  - Negative resting potential inside cell maintained by negatively charged protein molecules and ion pumps (−70mV; sodium out, potassium in).
  - Electrical stimulus causes depolarization to threshold (−55mV, Sodium gates open allowing sodium in and causing reversal of potential.
  - Potassium channels then open, allowing potassium out and restoring negative resting potential.
- **Nerve ending**: all axons end in peripheral branches.
  - One motor neuron supplies from 10 to 1000s muscle fibres, according to the dexterity required from the particular muscle (finer movements require smaller ratio).
  - Sensory neurons may acquire afferent signal from a single muscle spindle to a fairly large skin area; denser receptors providing greater discrimination.

- **Schwann cells**: active cells surrounding axons to produce a myelin sheath.
  - Facilitate conduction.
  - Active in nerve regeneration, producing new tubular conduit and neurotrophic factors.
- **Myelin**: surrounds all motor axons and large sensory axons (touch, pain, proprioception).
  - Multilayered lipoprotein membrane produced by Schwann cells.
  - Myelin sheath is interrupted every few millimetres, producing brief bare segments of axon (nodes of Ranvier).
  - Nerve impulses jump from node to node, increasing conduction speed considerably.
  - Ischaemia or compression depletes the myelin sheath, slowing conduction.
- **Endoneurium**: packing tissue around the axon/Schwann cell.
- **Perineurium**: surrounds groups of axons, usually with similar end function, to form a fascicle. The fascicles change composition along the length of a nerve.
- **Epineurium**: fascial layer, containing longitudinal vessels, surrounding the entire peripheral nerve.
  - Variable strength and thickness.
  - More robust where nerve glides around (e.g. ulnar nerve at elbow).
- **Neural vessels**: tiny vessels within endoneurium, link with larger longitudinal vessels within the epineurium.
  - Can be mobilized along some distance without risking ischaemia (e.g. ulnar nerve transposition).

Examination of the nerves of the upper limb

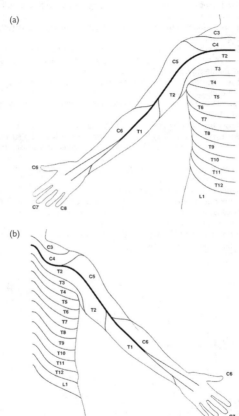

(a)

(b)

Fig. 11.1 Approximate distribution of dermatomes. (a) On the anterior aspect of the upper limb; (b) on the posterior aspect of the upper limb. Reprinted from *Aids to the Examination of the Peripheral Nervous System,* 4th edn, (2000), Elsevier, with permission from the Guarantors of Brain.

Table 11.1 Individual innervation

Muscle	Root	Nerve
Rhomboid	C4,C5	Dorsal scapular nerve
Serratus anterior	C5, C6, C7	Long thoracic nerve
Pectoralis major—sternal	C6 ,C7, C8	Lateral and medial pectoral nerves
Pectoralis major—clavicular	C5, C6	Lateral pectoral nerve
Pectoralis minor	C8	Branches to pec minor
Supraspinatus	C5, C6	Suprascapular nerve
Infraspinatus	C5, C6	Suprascapular nerve
Latissimus dorsi	C6, C7, C8	Thoracodorsal nerve
teres major	C5, C6, C7	Subscapular nerve
Deltoid	C5, C6	Axillary nerve
Biceps	C5, C6	Musculocutaneous nerve
Brachialis	C5, C6	Musculocutaneous nerve
Triceps	C5,C6, C7	Radial nerve
Brachioradialis	C5, C6	Radial nerve
ECRL	C5, C6	Radial nerve
ECRB	C5, C6	Posterior interosseous
Supinator	C6, C7	Posterior interosseous
Extensor carpi ulnaris	C7, C8	Posterior interosseous
Extensor digitorum	C7, C8	Posterior interosseous
Abductor pollicis longus	C7, C8	Posterior interosseous
Extensor pollicis longus	C7, C8	Posterior interosseous
Extensor pollicis brevis	C7, C8	Posterior interosseous
Extensor indicis proprius	C7, C8	Posterior interosseous
Pronator teres	C6, C7	Median nerve
Flexor carpi radialis	C6, C7	Median nerve
Flexor digitorum superficialis	C7, C8	Median nerve
Abductor pollicis brevis	C8, T1	Median nerve
Opponens pollicis	C8, T1	Median nerve
Lumbricals I, II	C8, T1	Median nerve
Pronator quadratus	C7, C8	Anterior interosseous
Flexor digitorum profundus II, III	C7, C8	Anterior interosseous
Flexor pollicis longus	C7, C8	Anterior interosseous
Flexor carpi ulnaris	C7, C8, T1	Ulnar nerve
Flexor digitorum profundus III, IV	C7, C8	Ulnar nerve
ADM, FDM, ODM	C8, T1	Ulnar nerve
Adductor pollicis	C8, T1	Ulnar nerve
Interossei (palmar, dorsal)	C8, T1	Ulnar nerve
Lumbricals III, IV	C8, T1	Ulnar nerve

Table 11.2 Movement of each joint

Movement	Muscle	Nerve	Root
Shoulder abduction	Deltoid Supraspinatus	Axillary Suprascapular	C5
Elbow extension	Triceps	Radial	C7
Elbow flexion	Biceps Brachialis Brachioradialis	Radial Musculocutaneous	C5
Wrist extension	ECRL ECRB	Radial Posterior interosseous	C6
Wrist flexion	FCR, PL FCU	Median Ulnar	C7 C8
Finger extension	EDC, EIP, EDM	Posterior interosseous	C7
Finger flexion	FDP, FDS	Anterior interosseous Median Ulnar	C8
Finger abduction	Adductor pollicis interossei, ADM	Ulnar	T1
Thumb abduction	Abductor pollicis brevis	Median (thenar)	T1

Clinical assessment

📖 See Chapter 1.

Tinel's test

This evokes peripheral tingling or dysaesthesia when a nerve is percussed. Useful in:

- Localizing site of compression
- Localizing neuroma-in-continuity
- Localizing end neuroma
- Monitoring progression of nerve recovery ('advancing Tinel's')
- Localizing nerve tumour (e.g. Schwannoma)

Motor testing

- wasting
- reflexes
- grip:
  - power
  - pinch
- MRC grading (📖 see Table 11.3)

Sensibility

- See Chapter 1.

Threshold tests

More sensitive and specific in compression neuropathy than density tests.

- Semmes–Weinstein monofilaments (slow-adapting fibres) provide best interobserver reliability.
- Vibrometry (pacinian corpuscles, fast-adapting fibres)

Density tests

These measure overlap and density of sensory endings. More useful in quantifying degree of functional recovery. Poor inter-observer reliability.

- Static two-point discrimination (Merkel cell, slowly adapting fibres)
- Moving two-point discrimination (Meissner corpuscles, fast-adapting fibres)

Sweating/dryness

Reduced sweating is a sign of reduced sympathetic innervation. Denervated skin will be drier. Useful in:

- Children
- Malingering
- Unconsciousness

Table 11.3 MRC grading

0	No contraction
1	A flicker of movement (this is usually palpated with the muscle contracting in its middle to outer range)
2	A small range of movement between middle and outer range with gravity eliminated
3	Some movement against gravity, but the muscle is still unlikely to contract through its full range
4	A full range of movement against gravity with some resistance
5	Normal movement and power as compared with the unaffected side

Neurophysiology tests

Two separate components
- Nerve conduction studies (NCS)
- Electromyography (EMG)

Terminology
The term 'EMG' is often used incorrectly instead of 'NCS', e.g. in carpal tunnel syndrome, EMGs rarely needed; NCS are the appropriate test.

Nerve conduction studies

Motor nerve conduction
- **Compound motor action potential (CMAP) or M-wave.** Wave form recorded from surface electrode over motor point of the muscle when the motor nerve to that muscle is stimulated with supramaximal stimulus. Measure onset latency, amplitude, area and duration.
- **Motor conduction veolocity (MCV):** stimulate motor nerve at two sites with supramaximal stimuli and calculate velocity by dividing the distance (mm) between the two sites by the difference (msec) in latency for proximal and distal sites. Affected by age and temperature.

Sensory nerve conduction
- **Sensory nerve action potential (SNAP).** Wave form recorded from a sensory nerve which has received supramaximal stimulation by surface electrode at another site along that nerve. May be recorded orthodromically (same direction as physiological nerve impulse) or antidromically (in opposite direction). Measure onset latency, amplitude, rise time. Affected by age and temperature. Not affected by pathology proximal to the dorsal root ganglion (therefore preserved in e.g. root avulsion).
- **Sensory conduction velocity (SCV).** Calculated by dividing the distance between stimulating and recording electrodes by the latency for the SNAP. Sensory conduction velocity and amplitude of SNAPs affected by age and temperature.

Mixed nerve conduction
Ulnar and median nerve trunks are stimulated distally, e.g. at wrist, and recordings made over the nerve more proximally, e.g. the elbow. Gives larger and more readily recordable potentials proximally than is achievable using SNAPs. Useful in localizing proximal nerve lesions, e.g. ulnar neuropathy at elbow.

Definitions
- **Latency:** the delay between the application of the stimulus and the first deflection on the wave form.
- **Amplitude of a SNAP** gives an estimate of the poportion of functioning sensory fibres in the nerve but is affected by distance between nerve and recording electrode. Amplitude of CMAP is an estimation of the number of muscle fibres activated by motor nerve stimulation.
- **Conduction block.** An abnormal fall in amplitude between distal and proximal stimulation suggests conduction block between the two sites.

Authorities differ in % drop required, from 20–50%, depending on circumstances.

Measures of proximal conduction

- **F wave:** when the motor nerve is stimulated supramaximally, an impulse will pass distally to produce M-wave response but also antidromically to anterior horn cell cells and excite some motor neurons to produce orthodromic nerve impulse giving a second, late and much smaller motor response (5% of M-wave). F-wave latency may sometimes help identify disease of roots, plexus and proximal nerve but is of greatest value in diagnosis of peripheral neuropathy and especially of demyelinating neuropathy, e.g. Guillain Barré, CIDP.
- **H reflex:** submaximal stimulation of afferent fibres from stretch receptors which stimulates anterior horn cell and produces a measurable motor response. Absent or delayed in radiculopathy, polyneuropathy. In upper limb, H-reflex may be attempted from the FCR muscles and unilateral absence or delay can provide evidence for C6, C7 radiculopathy.

Factors influencing conduction velocity

- **Temperature.** Conduction velocity changes by about 2 metres/sec/ degrees C but may not be strictly linear. Ideally hand temperature should be measured and maintained above 30°C.
- **Age.** Nerve conduction velocities at birth are around 50% of adult values which are reached by age 3–4. From midlife onwards there is a gradual reduction in amplitudes and velocities.

Electromyography

The measurement of the electrical activity of muscle by insertion of a needle electrode into a specific muscle. Useful in defining cause for loss of motor function.

- **Concentric needle electrode:** hollow steel cannula containing central wire which is the active elctrode with cannula as the reference. Most commonly used type of needle electrode.
- **Monopolar needle electrode:** solid steel needle acts as active electrode, a second needle or surface electrodes serves as reference.
- **Single fibre electrode:** cannula with central wire exposed at a side port behind the tip. Used to assess jitter in neuromuscular disease, e.g. myasthenia gravis.
- **Motor unit:** The anterior horn cell (motor neuron), nerve fibre and target muscle fibres (20 to 1000).
- **Motor unit potential (MUP)** A triphasic wave form generated in the muscle either by asking the subject to contract voluntarily or evoked by an artificial stimulus. The amplitude, duration and phases help distinguish between myopathy and neurogenic pathology. Large MUPs (high amplitude, long duration) with a reduced interference pattern (see below) usually indicate collateral reinnervation of previously denervated motor units but can occur in some chronic myopathies. Small highly polyphasic MUPs with reduced interference pattern occur as early sign of reinnervation by axon regeneration after nerve injury. Small short duration polyphasic motor units recruited rapidly to a full interference pattern on weak effort are typical of myopathy.

- **Insertional activity** When the needle is placed into the muscle a brief burst of muscle activity is recorded. Abnormally prolonged insertion activity may be early sign of denervation before spontaneous fibrillations appear. Loss of normal insertion activity may occur in muscle fibrosis or infarction.
- **Spontaneous activity** At rest, the muscle is quiet with no activity recordable (after the initial insertional activity). After denervation (may take 2 to 5 weeks), there are fibrillation potentials and positive sharp waves. These will disappear if reinnervation occurs successfully. Fibrillations and positive sharp waves may also occur in some myopathies.
- **Interference pattern** Motor units are recruited in increasing numbers as an increasing contractile force is needed. At full effort separate motor units become no longer separately distinguishable as so many are recruited and baseline is obsured by motor unit activity, this is termed the *interference pattern*.

In neurogenic disorders motor unit numbers are decreased and interference pattern is reduced and with large MUPs if disorder is chronic. In a muscle affected by myopathy, typically a full interference pattern of low amplitude appears on only weak effort.

Typical findings in various conditions

Normal values

Dependent on age, temperature, laboratory. The values below from our own laboratory are given as a guide. What is is normal depends on height and limb length (🕮 see Table 11.4).

Table 11.4 Normal values

Motor nerve conduction velocity, arms	>50M/sec
Motor nerve conducion velocity, legs	>40M/sec
Sensory/mixed nerve conduction, arms	>50M/sec
Sensory nerve conduction, thumb/fingers	>45M/sec
Sensory/mixed nerve conduction,legs	>40M/sec
Intersegment (e..g. elbow/ forearm) or internerve (e.g. median/ ulnar) or interside difference	<10M/sec
Distal motor latency, hand	<4.5msec
Distal motor latency, foot	<7msec
Sensory nerve action potential median (digit 2 or 3 to wrist)	<4.5msec
Sensory nerve action potential ulnar (digit 5 to wrist)	<7msec
Compound muscle action potential (baseline to negative peak) APB/ADM/FDIO	>5mV
F wave shortest latency: arm	<31msec
F wave shortest latency: leg	<57msec

Chronic compression/entrapment neuropathy

E.g. carpal tunnel syndrome, cubital tunnel syndrome

- Slow SCV and MCV and/or conduction block across site of lesion
- Sensory studies generally more sensitive than motor
- 'Inching' technique may give more precise localization
- Reduced or absent sensory and motor amplitudes to distal stimulation are evidence for axonal degeneration and a more severe lesion.
- EMG evidence for denervation if there is motor axonal degeneration

Carpal tunnel syndrome

- *Mild* sensory conduction digits 1, 2, 3 to wrist slowed and >10M/sec slower than ulnar sensory conduction digit 5 to wrist.
- *Moderate* as above plus median nerve distal motor latency > 4.5msec.
- *Severe* absent median SNAPs, delayed distal motor latency.
- *Very severe* as above plus thenar wasting, denervation in abductor pollicis brevis (APB).

Cubital tunnel syndrome

- Conduction block at elbow provides best evidence of localization
- Focal slowing (>10Msec) around elbow suggestive but not sole criterion
- Around 50% of cases show neither focal slowing nor block but diffuse slowing and reduced ulnar SNAP and CMAP amplitudes on distal stimulation below the elbow
- In mild ulnar neuropathy the ulnar mixed nerve conduction, wrist to above elbow, may be abnormal with ulnar motor nerve conduction normal.

Nerve trauma

Changes vary with time since injury and severity of lesion (neurapraxia, axonotmesis, neurotmesis).

Segmental demyelination (e.g. tourniquet paralysis, Saturday night palsy)
- conduction block across the lesion with normal conduction distally.

Axonotmesis and neurotmesis
- Immediate loss of sensory and motor conduction across the lesion
- Decline in sensory and motor amplitudes on distal stimulation to electrical inexcitability after 7 days
- Denervation on EMG after 2–5 weeks dependent on distance of muscle from the lesion
- Surviving motor units on EMG indicate at least partial nerve continuity
- In partial lesions collateral reinnervation may appear after 6–8 weeks
- Axon regeneration in axonotmesis occurs at 1–2mm per day.
- Findings in neurotmesis same as complete axonotmesis but regeneration does not occur
- Nerve conduction/EMG in first week may not differentiate neurapraxia from nerve division
- if recovery occurs, neurophysiological recovery precedes clinical

Radiculopathy

- EMG evidence of acute or chronic denervation in single myotome
- SNAPs normal (as the lesion is proximal to the sensory ganglion)
- Motor nerve conduction usually normal
- F-waves usually normal, sometimes mildly delayed

Nerve injury

Mechanism of injury

- Avulsion
- Crush
- Laceration
- Thermal
- Chemical
- Iatrogenic

Grading of injury

Seddon (1943)

- **Neurapraxia:** temporary conduction block
- **Axonotmesis:** variable damage to internal architecture, recovery variable
- **Neurotmesis:** division of nerve, no spontaneous recovery possible

Sunderland (1951)

- **First degree injury:** transient ischaemia and neurapraxia, readily reversible.
- **Second degree injury:** axonal degeneration takes place but endoneurium is preserved so able to regeneration completely once compression released.
- **Third degree injury:** endoneurium disrupted but perineurial sheaths intact. Regeneration possible but fibrosis and crossed connections limit recovery.
- **Fourth degree injury:** only epineurium intact. Nerve trunk still in continuity but internal damage severe. Recovery unlikely; injured segment should be excised and the nerve repaired or grafted.
- **Fifth degree injury:** nerve is divided and needs repair.

Sunderland's 2nd, 3rd and 4th degree injuries are all types of Seddon's axonotmesis. Recovery good in 2nd degree, poor in 4th degree.

Pathophysiology

Neurapraxia

- Note spelling!
- Reversible physiological nerve conduction block, loss of some types of sensation and muscle power, followed by spontaneous recovery after a few days or weeks.
- Caused by mechanical pressure, leading to segmental demyelination, typically seen in:
  - 'crutch palsy'
  - 'Saturday night palsy' (pressure paralysis when drunk)
  - milder tourniquet palsy
  - surgical retraction
  - displaced fractures

Axonotmesis

- More severe, typically after closed fractures and dislocations.
- Means, literally, axonal division.
- Loss of axonal conduction but endoneural and perineural structure intact.

- Pathophysiology:
  - Distal to the lesion, and for a few millimetres proximal, axons disintegrate and are resorbed by phagocytes.
  - Wallerian degeneration (physiologist, Augustus Waller 1851) takes only a few days, accompanied by marked proliferation of Schwann cells and fibroblasts lining the endoneurial tubes.
  - Denervated end organs (motor endplates and sensory receptors) gradually atrophy, and if not reinnervated within 2 years are unable to recover.
  - Within hours of nerve damage, axonal regeneration starts, probably encouraged by neurotropic factors produced by Schwann cells distal to the injury.
  - Numerous fine unmyelinated tendrils grow from the proximal stumps into endoneurial tubes.
  - These axonal processes grow at 1–2mm per day, the larger fibres slowly acquiring a new myelin sheath. Eventually they arrive at the end-organs, which enlarge and recover function.

Neurotmesis
- Means division of nerve, e.g. open wound or severe traction.
- Pathophysiology:
  - Rapid Wallerian degeneration, but the endoneurial tubes are destroyed over a variable segment and fibrosis prevents regenerating axons from entering the distal segment and regaining their target organs.
  - Rather, regenerating fibres mix with proliferating Schwann cells and fibroblasts at site of injury, forming a 'neuroma'.
- Even with surgical repair, recovery is never normal; axons will often fail to reach the distal segment. Even if they do, may fail to find suitable Schwann tubes or may not innervate the appropriate end-organ.
- If repair delayed, or regenerating distance too long, end-organs may degrade irrecoverably approximately 18 months after injury as the motor endplates fail. Regenerated fibres may remain incompletely myelinated.

Treatment of nerve injuries
Observation
- If low-energy injury or short-duration crush, then spontaneous recovery of the conduction block or segmental demyelination likely.
- Watch for advancing Tinel's and motor recovery at the expected rate.
- Usually a delay of a few weeks before advance.
- Sometimes difficult to decide whether grade 2, 3 or 4 injuries—mechanism of injury and delay in expected recovery are indications.

Early exploration
- If high-energy injury or open wound, then neurotmesis is likely.
- The earlier a divided nerve is explored and either repaired or grafted, the better the result.
- Surgical finding of a 'neuroma in continuity' is a challenge—will it recover or will it do better with a graft?
- Intra-operative nerve stimulation helpful—look for distal twitch. Ask anaesthetist not to use a paralysing agent or an axillary block.

Nerve repair
- Operating microscope, very fine instruments and micro-sutures needed. Align nerve using epineural vessels and perinerial bundles as clues.
- Loose circumferential apposition of epineurium.
- No tension in repair. No bunching of repair.
- No need for internal perineural sutures.
- Postoperative management—if repair reliable, aim for early movement to encourage gliding planes around the nerve.

Nerve grafting
- Nerves must not be repaired under tension.
- If surgery delayed then ends retract and fibrotic stumps need excision.
  - Use 11 blade or special nerve trimmer and not scissors (which crush nerve fibres).
- Interposition nerve grafting:
  - Traditionally, fill the gap using autologous nerve graft (sections of nerve are known as cables) held with a few positional micro-sutures and fibrin glue.
  - The cables undergo Wallerian degeneration too, and provide a tubular structure to guide regenerating proximal axons.
- Donor nerves:
  - sural nerve
  - lateral cutaneous nerve of forearm
  - posterior interosseous in 4th compartment just proximal to extensor retinaculum for digital nerve.

Entubulation
To avoid nerve grafting, the external environment is excluded. The space will fill with regenerating nerve. Freeze-dried muscle, silicone and vein have all been used with unclear results. Biodegradable tubes are the most recent suggestion, with promising results (in digital nerves, at least equivalent to nerve graft).

Neurotization
Transferring a proximal nerve into a different distal nerve stump. Used in brachial plexus surgery.

Neurolysis
Recovery of a nerve-in-continuity can be inhibited by circumferential fibrosis. Release of this may enhance recovery. May be a role for applying anti-adhesion gel, or membrane around the neurolysed segment.

Tendon transfers
Can be performed early (e.g. pronator teres to ECRB to provide wrist extension whilst awaiting radial nerve recovery, or late (failed recovery of an injured nerve). Discussed below.

Prognosis after nerve injury
- **Grade** Neurapraxia always recovers fully; axonotmesis may or may not; neurotmesis will not unless the nerve is repaired.
- **Level** The higher the lesion, the worse the prognosis.

- **Nerve type** Purely motor or purely sensory nerves recover better than mixed nerves, because there is less likelihood of axonal confusion.
- **Gap size** Above the critical resection length, suture is not successful.
- **Age** Children do better than adults.
- **Delay to repair** Crucial adverse factor. Best results obtained with early nerve repair. After a few months, recovery becomes progressively less likely.
- **Associated lesions** Damage to vessels, tendons and other structures makes it more difficult to obtain functional recovery even if the nerve itself recovers.
- **Surgery** Skill, experience and suitable facilities are needed to treat nerve injuries. If lacking, perform essential wound lavage and then transfer patient to specialized centre.

Postoperative rehabilitation

Splinting

- Even if splint required, design to allow some movement distally without stressing repair to allow a gliding plane to form around the repair.
- *Digital nerve:* If repair is not under tension and no gapping is present, splinting is not indicated. Where splinting is indicated 2 weeks protection is required.
- *Major nerve:* If no tension (e.g. graft, nerve tube), no splint needed. Splintage will reduce glide and have a detrimental effect (local traction due to adhesions). May need splinting to prevent or correct the secondary effects of the nerve injury to prevent contractures or enhance function (i.e. anti-claw splint, opponens splint).

Patient education

- Skin care
- Prevention of further injury
- Reassurance regarding nerve pains/regeneration symptoms experienced by the patient

Exercise advice

- Maintaining active motion of remaining innervated muscles
- Maintaining passive motion of paralysed muscles (no passive extension until 8 weeks post surgery)

Other aspects

- Assessment to establish baseline
- Scar management
- Sensory re-education
- Desensitization
- ADL advice not until 4 weeks after surgery

Compression neuropathy

Cause

Nerves can be compressed when:

- Traversing fibro-osseous tunnels
- Passing between muscle layers.
- Through traction as they cross joints (e.g. ulnar nerve behind the elbow in flexion, median nerve in front of the wrist in extension).
- Buckling (e.g. median nerve in front of the wrist in flexion).
- Distortion (e.g. median nerve after Colles' fracture, ulnar nerve after supracondylar fracture, radial nerve after humeral shaft fracture
- Space-occupying lesion (e.g. ganglion, osteophyte)
- The nerve may be more predisposed to compression if the soft tissues are swollen (rheumatoid, pregnancy)
- Direct pressure (e.g. radial nerve in Saturday-night palsy)

Certain conditions enhance the risk

- Rheumatoid—synovitis compromising the volume of the carpal tunnel
- Pregnancy
- Hypothyroidism
- Diabetes
- Cervical spondylosis—double-crush phenomenon in which the synthesis and transport of neural structural protein and transmitters is impaired by proximal compression
- Alcoholism

Pathophysiology

- Nerve compression/traction impairs epineural blood flow and axonal microtubular transport (causing numbness, paresthaesia, and muscle weakness).
- Relief of ischaemia explains the sudden improvement in dysaesthesia after surgical decompression.
- Prolonged or severe compression causes segmental demyelination, target muscle atrophy and nerve fibrosis; symptoms of numbness and weakness are therefore less likely to resolve after decompression.
- Sensory fibres affected before motor fibres.
- Even after relief of compression and regeneration, nerves may not restore efficient myelin sheath and nodes of Ranvier—permanent nerve conduction defects on electrophysiology even if symptoms much improved.

Carpal tunnel syndrome

Anatomy

The carpal tunnel runs beneath the transverse carpal ligament which transversely connects the pisiform, hamate, scaphoid and trapezium and longitudinally connects the deep fascia of the forearm (+/− palmaris longus) and the palmar fascia. It contains:

- Median nerve
- Motor branch of median nerve variable take-off:
  - extraligamentous 50%
  - subligamentous 30%
  - transligamentous 20%
- FPL, FDSx4, FDPx4

Carpal tunnel pressure

Lowest at rest with wrist in neutral (2.5mmHg). Rises to 30mmHg in full wrist flexion. In CTS pressures rise to 30mmHg and 90mmHg respectively (Phalen's test provokes this rise in pressure).

Anomalies

These can confuse clinical assessment, explaining discrepant signs (e.g. little finger numbness in carpal tunnel syndrome)

- **Martin Gruber:** Motor interconnections from median to ulnar in forearm
- **Riche-Cannieu:** Motor and sensory interconnections from median to ulnar in the hand

Causes

- Idiopathic—most common, typically female 35 to 55
- Traumatic—5% of wrist fractures, 60% of lunate dislocations
- Metabolic—pregnancy (common), renal failure and haemodialysis, hypothyroidism (rare)
- Vibration
- Repetitive use (controversial, abnormal load, repetition and posture all required; proposed by some, denied by many).
- No good evidence to link typing with CTS
- Synovitis—rheumatoid flare-ups, OA wrist
- Very rare—mucopolysaccharidosis, mucolipidosis, amyloidosis, space occupying lesion (ganglion, nerve tumour, anomalous flexor digitorum brevis)

Diagnosis

Symptoms

- Nocturnal dysaesthesia inducing a reflex to shake or hang the hand
- Reduced sensation or tingling in the median nerve distribution:
  - Holding car steering wheel produces tingling
  - Holding telephone produces tingling
- Reduced dexterity between thumb and fingers:
  - Difficulty undoing/doing up shirt buttons
  - Inability to pick up small objects (e.g. coins)
  - Inability to hold needle to sew

Signs
- Tinel's sign percussion positive:
  - sensitivity 60%, specificity 67%
- Phalen's flexion test positive within 60 seconds:
  - sensitivity 75%, specificity 47%
- Direct *nerve compression test* (pressure on nerve by examiner, tingling within 30 seconds:
  - sensitivity 87%, specificity 90%
- Threshold tests (monofilaments and vibration) do not aid diagnosis but can quantify severity.
- Density tests (2-point discrimination) not sensitive or specific. Show advanced sensory failure.

Electrophysiology
- NB NOT REQUIRED when clinical picture is typical
- Can mislead—10% of those with typical CTS, cured by surgery, have normal studies, especially younger females.
- Diagnostic findings: terminal sensory latency >3.5ms or sensory conduction velocity>0.5ms cf. other side.; motor latency >4.5ms or motor conduction velocity >1.0ms cf. other side.
- EMG shows fibrillation and positive sharp spikes in severe compression with muscle atrophy.
- Values do not return to normal even after successful decompression, so of little value for diagnosis of persistent or recurrent carpal tunnel syndrome.

Differential diagnosis
- C6 radiculopathy
- Pronator syndrome
- Proximal median nerve compression in brachial plexus

Non-operative treatment
- *Observation*: may settle, e.g. pregnancy, untreated rheumatoid flare-up.
- *Splintage*: Effective for night-only symptoms. If muscle failure, Opponens splint or C-bar (1st webspace contractures)
- *Steroid injection*: may help temporarily, rarely curative except early symptoms or demonstrable synovitis. Danger of iatrogenic nerve injury. Transient response helps confirm diagnosis.

Carpal tunnel release
Open release
Longitudinal scar in 4th ray (in line with radial border of ring finger to mid-point of distal wrist crease) over carpal tunnel avoiding damage to cutaneous nerves, divide palmar fascia, divide transverse carpal ligament towards ulnar side to avoid thenar branch and to allow subsequent cover of nerve, ensure ligament and fascia divided distally and well-proximally under direct vision, direct visual confirmation of position and integrity of motor branch. No added benefit from internal neurolysis.

Endoscopic release

One portal or two portal. Slightly quicker return to function and work, greater risk of iatrogenic nerve/tendon/superficial arterial arch damage and incomplete decompression especially early in learning curve.

Results

95% prompt cure of nocturnal dysaesthesia, regardless of age, pre-operative severity, duration of symptoms. Numbness and motor weakness may not recover, especially in older age and longer duration. Takes 4 to 6 weeks for scar to settle and good power grip to return.

Complications

* Complex regional pain syndrome (📕 see also p. 41)
* Scar pain (common for several weeks, usually settles, helped by therapy)
* Pillar pain (cause unclear, pain over bone border, may be refractive and last for several months, when it usually resolves)
* Infection.
* Recurrence: less than 1%. Re-operation only about 70% successful. NCS not helpful for diagnosis as remain abnormal even after successful decompression.

Salvage

If poor opposition due to APB failure consider opposition transfer either at time of surgery (if older than 70 or long duration of compression) or if no recovery within 6 months of release (if younger than 70 and compression of short duration). Donor options:
* FDS IV
* EIP
* Palmaris longus with fascia (Camitz):
  * can do at same time as carpal tunnel decompression through same incision, although not as strong as FDS IV or EIP.
* ADM (Huber):
  * good in children.
  * provides thenar muscle bulk.
  * can immobilize postoperatively without adverse consequences; it relies on muscle contraction and not tendon glide.

Proximal compression of the median nerve

Anatomy

The median nerve enters the forearm through the antecubital fossa. It can be compressed at:

- Ligament of Struthers (connects medial epicondyle with a supracondylar process of humerus)
- Lacertus fibrosus (fascial sheet attached to biceps tendon)
- Fibrous bands between deep and superficial origin of pronator teres
- Arched origin of FDS

Symptoms and signs

- Tingling, numbness and dysaesthesia in the median nerve distribution. No nocturnal preference (cf carpal tunnel syndrome)
- Aching in the front of the forearm, especially on activities needing rotation or grip.
- Weakness and wasting in APB and FPL, FDS, FDP II, III.
- Reduced sensation and sweating in the median nerve cutaneous distribution.
- Tinel's sign positive at site of proximal compression, over the median nerve within the antecubital fossa, negative over the carpal tunnel.
- Phalen's test negative.
- Resisted contraction may evoke symptoms:
  - FDS
  - Pronator teres
  - Biceps
- 'Monkey hand': thumb is held in adduction and extension (if complete failure of thenar muscles and anterior interosseous nerve)
- Trick movements:
  - Radial abduction using abductor pollicis longus
  - Thumb grip is performed by adductor pollicis and FPL

Investigation

- Plain X-ray (supracondylar spur)
- MRI (space-occupying lesion within antecubital fossa, ligament of Struthers, muscle oedema on T1 image)
- Nerve conduction studies and insertional EMG.
  - Usually normal.
  - Severe failure—fibrillations and sharp positive spikes in pronator quadratus and FPL.

Management

- Observation. Avoid provocative manoevres
- Surgery:
  - If space-occupying lesion or if motor signs, explore antecubital fossa and release nerve
  - If no recovery of motor function, tendon transfers.

Anterior interosseous nerve syndrome

Innervation

- Flexor digitorum profundus (index)
- Flexor pollicis longus
- Pronator quadratus

Causes of failure

- Spontaneous failure (most common). Probably due to brachial neuritis (Parsonage–Turner syndrome)
- Compartment syndrome affecting the deep flexor compartment of the forearm
- Compression by deep head of pronator teres (PT), arch of FDS, FCR, Gantzer's muscle (accessory head of FPL)
- Space-occupying lesion
- Iatrogenic
- Open fracture
- Elbow dislocation

Symptoms and signs

- Unable to bend tip of thumb and tip of index finger (cannot make an 'O' sign by apposing the tip of the thumb and index
- Unable to pronate against resistance (with the elbow fully flexed to delete pronator teres)
- APB power and bulk preserved, median nerve sensation and sweating preserved
- Recent history of viral illness or shoulder pain

Investigation

- Insertional EMG to confirm denervation
- MRI (muscle denervation, space-occupying lesion)

Management

- If spontaneous onset and no lesion on MRI, wait for several months
- If no recovery clinically or electrically, consider tendon transfer (FDS IV to FPL, side to side FDP III to FDP II).

Ulnar nerve compression at the elbow

Synonym

Cubital tunnel syndrome.

Differential diagnosis

- Thoracic outlet syndrome (TOS) which also can present with tingling over the ulnar side of the upper arm (T1) forearm and hand (C8). However, in TOS: involvement of long flexors (C8) and all small muscles of hand (T1); absent Tinel's sign over ulnar nerve; cervical rib sometimes on imaging.
- Pancoast tumour (apical lung tumour compressing T1).
- C8 and T1 radiculopathy. Have neck pain. MRI changes, delayed H-reflex, prolonged F-wave latency.

Ulnar paradox: 'High' ulnar nerve lesion at the elbow causes less clawing than 'low' ulnar nerve lesion at wrist, even though more muscles involved. FDP IV and V still intact in distal palsy, so more apparent PIP and DIP flexion from tenodesis effect.

Causes

The ulnar nerve at the elbow can be affected in many ways.
- Direct pressure
- Traction/compressionfrom elbow flexion. The volume of the cubital tunnel reduces in flexion and the nerve is stretched behind the epicondyle
- Irritation from subluxation over the medial epicondyle
- Traction from cubitus valgus
- Pressure from external swelling—synovium, osteophytes, lipoma
- Arcade of Struthers, 8cm proximal to to medial epicondyle of humerus, arching over the ulnar nerve from the medial intermuscular septum to the medial head of triceps) (cf. ligament of Struthers involved in pronator syndrome)
- Inadequate space in the cubital tunnel (the roof is formed by the cubital tunnel retinaculum or arcuate ligament of Osbourne).
- Compression between the two heads of FCU.
- Flexor-pronator aponeurosis, distal to the heads of FCU
- Aponeurosis between FDS IV and humeral head of FCU

Symptoms

- Often postural—leaning on the elbow or prolonged flexion of the elbow causes tingling in the little and ring finger promptly relieved by extending the elbow.
- More *established compression*: numbness in the little and ring finger and weakness of the hand.
- In late-middle-aged men in particular, sudden onset of symptoms with no obvious predisposing cause.

Predisposition: cubitus valgus (previous condylar fracture or radial head excision with medial collateral instability); rheumatoid elbow, osteoarthritis (swelling, osteophytes)

Physical signs

- Usually no signs in postural cubital tunnel syndrome.
- Tinel's percussion test positive over cubital tunnel (but may be positive also on other side).
- Subluxation of nerve forwards over medial epicondyle on elbow flexion (but found in about 17% of normal people).
- Reduced sensation over front and back of ulnar side of palm, little finger and half of ring finger.
- Wasting and weakness of FCU, hypothenar eminence, interosseous space, first dorsal interosseous and adductor pollicis.
- Weakness of ring and little FDP.
- Positive Froment's sign:
  - thumb tip flexes as card grasped between the pulp of thumb and radial side of 2nd metacarpal head
  - the patient uses FPL (anterior interosseous nerve) to grip as adductor pollicis and 1st dorsal interosseous muscles are not functioning to provide pinch grip.
- Clawing of little and ring fingers (due to weakness of FDM and interossei); index and middle not clawed as lumbricals preserved).
- Wartenburg's sign: abduction of little finger due to ADM inadequately opposed by 3rd palmar interosseous.
- Trick movements:
  - Some adduction/abduction by the long finger flexors and extensors
  - Adduction of the thumb by the long extensors and/or gravity
  - Lateral key grip via FPL.

Investigation

- X-rays to define osteoarthritis.
- MRI if space occupying lesion suspected (very rare).
- Nerve conduction studies: usually negative for postural symptoms. Conduction block with established compression although site not always clear.

Non-operative treatment

- Postural symptoms: advice to simply avoid flexing the elbow or leaning on the inner side of the elbow.
- Splinting the elbow at 45° extension at night.
- Cortisone injection not recommended.
- Prompt surgery must be considered if any numbness or weakness in the hand (representing axonal demyelination; long regeneration distance).
- Splinting: Anti-claw splint (MCPs in some flexion permitting IP joint extension).

Indications for surgery

- Intrusive sensory symptoms for more than 3 months despite postural care
- Motor weakness or loss of senstion/sweating
- Subluxing ulnar nerve: medial epicondylectomy or anterior transposition
- Valgus elbow, articular swelling: anterior transposition

- Compression in cubital tunnel: simple decompression is preferred as it preserves the epineural blood supply and the gliding plane of the nerve.

Technique of ulnar nerve decompression

Simple decompression

Tourniquet; incision between medial epicondyle and olecranon (not over bone prominence). Respect posterior branch of medial cutaneous nerve of forearm which runs across the field to avoid troublesome cutaneous neuroma. Identify ulnar nerve proximal to medial epicondyle. Carefully trace distally, preserving mesentery containing blood vessels. Develop space between two heads of FCU, preserving nerve branches to FCU. Follow distally for a few centimetres, and check for flexor–pronator aponeurosis and under FDS IV. Check elbow flexion–extension—if nerve stable then close. If unstable and stretches by subluxating forward over the epicondyle, then transpose. Early movement to prevent adhesions.

Anterior transposition

Mark skin just anterior to epicondyle. Release nerve more proximally. Carefully and thoroughly excise distal part of medial intermuscular septum, bipolar diathermy to leash of vessels alongside septum. Elevate nerve from bed and move anterior to epicondyle, no kinking. Suture subdermal fascia at level marked on skin to the fascia just distal to the medial epicondyle, preventing nerve from subluxing backwards. Ensure unrestricted passage. Deflate tourniquet, haemostasis, close skin. Early movement.

Submuscular transposition

This involves a greater dissection and not recommended for primary surgery. Elevate flexor-pronator origin from the medial epicondyle, pre-serving medial collateral ligament insertion. Free ulnar nerve from its bed, maintaining epineural blood vessels. Excise intermuscular septum. Lay nerve alongside median nerve. Re-attach flexor-pronator origin. Splint wrist postoperatively for 4 weeks to allow healing of muscle.

Medial epicondylectomy

Leave ulnar nerve in bed, release compression. Remove tip of medial epicondyle subperiosteally, preserving medial collateral ligament.

Percutaneous release

Technically possible, not generally recommended

Endoscopic release

Technically possible, not generally recommended

Complications
- Haematoma
- Infection
- Neuroma or CRPS from damage to medial cutaneous nerve of forearm.
- Devascularization of the ulnar nerve during anterior transposition (devastating, a reason to avoid routinely performing this procedure).

Outcome
- Dysaesthesia usually promptly relieved.
- Numbness and muscle wasting in the hand can take several months to recover as the axons regenerate along the forearm.

- After severe or prolonged compression, particularly in the elderly, the sensory receptors and motor end plates may not recover.
- As the ulnar nerve recovers, the little finger can assume an ulnar-abducted posture (Wartenburg's sign) due to unbalanced recovery of the 3rd palmar interosseous muscle and ADM.

Ulnar nerve compression at the wrist

This is much less common than cubital tunnel syndrome. It is possible (but very rare) to get compression both in the cubital tunnel and in Guyon's canal.

Anatomy of Guyon's canal

Borders
- Ulnar border: pisiform/ADM
- Floor: flexor retinaculum, ADM, FDM, ODM
- Radial border: hook of Hamate
- Roof: palmaris brevis and volar carpal ligament (continuation of distal forearm fascia)

Zones of nerve
- I   Proximal to bifurcation of nerve into deep motor and superficial sensory
- II around deep motor branch
- III around superficial sensory

Course of nerve
The ulnar nerve runs just radial and dorsal to the FCU tendon, then immediately radial to the pisiform. It gives of a branch to palmaris brevis and then bifurcates into 3 branches—sensory (which splits to the ulnar side of the little finger and the common digital nerve to the little and ring finger) and the deep motor branch. The latter dives dorsally beneath the pisohamate ligament then winds around the base of the hamate hook to supply the interosseous muscles, ending in the radial side of the hand with the adductor pollicis and first dorsal interosseous muscles.

Causes of compression
- Ganglion from pisotriquetral joint
- Osteophyte from pisotriquetral joint
- Fracture hook of Hamate
- Ulnar artery aneurysm
- Prolonged pressure (e.g. cyclist resting on handlebars)

Symptoms
Similar symptoms to cubital tunnel syndrome. Not related to position of the elbow. Ulnar artery thrombosis can be confused for Zone III sensory symptoms.

Physical signs
- Sensation preserved over back of ulnar border of hand preserved (as the dorsal sensory branch of the ulnar nerve has taken off 5 to 10cm proximal to Guyon's canal).
- FCU and FDP (IV, V) preserved.
- Ulnar paradox: clawing may be worse as FDP (IV and V) preserved, accentuating the flexion of the PIPJ and DIPJ by the tenodesis effect, especially when the MCPJs are extended by loss of lumbrical (MCPJ flexion) action
- Variable; depends on the level at which the nerve is compressed.

- Zone I sensory and motor failure
- Zone II sensation preserved, motor affected
- Zone III sensory only affected

Investigation

- Pisotriquetral X-ray (lateral in 20° supination) if pisotriquetral OA suspected
- Ultrasound: if ganglion suspected
- Arteriogram or duplex ultrasound: if ulnar artery aneurysm suspected
- MRI: if ganglion suspected and precise location needs definition
- NCS and EMG to confirm level of conduction block

Treatment

- Avoid pressure on canal (gloves, alter cycling position etc.)

Surgical

- Find nerve just proximal to pisiform
- Explore canal, trace branches of nerve distally
- Divide pisohamate ligament.
- Treat pathology as identified (e.g. excise ganglion, pisiform, hamate)

Outcome

Short distance for regeneration of nerve, usually recovers unless left for too long.

Radial nerve

This can present in various ways.
- High radial nerve
- Posterior interosseous nerve compression
- Radial tunnel syndrome
- Wartenburg's syndrome

High radial nerve

Causes
- Crutch palsy (pressure in the axilla)
- Saturday-night palsy (sleeping with arm slumped over a chair back, compressing the radial nerve in the axilla)
- Traumatic division
- Iatrogenic injury (e.g. plate fixation of proximal radius or ulna)
- Traction (e.g. Holstein–Lewis fracture = oblique fracture distal third humerus)

Symptoms and signs
- Slight weakness of elbow flexion—brachioradialis (BR)
- Marked weakness of elbow extension (triceps), wrist extension (ECRL, ECRB), finger elevation (EDC, EDM, EIP), thumb retroposition (EPL). Numb over back of thumb base. (Superficial radial nerve)
- Still able to extend thumb tip (ADM and add. poll. via extensor expansion)

Treatment
- *Pressure palsy*: observation. Recovers sometimes in hours, sometimes over several weeks or months. In event of recovery, tendon transfer.
- *Division*: urgent repair or graft.
- *With humerus fracture*::
  - Wait: if closed low-energy injury/unfit for surgery. If no recovery by 6–12 weeks, EMG. If denervation then consider exploration.
  - Operate: open injury; high-energy injury; failure if initially intact then palsy after manipulation of humerus fracture.
- *Failed* nerve repair: tendon transfer.

Posterior interosseous nerve compression

Anatomy
Radial nerve divides into posterior interosseous nerve (motor) and superficial radial nerve (sensory) at a variable distance proximal to the ECRB. Passes under the arch formed by origin of ECRB (radial tunnel).

Causes
- Brachial neuritis (Parsonage–Turner syndrome): not a compressive neuropathy in the forearm, but failure of part of the brachial plexus, often preceded by a viral illness and shoulder/neck pain.
- Spontaneous compression in radial tunnel:
  - Fibrous bands anterior to the radial head

- Fibrous proximal edge of ECRB
- Arcade of Frohse (proximal edge of supinator)
- Distal edge of supinator
- Recurrent radial leash of vessels
- External compression:
  - Lipoma
  - Synovitis from proximal radioulnar joint or radiocapitellar joint.

Symptoms and signs

- Weakness of the hand and wrist, often rapid onset. Shoulder pain or viral illness (brachial neuritis)
- Wrist extension preserved but moves radialwards (ECRL innervated proximal to the elbow, ECRB and ECU failed); no elevation of the MP joints. No retropostion (weak EPL).
- Trick movements:
  - Able to extend PIP with intrinsic muscles—ulnar nerve
  - Still able to extend thumb tip (FPB, APB, opponens pollicis and adductor pollicis via extensor expansion)
  - Finger extension using gravity to recruit passive tenodesis effect as wrist falls into flexion
  - Wrist extension by relaxing wrist flexors, gravity eliminated

Investigation

- MRI or ultrasound of antecubital fossa to exclude lesion compressing nerve
- Nerve studies—insertional EMG

Non-operative treatment

Observation: if no space-occupying lesion, and brachial neuritis possible, then observe. May take 12 months.
Splinting:
- Wrist extension support
- Dynamic extension splint (holding wrist in extension and MCPs in neutral)
- Tenodesis splint (relies on natural tenodosis action)

Surgery

- Dorsoradial approach. Cosmetically preferable. Find interval between EDC and ECU distally, develop proximally. Divide superior slip of supinator, release edge of ECRB, ligate vessels crossing nerve.
- Anterior: S incision across antecubital fossa. Identify PIN between brachialis and brachioradialis, trace distally; divide ECRB edge and superior leaf of supinator; ligate vessels crossing nerve. Leaves large scar prone to hypertrophy.
- Tendon transfer: if no recovery, then radial nerve tendon transfers.

Radial tunnel syndrome

Cause

Controversial, existence of this syndrome denied by some. Pathology not clear. The PIN, although providing only motor function, contains a high proportion of sensory nerve fibres.

Symptoms
- Pain within the wad of extensor muscles (upper outer forearm) just beyond the lateral epicondyle.
- Aggravated by use, helped by rest.
- No specific extensor weakness.
- Can be confused with (and ? coexist with) tennis elbow.

Signs
- No motor signs.
- Tenderness in the extensor wad.
- Sometimes pain reproduced by resisted wrist extension or supination or middle finger extension.

Investigation
- Nerve studies: normal, not indicated.
- Local anaesthetic beneath the extensor wad—temporary reduction in symptoms supports the diagnosis

Treatment
- *Observation:* may spontaneously recover and other treatment uncertain
- *Treat coexistent tennis elbow* (cortisone injection, stretches, clasp, ultrasound)
- *Surgery* for symptoms which persist, are intrusive and can be reasonably attributed to this syndrome. Dorsoradial surgical approach (described above). Improvement not guaranteed.

Wartenburg's syndrome
Very rare.

Cause
- Compression of superficial radial nerve as it emerges from beneath brachioradialis to reach the subcutaneous plane over the radial border of the distal forearm.
- Causes: Spontaneous; pressure from wrist watch or bangles; handcuffs; direct blow
- Differential diagnosis: de Quervain's, cross-over syndrome (peritendonitis crepitans), basal thumb arthritis

Symptoms and signs
- Tingling over back of thumb base
- Tinel's percussion test positive over nerve (more than normal side—this nerve is always very irritable)
- Reduced conduction on electrophysiology testing

Treatment
- Avoid pressure from watch or bangles
- Surgical decompression. Dorsoradial approach. Superficial radial nerve identified ands released as it emerges beneath brachioradialis tendon.

Complications
Causalgia.

Thoracic outlet syndrome

Anatomy

The thoracic outlet defines a space bordered proximally by the scalenus medius, scalenus anterior, first rib, distally by the clavicle and first rib. The brachial plexus and subclavian artery run through the interscalene space; the vein runs anterior.

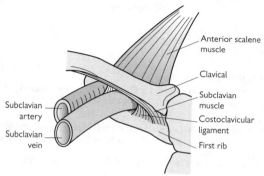

Fig. 11.2 Vascular anatomy in the costoclavicular space.

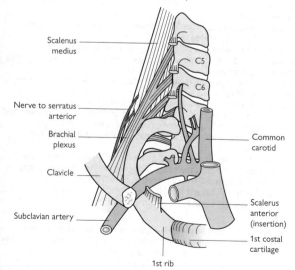

Fig. 11.3 Anatomy of the thoracic outlet.

Cause
- Poor posture, allowing the clavicle to droop down onto the neurovascular bundle as it passes through the thoracic outlet
- Scarring of scalene muscles after trauma
- Cervical rib—extra rib either bone or cartilaginous–fibrous
- Anomolous insertion of scalene muscles
- Clavicle and first rib fractures
- Pressure on plexus, e.g. apical lung tumour

Types
- Neurological
- Venous
- Arterial

Neurological compression

The T1 nerve roots, and sometimes C7 nerve roots, are compressed. The diagnosis is usually clinical and not confirmed by tests.

Symptoms
- Typically female in 30s. Discomfort and tingling in the inner side of the arm, often precipitated by elevating the hand above shoulder height or using a back pack.
- If severe compression, reduced grip and dexterity in the hand.

Examination
- In most patients there are no clear physical signs to support the diagnosis.
- Slouched posture.
- Reduced sensation over the T1 dermatome (upper inner arm) and sometimes C7 (ulnar side of arm).
- If very severe: muscle wasting of all the intrinsics, hypothenar eminence). and thenar eminence (cf. ulnar nerve compression—thenar eminence preserve)
- Clawing of all fingers (cf. ulnar nerve compression—only little finger and ring finger clawed)
- Provocative tests are non-specific and of limited value.
  - **Adson's test:** patient's neck extended and turned towards affected side while breathing in deeply; compresses interscalene space, causing paraesthesia and obliteration of the radial pulse. Poor specificity.
  - **Wright's test:** arm abducted and externally rotated; again the symptoms recur and the pulse disappears on the abnormal side causes paraesthesia and obliteration of radial pulse.
  - **Roos' test:** ask patient to hold arms high above head and then open and close fingers rapidly; symptoms reproduced on affected side.

Investigation
- Plain X-ray and thoracic outlet X-rays—cervical rib may show (but usually cartilaginous-fibrous so radiolucent). Long C7 transverse process.
- Chest X-ray to exclude apical tumour of lung
- MRI scan most sensitive for diagnosing cervical rib
- Electrophysiology tests usually of no value

Differential diagnosis
- *Ulnar nerve compression* (little finger and half of ring involved, rather than inner side of arm)
- *Tumour* at apex of lung—pancoast tumour (chest X-ray excludes)
- *Cervical spondylosis* impinging on the T1 nerve root (unusual level for cervical spondylosis; cervical spine X-rays should show; Horner's syndrome)
- *Nerve tumour* impinging on the T1 nerve root (very rare, cervical spine MRI should show)
- *Rotator cuff pain* (radiates to outer rather than inner side of arm. Shoulder signs)

Treatment
Postural: physiotherapy advice and exercises to strengthen the shoulder girdle and thus open the space. Great majority respond to therapy; surgery rarely required.

Surgery: this is reserved for symptoms which persist despite physiotherapy, are intrusive and can be clearly explained only by thoracic outlet syndrome. The approaches:
- Supraclavicular. The interscalene space is explored and compressive elements removed.
- Transaxillary. The arm is abducted. The axillary soft tissues are swept aside and the first rib is exposed. Removal of the rib creates space in the thoracic outlet. More hazardous than the suprascalene approach.
- Thoracoscopic. The first rib is excised from the underside through the chest.

Venous compression

Rare. The subclavian vein is compressed.
Presents with swelling and pain in the arm on overhead use.
Occasionally presents as axillary vein thrombosis.

Investigation
- Venogram
- Duplex ultrasound

Treatment
- Anticoagulation for axillary vein thrombosis
- Surgical release of obstruction

Arterial compression

Rare. Caused by pressure on the artery or an aneurysm
Presents with unilateral Raynaud's phenomenon (intermittent white–red–blue discolouration in the fingertips) or occasionally splinter haemorrhages (from small emboli).

Diagnosis
- Bruit in the subclavian artery
- Obliterated peripheral pulse

Investigation
- Arterigram.
- Duplex studies

Treatment
Release of compression. Grafting of aneurysm if present.

Brachial plexus injuries

Anatomy

The dorsal root ganglion is outside the verteba. Lesions proximal to this are 'preganglionic' and not repairable. Injuries distal are 'postganglionic' and may be repairable.

Clavicle arbitrarily separates plexus into supraclavicular inuries (e.g. motorcycle distraction) and infraclavicular (e.g. shoulder dislocation).

Causes of injury

Injury

Traction

- Typically motorcycle rider or fall from a height.
- Side of head and top of shoulder distracted.
- Mixed injury—avulsion of roots, traction on cords.
- When severe traction, subclavian artery also injured (intimal tear or rupture).
- Also vulnerable in shoulder dislocations (axillary nerve, radial nerve, musculocutaneous nerve).

Stab wounds

Iatrogenic

- Axillary or supraclavicular node dissection.
- Clavicular fracture.
- First rib resection.

Radiation

Brachial plexus is in the field for breast and axillary irradiation.

Clinical findings

High-energy transfer injuries, so other systemic injuries are likely (chest, pelvis, abdomen, spine).

Bruising over the top of the shoulder or side of face.

Localization of injury

Establish level of injury by systematic examination of neurological function aided by wiring diagram of plexus or functional chart. Often mixed pattern of injury (rupture and in-continuity), neurapraxia, axonotmesis and neurotmesis. Anatomical distribution may change as recovery.

Beware worsening neurology—? Haematoma.

C5 avulsion

- Loss of rhomboids and long thoracic nerve.
- Loss of shoulder abduction and external rotation (C5 deltoid and suprascapular nerve).

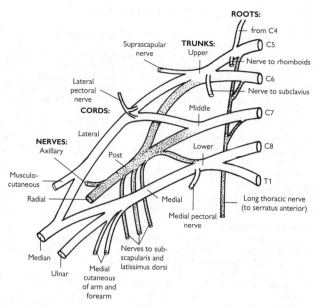

Fig. 11.4 Brachial plexus: schematic diagram of trunks, cords, and branches. Reproduced with permission from MacKinnon P and Morris J (2005). *Oxford Textbook of Functional Anatomy, Vol. 1,* 2nd edn, Oxford University Press, Oxford.

Sensory loss over lateral shoulder and upper arm

Upper trunk (C5,C6)

- *Preservation* of the dorsal scapular nerve (C5 rhomboids), long thoracic nerve (C5, 6, 7 serratus anterior)
- *Motor loss:* abduction (axillary nerve, suprascapular nerve), external rotation (suprascapular nerve) elbow flexion (C5, C6 biceps via musculocutaneous nerve, brachioradialis and brachailis via radial nerve); supination (C6 biceps via musculocutaneous nerve, supinator via radial nerve) pronation (C6 pronator teres and pronator quadratus via median nerve).
- *Sensory loss:* over lateral side of shoulder, arm, forearm and thumb

C7, C8 avulsion or lower trunk

- Rare. Weak wrist and finger flexors are weak; absent intrinsic muscle function. Clawing of all fingers.
- Sensory loss: ulnar side of arm, forearm and hand.

Pan-plexus

- Usually associated vascular injury
- Loss of: all muscle function and sensation.

Pre- or postganglionic?

Preganglionic lesions (root avulsions) are irreparable. Features include:

- Burning pain in anaesthetic hand
- Paralysis of scapular muscles
- Paralysis of diaphragm
- Horner's syndrome: ptosis, miosis (small pupil), enopthalmos and anhidrosis
- Severe vascular injury
- Associated fractures of the cervical spine
- Spinal cord dysfunction (e.g. hyperreflexia in the lower limbs).
- Positive histamine test: intradermal injection of histamine usually causes triple response in surrounding skin (central capillary dilatation, a wheal and surrounding flare). If the flare reaction persists in an anaesthetic area of skin, the lesion is proximal to the posterior root ganglion
- CT myelography or MRI, may show pseudomeningocoeles produced by root avulsion (false positive rate if dura torn without root avulsion)
- Nerve conduction studies: need careful interpretation.; if sensory conduction from anaesthetic dermatome, suggests a preganglionic lesion (i.e. the nerve distal to the ganglion is not interrupted). This test becomes reliable only after a few weeks, when Wallerian degeneration in a postganglionic lesion will have blocked nerve conduction.

Postganglionic lesions: may recover (neurapraxia or axonotmesis) or may be amenable to repair.

Management

Priorities

- Resuscitation and treatment of life-threatening injury takes priority.
- Repair vascular lesion
- Stabilize associated skeletal injuries
- Transfer to a specialist centre

Open injuries
Urgent surgical exploration indicated

High-energy injuries
- More likely to be severe (4th or 5th degree).
- Surgery technically much less difficult in first week; better results from early surgery.

Low-energy closed injuries
- More likely to be mild (1st or 2nd degree) and so will probably recover. Period of observation justified. Since there may be different degrees of injury within the plexus, some muscles may recover while others fail to do so.
- If recovery proceeds at expected rate, continue observation.
- Repairs performed after 6 months are unlikely to succeed.

Surgical strategy
- If one nerve root available (e.g. C5) graft to lateral cord which will supply elbow flexion, finger flexion and sensation over the radial side of the hand.
- If two roots available (e.g. C5, C6) these graft to lateral and posterior cords.

These procedures bypass the suprascapular nerve which is neurotized by the spinal accessory nerve.

Nerve grafting
Direct repair only possible in laceration; otherwise nerve grafting usually needed as segment of nerve affected by traction injury.

Donor sites
- Sural nerve
- Lateral cutaneous nerve of forearm
- Pedicled ulnar nerve (if T1 avulsion)

Nerve transfer
If C5 and C6 are avulsed, then spinal accessory nerve transferred to the suprascapular nerve; or two or three intercostal nerves transferred to musculocutaneous nerve.

Outcomes of nerve surgery
- Distance for regeneration means that lower trunk/medial cord injuries will not regenerate to the motor end plates before atrophy of the muscle and loss of sensory receptors.
- Shorter distance allows more favourable outcome for upper roots or trunk lesions.
- Therefore effort of repair or later reconstruction concentrated on C5 and C6 lesions, to to regain shoulder abduction, elbow flexion, wrist extension, finger flexion, and sensibility over the lateral (radial) side of the hand.
- Two or three years until final outcome apparent.

Three typical patterns
- *C5, 6(7) avulsion or rupture with C(7) 8, T1 intact:* most favourable outcome as hand function (C8, T1) preserved and muscles innervated from the upper roots can get reasonable function from early repair or later reconstruction.
- *C5, 6(7) rupture with avulsion of C7, 8, T1:* may recover shoulder and elbow movement after early repair or later reconstruction repair but hand function usually irrecoverable.
- *C5–T1 avulsion:* poor outcome. Few donor axons available to neurotize the upper levels (shoulder and elbow function) and hand function usually irrecoverable.

Late reconstruction
Best results after very early operation. If the patient is not seen until very late after injury, or if nerve surgery has failed, then reconstruction considered. Functional return is prolonged and limited but as Sterling Bunnell stated 'to someone who has nothing, a little is a lot'.

Priorities in order
- Elbow flexion
- Shoulder abduction
- Grasp (sensitivity and thumb-finger movement)

Options include:

Tendon transfer to achieve elbow flexion
- Pectoralis major (Clarke's transfer)
- Common flexor origin (Steindler transfer)
- Latissimus dorsi
- Triceps

The nerve supply to these muscles must remain intact, so they are suitable only for certain patterns of injury.

Free muscle transfer
- Aim: to regain elbow flexion and wrist extension when original muscle has irreversible failure due to prolonged denervation.
- Gracilis, rectus femoris or the contralateral latissimus dorsi can be transferred as a free flap, innervated with two or three intercostal nerves (with or without sural nerve graft extensions), or Oberlin transfer (fascicles of intact ulnar nerve to FCU).

Nerve transfer (neurotization)
- Intercostal to biceps
- Sensory intercostals to lateral cord (C6, C7)
- Contralateral C7 root extended with nerve grafts
- Spinal accessory nerves
- Vascularized ulnar nerve

Shoulder arthrodesis
Indications: unstable or painful shoulder. After failure of re-innervation of supraspinatus. No ideal position—tailored to individual patient needs.

Obstetrical brachial plexus palsy

Cause
Excessive traction on the upper limb (and brachial plexus) during childbirth.

Clinical features
Usually obvious at birth: following difficult delivery. Baby has floppy or flail arm. Further examination a day or two later will define the type of brachial plexus injury.
- *Upper root injury (Erb's palsy)*, typically overweight babies with shoulder dystocia at delivery.
- *Complete plexus injury (Klumpke's palsy)*, typically after breech delivery of smaller babies.

Erb's palsy
Iinjury of C5, C6 and (sometimes) C7. Abductors and external rotators of shoulder and supinators are paralysed. Therefore arm held to the side, internally rotated, elbow extended and forearm pronated. Sensation cannot be tested in a baby.

Klumpke's palsy
Much less common, but more severe. Complete plexus lesion. Arm flail and pale; all finger muscles are paralysed. May also be vasomotor impairment and unilateral Horner's syndrome.

Management
Specialist advice must be sought.

X-rays
To exclude fractures of shoulder or clavicle.

Observation
Over the next few months, prognosis becomes apparent:
- *Complete recovery* Many (perhaps most) upper root lesions recover spontaneously. Return of biceps activity by 3rd month is good prognostic factor. However, absence of biceps activity does not completely rule out later recovery.
- *Partial recovery* A total lesion may partially recover, leaving the infant with either an upper or a complete root syndrome which is unlikely to change.
- *No recovery* Paralysis may remain unaltered. This is more likely with complete lesions, especially in the presence of a Horner's syndrome.

Physiotherapy
While waiting for recovery, physiotherapy is applied to keep the joints mobile.

Operative treatment
If no biceps recovery by 3 months, consider surgical exploration of the brachial plexus.
- *Nerve transfer* : for root avulsion e.g. accessory to suprascapular.
- *Nerve grafts.* extraforaminal rupture.
- *Subscapularis release*: fixed internal rotation and adduction deformity.
- *Latissimus dorsi transfer, pectoralis transfer*; to restore active shoulder control
- *Derotation ostotomy of the humerus* for fixed deformities in later childhood.

Tendon transfers

Indications
- Tendon rupture
- Nerve failure
- Muscle weakness
- Muscle imbalance (head injury, cerebral palsy, cerebro-vascular accident)

Planning
- The patient should be:
  - Motivated
  - Fit for surgery
- Assess the problem.
  - Which muscles are missing?
  - Which muscles are available?
  - Does the primary cause need addressing (e.g. bone impingement from radius, STT Joint—Mannerfelt Syndrome—or ulnar head (Vaughn–Jackson).
- The donor muscle should:
  - Be expendable
  - Have adequate power
  - Have similar excursion
  - Be an agonist or synergist.
- The traversed structures should have:
  - Mobile but stable joints
  - Pain-free joints
  - Supple tissues
  - Good soft tissue cover.
- The transferred tendon should:
  - Be routed subcutaneously
  - Have a straight line of pull
  - Be capable of firm fixation
  - Avoid traversing interosseous membrane
  - Have a single function.

Surgical technique
- Minimal skin incision
- Gentle subcutaneous tunnel
- Avoid traversing interosseous membrane when possible
- Distal reattachment.
  - Intraosseous tunnel (drill hole +/– suture anchors, +/– transosseous suture)
  - Interference screw
  - Weave suture (Pulvertaft weave: through-and-back grasping sutures across crux, (not strangulating through-and-round); non-soluble suture; repeat 3 to 4 times
  - Avoid end-to-end (weak, does not allow early movement)
- Tension: slightly overtight to allow for stretch. Passive tenodesis of wrist will show posture of flexor or extensor transfer.

Rehabilitation

Experienced Hand Therapist.

Splintage

If distal insertion robust, then protect against excess passive tension but allow early excursion (e.g. EIP to EPL transfer: wrist extended to 20 degrees, thumb base retroposed to neutral, IPJ free).

Movement

Encourage synergistic combined movements (e.g. oppose tip of thumb to tip of ring after FDS opposition transfer; wrist flexion and simultaneous MCP extension after FCR to EDC transfer).

Low median nerve

At level of wrist. Thumb opposition lost, Sensation in median nerve territory and proprioception in thenar eminence lost ('blind hand')— compromises functional outcome of transfer.

Principles

Attach distal end into abductor tubercle of thumb metacarpal or overlying soft tissues. Runs obliquely across palm from region of pisiform.

Options

- *Camitz:* palmaris longus prolonged with strip of palmar fascia. Not always available if congenitally absent.
- *Huber:* abductor digiti minimi, raised on neurovascular pedicle. Restores some pulp in thenar eminence but some donor functional loss.
- *FDS (ring):* should loop around FCU or palmar fascia which alters line of pull. Synergistic transfer.
- *EIP:* remains available even with high median nerve loss or simultaneous ulnar nerve loss. Re-routed around ulnar side of wrist.

High median nerve palsy

- EIP transfer or Huber transfer (FDS and PL not available).
- FDS (III, IV) to FDP (II, III)
- BR to FPL

Radial nerve palsy

Wrist extension

- *ECRL preserved:* transfer insertion of ECRL distally into ECRB or base of 3rd/4th metacarpal to centralize wrist extension.
- *ECRL absent:* pronator teres with periosteal extension into adjacent ECRB.

MCP extension

- FCR into EDC and EPL (good synergistic transfer, as wrist flexes, fingers extend
- Or FCU into EDC (but reduces grip as ulnar deviation lost so generally avoided)
- Or FDS (III) and FDS(IV) into EDC (antagonistic)

Thumb abduction

- FCR into APL (then needs FDS transfer for MP extension)
- Re-routed PL into APL

Low ulnar nerve palsy

- *Thumb adduction:* ECRB extended with graft, through interosseous space and across to adductor tubercle. Synergistic—as wrist extends, thumb adducts.
- *Intrinsic minus posture:* FDS (II) and (IV) split into 2 each. Passed through interosseous space anterior to axis of MCPJ, attached to lateral bands (causes swan neck if too tight).
- *Claw deformity:* Bouvier manoeuvre—if clawing corrected by pushing base of proximal phalanx palmarwards, then Zancolli lasso— divide one slip of FDS at distal edge of A2 pulley, retrieve between A1 and A2, loop around palmar surface of A1 and reattach to itself, inducing some flexion at MCPJ.
- *Thumb adduction:* ECRB elongated with graft through intermetacarpal space to adductor pollicis tendon.

High ulnar nerve palsy

As above, also:
- *Finger flexion:* FDP (IV, V): side to side tenorrhaphy to FDP (II, III)

Low median nerve and low ulnar nerve

All four fingers clawed as no lumbrical or interosseous function.
- *Opposition:* EIP or FDS(IV) opposition transfer
- *Clawing:* Zancolli lasso or split FDS to intrinsic transfer
- *Thumb adduction:* ECRB plus graft to adductor pollicis tendon

High median nerve and high ulnar nerve

- *Thumb flexion:* BR or EIP to FPL
- *Finger flexion:* ECRB to FDP via interosseous membrane.
- *Clawing:* static lasso for clawing

Tendon ruptures in rheumatoid

📖 See Chapter 12.

Flexor tendon rupture

📖 See Chapters 12 and 13.

Alternatives to tendon transfer

Other options are sometimes suitable, such as:
- Arthrodesis (e.g. FPL rupture, FDP rupture)
- Primary repair
- One-stage graft
- Two-stage graft

Nerve tumours

Classification

The histology of nerve tumours is complex. They are classified as follows.

Table 11.5 Classification of nerve tumours

	Benign	Malignant (MPNST)
Nerve sheath tumour	Schwannoma (neurilemmoma)	Malignant peripheal nerve sheath tumour (malignant schwannoma, neurofibrosarcoma, nerve sheath fibrosarcoma)
	Solitary neurofibroma	Malignant neurofibroma
	Plexiform neurofibroma (NF1)	Primitive neuroectodermal tumour
	Lipoma, angioma, fibroangioma	
Neural tumour	Ganglioneuroma	Neuroblastoma, ganglioneuroblastoma
Tumour-like conditions	Intra-neural ganglion	
	Haemangioma	

Clinical features

- Swelling, in line of nerve
- Increasing size
- Percussion test may be positive
- Mobile from side to side but not in line of nerve

Investigation

Ultrasound and MRI

- Not specific for histology
- Close association with nerve confirms likely neural tumour

Biopsy

- Large trucut risks nerve damage and also false sample (i.e. false negative)
- Fine needle aspiration not reliable
- Open biopsy can spoil subsequent surgical field

Schwannoma

Clinical findings

- peak age 30 to 60, male = female,
- Usually solitary, slow-growing. Present with lump, rarely pain, almost never weakness or numbness (unless within the carpal tunnel).
- Rarely multiple (e.g. in association with bilateral VIIIth nerve tumours = NF2).

- Tinel's percussion test may be very strongly positive, but sometimes negative.
- Malignant transformation is exceedingly rare.
- *NB these tumours are sometimes mistaken pre-operatively for ganglia or lipomata, then excised with damage to the host nerve. High index of suspicion!*

Histology

- Usually solitary, arise from the nerve sheath Schwann cells. Fibrous capsule. Well-differentiated spindle-like cells, stain for S100. Arranged into compact bundles (Antoni A tissue) or disordered matrix (Antoni B tissue).

Treatment

- Meticulous enucleation under operating microscope. Nerve fibres are stretched over the lesion and in larger trunks intra-operative nerve stimulation can aid dissection.
- Separation from the host nerve without subsequent defect usually possible. Much more difficult if previous biopsy.
- A small 'feeding' attached vascular bundle may need division.

Neurofibroma

Clinical findings

- Rare.
- Usually solitary, occasionally multiple.
- May undergo malignant transformation (usually when associated with von Recklinghausen's disease).
- Painless and slow-growing. Occasionally pressure symptoms if in carpal tunnel.

Histology

Interlaced bundles of long cells. Stain less intensely than Schwannoma for S100. Cutaneous nerves more commonly involved. No capsule.

Treatment

These lesions are usually asymptomatic. There is no surgical plane so the host nerve is damaged by removal. Sudden growth or pain, especially in NF1, consider malignant change and therefore biopsy.

Neurofibromatosis

Type 1

Von Recklinghausen's, one of the most common inherited diseases (1:4000). Autosomal dominant mutation on chromosome 17, 50% occur spontaneously. Range of presentation from very minor to widespread manifestations: 'Elephant man'. Café-au-lait spots (light brown patches in axilla, trunk and inguinal area). Multiple Schwannomata.

Type 2

Much rarer. Mutation on long arm of chromosome 22. Associated with cataracts, brain tumours, spine tumours, acoustic neuroma. Peripheral nerve tumour, usually plexiform neurofibroma.

Other nerve tumours

These tumours are all very rare.
- Intra-neural ganglion (rare in hand, usually common peroneal nerve)
- Lipoma
- Angioma

Malignant PNST

Highly malignant. Associated with Neurofibromatosis Type 1. Exceedingly rare in the hand. Cardinal feature is pain, with a developing neurological deficit. Diagnosis is difficult, biopsy can damage the nerve and then spoil the surgical field for subsequent excision. Radical surgery required. Prognosis very poor. No effect from chemotherapy or radiotherapy.

Spasticity

Causes

Motor disorder with increased muscular tone due to reduced central inhibition.

- Cerebral palsy
- Head injury
- Cerebrovascular accident

Features

General

- Increased muscle tone
- Reduced or absent motor control
- May be reduced sensibility
- Exaggerated tendon reflexes.
- Incoordinated agonist–antagonist (athetoid movements)

Various deformities

General similarity with different aetiology.

- Elbow flexion
- Forearm pronation
- Wrist flexion
- Wrist ulnar deviation
- MP flexion
- Swan neck deformity
- Thumb-in-palm

Deformity due to

- Muscle hypertonia
- Secondary joint contracture
- Secondary muscle shortening
- Secondary joint deformities

Symptoms

- Reduced function
- Painful posture (forced extension of DIPs against palm, nails protruding into palm, median nerve compression)
- Poor hygiene (maceration in hand)
- Difficulties dressing
- Cosmetic
- Psychological

Functional classification

- *Good function:* independent grasp and release
- *Simple function:* grasp and release present, poor control
- *Assist function:* no grasp
- *No function*

General management

- Splintage
- Passive stretching
- Hand hygiene
- Medication:

- Diazepam
- Baclofen
- Dantrolene Sodium
- Clonidine

Neural interruption

- *Botulinum toxin.* Neurotoxin, Type A *Clostridium Botulinum.* Inhibits release of acetylcholine at the motor endplate. Injected into the target muscle belly. Latency 1 day to 2 weeks. Lasts few months. Repeated use—formation of antibodies. Can aid splintage and stretching programme. Helps distinguish between contracture and spasticity.
- *Phenol injection.* Lasts several months, e.g. motor branch of ulnar nerve for passively reversible intrinsic tightness.
- *Surgical neurectomy.* Permanent paralysis, e.g. motor branch of ulnar nerve, branches to FDS.

Surgery

Reduce muscle tone

- *Lengthen muscle unit* to reduce tone:, if voluntary control:
  - Fractional lengthening (dividing tendon within the muscle belly)
  - Z-lengthening of tendon.
- *Tenotomy* (if no voluntary control).
- *Fascial release* e.g. pronator–flexor fascia for mild, passively correctible pronation–flexion deformity

Reposition joint

- *Tendon transfer,* if volitional control still present and passively correctible deformity:
  - FCU to ECRB (to correct a reversible ulnar deviation deformity)
  - FDS to FDP (lengthens the flexors but maintains some active control, avoid if fairly good volitional control)
- *Tenodesis,* e.g. BR to APL for thumb in palm deformity, if passively correctible
- *Fusion.* Indications: if no volitional control; unable to correct passively; athetosis, extreme joint position, inability to otherwise reliably rebalance a joint; cosmesis; joint pain
- *Wrist fusion* may need proximal row carpectomy if extreme fixed flexion
- Thumb base fusion into abduction

Elbow flexion

- Less than 30°
  - Leave alone
- *Greater* deformities
  - Z-lengthen biceps
  - Elevate brachioradialis origin
  - Myotomy of brachialis
  - Anterior capsular release
  - Skin Z-plasty

Forearm pronation

- Tenotomy:
  - Pronator quadratus release
  - Pronator teres tenotomy

- Flexor pronator slide
- Transfer:
  - Re-route PT from radius to ulna
- Bone:
  - Radial de-rotation osteotomy
  - Radioulnar fusion

Wrist deformity
- Transfers
- If hypertonic rather than contracted +/− functional:
  - FCU to ECRB
  - ECU to ECRB
  - PT to ECRB
- Tenotomy (if no function):
  - FCR, FCR, PL
- Fractional lengthening (if functional and actively partially correctible)
- Bone (if soft tissue correction inadequate):
  - Proximal row carpectomy
  - Radiocarpal fusion

Thumb-in-palm
- Tenotomy:
  - Adductor pollicis
  - First dorsal interosseous
  - FPL tenotomy (no function), fractional lengthening (function)
- Tenodesis:
  - APL to brachioradialis
- Transfer:
  - EPL to EPB
- Fusion:
  - Thumb MCPJ
  - Sesamoid fusion of thumb MCPJ
  - Occasional CMCJ or IPJ
- First web space z-plasty

Finger deformity
- Flexed fingers
- Transfer (if passively correctible and volitional control):
  - FDS to FDP
  - FCU to EDC
- Tenotomy (if not):
  - FDP, FDS
- Swan neck/intrinsic+:
  - if contracted—intrinsic release
  - if functional—lateral band transfer
  - no function, passively correctible—ulnar neurectomy

Tetraplegia

- Transection of the spinal cord above C4 is fatal due to phrenic nerve failure. Below this level patients can survive. Caring for tetraplegic spinally injured patients requires a multidisciplinary approach, and surgical procedures should be performed in conjunction with specialist nursing and postoperative therapy.
- Below C5 there will be some efferent motor supply from the cord. This can be redistributed to reanimate the arm, and this can make a dramatic difference to these patients' lives, allowing independent transfer in and out of a wheelchair, and providing grip for the hand.
- The assessment is difficult, and patient selection is very important in determining a successful outcome after surgery for tetraplegia. There are many patient factors to consider (psychological adjustment to the spinal injury, age, occupation, family support).
- The neurological function changes (and sometimes improves) for up to approximately a year after the injury. Cord lesions are often of mixed or partial levels (ie not purely C5 or C6), and the levels can be different on each side (asymmetrical). They may be different from the level of the bony injury to the spine. There may be unusual patterns of sparing of motor and/or sensory function, from which the **International Classification for Surgery of the Hand in Tetraplegia** has been developed.

Table 11.6 The International Classification for Surgery of the Hand in Tetraplegia

Sensibility (O or Cu) Group	Motor Characteristics	Description Function
0	No muscle below elbow suitable for transfer	Flexion and supination of the elbow
1	BR	
2	ECRL	Extension of the wrist (weak or strong)
3	ECRB	Extension of the wrist
4	PT	Extension and pronation of the wrist
5	FCR	Flexion of the wrist
6	Finger extensors	Extrinsic extension of the fingers (partial or complete)
7	Thumb extensor	Extrinsic extension of the thumb
8	Partial digital flexors	Extrinsic flexion of the fingers (weak)
9	Lacks only intrinsics	Extrinsic flexion of the fingers
X	Exceptions	

Sensory classification

This has two categories; 'O' for ocular (visual) afferent input, and 'Cu' for cutaneous afferetnt input (they need 2PD less than 10mm to qualify as Cu).

Motor classification

The motor function is classified according to the International Classification Group (□ see Table 11.6). Muscles are only included if they are of Medical Research Council Grade 4 or above. It is important to be able to distinguish between the function of ECRL and ECRB for classification and planning of tendon transfers. The *Bean* sign can be used to test these muscles (a groove if felt between the muscle bellies of ECRL and ERCB distal to their origin from the lateral epicondyle if they are both of MRC Grade 4 or 5).

Most patients who become tetraplegic following injury are graded into the first half of the International Classification.

Medical Research Council grading of motor function (1943)

0 No contraction
1 Flicker or trace of contraction
2 Active movement with gravity eliminated
3 Active movement against gravity
4 Active movement against gravity and resistance
5 Normal

Surgical planning

- Usually at least one year after injury, when any spontaneous recvovery has ceased.
- Main goal of surgical reconstruction is to achieve a lateral pinch (key grip), taking advantage of the natural tenodesis effect of wrist extension to cause the (intact) digital flexors to flex the fingers (the paralysed extensors provide no resistance) and the thumb to adduct against the index finger.
- Restoration of triceps function using a deltoid to triceps transfer can allow transfer in an out of a wheelchair, and with it independence.

There are many variations on the tendon transfers which are available.

Surgical procedures

Elbow extension (Moberg)

- The posterior part of the deltoid is mobilized and connected to the triceps aponeurosis using a graft—autologous (fascia lata)—or artifical (Dacron).
- The elbow is splinted in extension, and then a cast brace is applied approximately 2 weeks following surgery, to gradually bring the elbow into flexion, by about 10° per week..

Key pinch restoration

- Brachioradialis to FPL
- Split FPL distal tenodesis (the New Zealand split)
- EPL tenodesis

Digital grip
- ECRL to FDP I–IV
- Use reverse cascade, with index more flexed than little finger
- May be helped by Zancolli lasso

MCPJ flexion or anti-claw procedure (Zancolli lasso)
- Transverse incision across volar MCPJ crease
- Incise flexor tendon sheath between A1 and A2 pulley, and proximal to A1 pulley
- Retrieve FDS and divide both slips distally
- Loop the FDS over the A1 pulley and suture back onto itself with correct tension (ie MCPJ flexion with wrist extended).

International Classification Group surgical options
Each group needs:
- Elbow flexion
- Elbow extension
- Wrist flexion
- Wrist extension
- Thumb flexion
- Thumb extension
- Finger flexion
- Finger extension
- Intrinsics

Group 0	all C5 ocular
Has	**Available**
Biceps	Deltoid

Group 0 solution

Needs	**Solution**
Elbow flexion	Biceps
Elbow extension	Deltoid to triceps
Wrist flexion	None
Wrist extension	None
Thumb flexion	None
Thumb extension	None
Finger flexion	None
Finger extension	None
Intrinsics	None

Group 1	Strong C5	2/3 Ocular, 1/3 O, Cu
Has		**Available to transfer**
Biceps		Deltoid
		BR

Group 1 solution

Needs	**Solution**
Elbow flexion	Biceps
Elbow extension	Deltoid to triceps
Wrist flexion	Gravity
Wrist extension	BR to ECRL
Thumb flexion	FPL tenodesis, pulley release

Thumb extension
Finger flexion
Finger extension
Intrinsics

IP stabilization
Tenodesis (natural)
Tenodesis (natural)
Tenodesis (lasso) ? thumb CMCJ fusion

Group 2   *Weak C6*

Has
Biceps
ECRL

90% O, Cu
Available to transfer
Deltoid
BR

Group 2 solution

Needs
Elbow flexion
Elbow extension
Wrist flexion
Wrist extension
Thumb flexion
Thumb extension
Finger flexion
Finger extension
Intrinsics

Solution
Biceps
Deltoid to triceps
Gravity
ECRL
FPL tenodesis
IP stabilization
Tenodesis (natural)
Tenodesis (natural)
Tenodesis (lasso) ? thumb CMCJ fusion

Group 3   *C6*

Has
Biceps
ECRB

ECRL

90% O, Cu
Available to transfer
Deltoid
BR

Group 3 solution

Needs
Elbow flexion
Elbow extension
Wrist flexion
Wrist extension
Thumb flexion
Thumb extension
Finger flexion
Finger extension
Intrinsics

Solution
Biceps
Deltoid to triceps
Gravity
ECRB
BR to FPL
IP stabilization
ECRL to FDP tenodesis (natural)
Tenodesis (natural)
Tenodesis (lasso) ? thumb CMCJ fusion

Group 4   *Strong C6*

Has
Biceps
Triceps
ECRB

All O, Cu
Available to transfer
Deltoid
BR
ECRL
PT

Group 4 solution

Needs
Elbow flexion
Elbow extension
Wrist flexion

Solution
Biceps
Triceps
Gravity

Wrist extension		ECRB
Thumb flexion		BR to FPL
Thumb extension		ECRL to EPL
Finger flexion		PT to FDP
Finger extension		ECRL to EDC
Intrinsics		Tenodesis (lasso) ? thumb CMCJ fusion

Group 5	*Weak C7*	*All O, Cu*
Has		**Available to transfer**
Biceps		Deltoid
Triceps		BR
FCR		ECRL
ECRB		PT

Group 5 solution

Needs	**Solution**
Elbow flexion	Biceps
Elbow extension	Triceps
Wrist flexion	FCR
Wrist extension	ECRB
Thumb flexion	BR to FPL
Thumb extension	ECRL to EPL
Finger flexion	PT to FDP
Finger extension	ECRL to EDC
Intrinsics	Tenodesis (lasso) ? thumb CMCJ fusion

Group 6	*C7*	*All O, Cu*
Has		**Available to transfer**
Biceps		Deltoid
Triceps		BR
FCR		ECRL
ECRB		PT
EDC		

Group 6 solution

Needs	**Solution**
Elbow flexion	Biceps
Elbow extension	Triceps
Wrist flexion	FCR
Wrist extension	ECRB
Thumb flexion	BR to FPL
Thumb extension	ECRL to EPL
Finger flexion	PT to FDP
Finger extension	EDC
Intrinsics	Tenodesis (lasso) ? thumb CMCJ fusion

Group 7	*Strong C7*	*All O, Cu*
Has		**Available to transfer**
Biceps		Deltoid
Triceps		BR
FCR		ECRL
ECRB		PT
EDC		
EPL		

Group 7 solution
Needs

Solution
Biceps
Triceps
FCR
ECRB
BR to FPL
EPL
PT to FDP
EDC
Tenodesis or transfer

Elbow flexion
Elbow extension
Wrist flexion
Wrist extension
Thumb flexion
Thumb extension
Finger flexion
Finger extension
Intrinsics

Group 8   C8
Has
Biceps
Triceps
FCR
ECRB
FPL (weak)
EPL
FDP (weak)
EDC

All O, Cu
Available to transfer
Deltoid
BR
ECRL
PT

Group 8 solution
Needs
Elbow flexion
Elbow extension
Wrist flexion
Wrist extension
Thumb flexion
Thumb extension
Finger flexion
Finger extension
Intrinsics

Solution
Biceps
Triceps
FCR
ECRB
FPL (augment)
EPL
FDP (augment)
EDC
Transfer(s)

Group 9   C8
Has
Biceps
Triceps
FCR
ECRB
FPL
EPL
FDP
EDC

All O, Cu
Available to transfer
Deltoid
BR
ECRL
PT

Group 9 solution
Needs
Elbow flexion
Elbow extension
Wrist flexion
Wrist extension

Solution
Biceps
Triceps
FCR
ECRB

Thumb flexion	FPL
Thumb extension	EPL
Finger flexion	FDP
Finger extension	EDC
Intrinsics	Transfer(s)

Painful neuroma

Complex problem, caused by disordered distal end of injured nerve, usually severed, sometimes crushed or stretched.

Clinical features

- Extreme local tenderness.
- Positive Tinel's test
- Cold intolerance
- Complex regional pain syndrome (qv)
- Features of chronic pain and psychological distress
- Disuse

Management

Non-operative

- Local over-stimulation: capsaicin cream, massage, percussion
- Transcutaneous nerve stimulation
- Medication: pregabalin, gabapentin, carbamezepine, amitryptilline
- Liaison with Pain Clinic

Surgery

- Excision and direct repair
- Excision and bridging with nerve graft, freed muscle, soluble nerve guide, vein graft
- End-to-end repair, e.g. digital nerve terminal neuroma
- Diversion of end away from likely pressure into muscle or bone tunnel, e.g.:
  - Digital nerve into base of P1 or MC neck
  - Palmar digital nerve, palmar branch of median nerve into pronator quadratus
  - Superficial radial nerve into brachioradialis
- Cryosurgery (ablation with very cold probe)

Focal dystonia

Clinical features

Spontaneous onset of cramping, uncontrolled fine movements in a complex, repetitive, dexterous task that was previously learned (writing, violin playing etc.). Co-contraction of agonist and antagonist muscles.

Treatment
- If any doubt about aetiology, neurological referral.
- Hand therapy
- *Botulinum* toxin
- Treatment often disappointing

Hyperhydrosis

Causes

Natural variation in activity of exocrine sweat glands. Can be generalized or confined to the palms. Seen as a feature of vasomotor instability in some people with CRPS (📖 see Chapter 2).

Treatment
- Hygiene
- Iontophoresis
- *Botulinum* toxin injections
- Thoracic sympathectomy

Clenched fist syndrome

Cause

Inexplicable flexion of the little, ring and middle fingers. Index and thumb usually preserved. Likely psychogenic cause. As secondary contractures occur, cannot be passively released even under anaesthesia. Differential diagnosis includes Dupuytren's, locked trigger finger, spasticity.

Treatment
- Establish diagnosis
- Usually no treatment required.
- Painful fixed flexion deformities—PIP fusion (rare)

Rheumatology

General principles

A number of rheumatological diseases affect the hand and wrist. Many are associated with considerable systemic inflammation. This produces chronic ill-health, poor wound healing and osteoporosis. Attempts to eliminate inflammation at the earliest opportunity are vital. Multiple involved joints with high acute phase markers (CRP and erythrocyte sedimentation rate [ESR] raised) and early morning stiffness are key features.

Inflammatory and rheumatological conditions affecting the wrist and hand

- Rheumatoid arthritis
- Psoriatic arthropathy
- Systemic lupus erythematosis
- Scleroderma
- Gout
- Pseudogout
- Juvenile rheumatoid arthritis

Rheumatoid arthritis

Pathology

Autoimmune disorder; females>males 3:1. Cause genetic and environmental. Inflammatory reaction in synovium causes attenuation/destruction of soft tissues and articular cartilage; systemic manifestations: pericarditis, vasculitis, pulmonary nodulosis, pulmonary fibrosis and scleritis. Many immune cell types involved: T cells, B cells and macrophage/monocytes. Damage driven by inflammatory cytokines. Particularly tumour necrosis factor α (TNFα) and interleukin-1β (IL-1β).

Diagnosis of rheumatoid arthritis

Key features are symmetrical involvement of small joints of hands and feet with early morning joint stiffness >30 minutes. Raised ESR and CRP. Positive rheumatoid factor (RF) in around 80% but not diagnostic. Anti-CCP antibodies very specific. Radiology shows erosions (X-ray, US, MRI) and synovitis (US, MRI).

Features

- Wrist and hand commonly involved in those with rheumatological conditions
- Typical deformities of wrist, fingers and thumb
- Pain and functional loss can be disabling
- Medical and surgical treatment often effective
- Systemic inflammation leads to osteoporosis, reduced lifespan and increased incidence of cardiovascular disease. Fatigue can be overwhelming.

Medical treatment

Cortisone injection

Intra-articular or peri-tendinous. Reduce inflammation, Can be repeated.

Splintage

- Support an established deformity or painful joint (e.g. wrist splint)
- Progressive correction, or at least resist deterioration (ulnar drift splint)
- Postoperative splintage, e.g. dynamic splints after MCP replacement, cast until wrist fusion united etc.

Hand Therapy

- Joint protection techniques to minimize pain, prevent deformity and maintain ROM. Principles include:
  - Respect pain
  - Use larger/stronger joints
  - Spread load over several joints
  - Minimize effort
  - Avoid tight gripping
  - Avoid deforming positions
  - Stabilize joints
- Education:
  - On condition
  - Self-management
  - Pacing

- • Prioritizing
- • Getting organized
- ADL:
  - • Identifying areas of difficulty
  - • Reinforcing joint protection techniques through alternative techniques
  - • Provision of adaptive equipment
  - • Referral to appropriate agencies for adaptations at home
- Exercise:
  - • To maintain range of motion
  - • Prevent deformities
  - • Hydrotherapy
  - • Wax

Drugs

Symptomatic

- • Analgesia
- • Anti-inflammatories

Disease-modifying

- • Corticosteroids
- • Methotrexate (first choice DMARD)
- • Sulfasalazine
- • Gold (rarely now)
- • Penicillamine (rarely now)
- • Biological therapy (TNF inhibitors, B cell inhibitors and a number of other therapies available and in development)

Principles of surgical treatment

Indications

- To delete active synovitis unresponsive to medical treatment.
- To treat pain despite non-operative measures
- To correct established deformity (e.g. swan neck, ulnar drift of MCPJ etc.)
- To improve function (e.g. tendon failure, lax thumb MCPJ etc.)
- To arrest progressive deformity (e.g. early ulnar drift treated by correction of radial tilt of wrist and soft tissue realignment of MCPJ; deletion of ulnar head prior to sequential tendon rupture)
- Cosmetic concerns (the appearance of MCP ulnar drift and severe finger deformities can be distressing).

Wrist first, MCPs second

Wrist surgery should, in general, precede MCP surgery. Examples:
- Correction of radial deviation of the wrist may improve ulnar drift of the MCPs.
- The requirements for rehabilitation of MCP realignment conflict with those for extensor tendon reconstruction at the wrist.
- Wrist fusion deletes the tenodesis effect that compliments MCP movement.

Functional demands

Some rheumatoid patients have good upper limb function, spoilt by one or two specific problems. Surgical correction of these problems (e.g. wrist fusion, thumb stabilization) can hugely improve function.

Other patients have a limb with diffuse problems; medical therapy and Hand Therapy have a greater role. However, the reduced overall function can give reliable results for procedures that in higher-demand individuals would carry uncertainty (Darrach's, elbow replacement, silicone PIP replacement etc).

Bone joint and soft tissue quality

- Bone in RhA often very osteopaenic (general effect of disease, disuse, corticosteroids). Standard fixation (e.g. wrist fusion plate) may be unreliable due to poor screw purchase.
- Wounds at greater risk of failure due to inflammatory process. Corticosteroids also impair wound healing. Methotrexate does not appear to worsen surgical outcome. TNF blockers increase surgical infection risk.
- Soft tissues often very fragile. Repair can be tenuous and unsatisfactory.
- Joints may spontaneously fuse. This can be an advantage, e.g. ease of wrist fusion with simple intramedullary rods.

Multidisciplinary practice

- Decision for surgery should involve all parties (patient, family, carers, GP, rheumatologist, Hand Therapist)
- Rheumatoid patients may have significant other musculoskeletal problems. Hand or wrist surgery may render them dependent on others (e.g. cannot use crutch after carpal tunnel release, cannot self-care after thumb surgery)
- Many procedures require specific hand therapy input—splintage, excercise, manipulation)
- Medication may need amendment prior to surgery. TNF inhibitors should be stopped temporarily for surgery. Corticosteroids should be reduced to lowest possible dose in the weeks before surgery. It appears that continuing methotrexate is does not cause problems.

Rheumatoid nodules

Subcutaneous nodules. Found over sides of PIPJ and DIPJ, ulnar border of proximal forearm and olecranon. Associated with methotrexate therapy and positive rheumatoid factor. Surgical excision if troublesome but beware high wound failure rate, recurrence and risk to digital nerves.

Rheumatoid wrist

Features in RhA

75% of RhA patients have wrist involvement. Usually bilateral. Wrist fails due to articular and bone erosion, ligamentous attenuation, tendon imbalance. Leads to pain, instability, weakness, deformity, tendon rupture.

Typical deformity

Radial deviation (contributes to ulnar drift of MCPJ); carpal supination; ulnar translocation of proximal row; palmar subluxation of carpus; volar intercalated instability, caput ulnae.

Caput ulnae

Palmar subluxation and supination of radius (rather than dorsal subluxation of ulna). Prominent ulna head and unstable DRUJ (piano-key sign). Synovitis of DRUJ. +/– tendon rupture, initially EDM then EDC, (Vaughn–Jackson syndrome) EIP usually spared; ECU subluxation.

Tendon rupture

- EDM (test by independent extension of little finger)
- EIP (test by independent extension of index finger)
- EIP (test by independent extension of index finger)
- EPL (test by independent extension of little finger); (test by elevation of thumb behind plane of hand)
- FPL (Mannerfelt lesion)
- ECRL, ECRB, FCU, FCR (rare)

Radiological findings

Erosions: base of styloid, scaphoid waist, lunotriquetral region
Spontaneous fusion of part or entire carpus common. Joint changes (📖 see classification)

Classification
Larsen

Grade	Definition	X-ray findings
0	Normal	Abnormalities not related to RhA
I	Slight abnormality	Peri-articular soft tissue swelling or osteoporosis or slight joint space narrowing
II	Definite early abnormality	Erosion and joint space narrowing
III	Medium destructive abnormality	Erosion and joint space narrowing, Bone deformation in weight-bearing joints
IV	Severe destruction	Loss of joint space
V	Mutilating abnormality	Original articular surfaces have disappeared. Gross bone deformation in the weight-bearing joints

Simmen

I	Ankylosing type
II	Osteoarthritic type
III	Disintegrating type

Wrightington

		Therapy
I	Architecture preserved	Synovectory
II	Radiocarpal and mid-carpal malalignment, minimal erosion	Soft tissue stabilization/partial fusion
III	Diffuse moderate joint erosions, early palmar subluxation	Arthroplasty or arthrodesis
IV	Severe erosion and deformity	Arthrodesis

Surgical treatment of the rheumatoid wrist

ECRL to ECU tendon transfer

Radial tilt of the wrist is a common deformity in rheumatoid. Reduces grip (which is most efficient in ulnar tilt) and predisposes to ulnar drift of MCPJ.

Indications

Consider in younger patients with correctible symptomatic deformity, minimal radiological changes.

Wrist synovectomy

Indications

Active symptomatic synovitis unresponsive to medical treatment for 6 months, minimal radiological changes; correctible deformity.

Technique

Open (limited access but other procedures can be performed concomitantly) or arthroscopic (much better access). Portals: 3–4, 6U, radial mid-carpal, ulnar mid-carpal. Shaver or preferably thermocoagulation.

Outcome

Reduces pain and improves movement in short and intermediate term.

Extensor tendon surgery

Rupture due to:
- Erosion from synovitis of DRUJ (Vaughan–Jackson syndrome)
- Erosion from infiltration of tenosynovium
- Intratendinous lesions
- Erosion from bone prominence
- Ischaemia within fibro-osseous tunnel (e.g. EPL rupture)

Examination

- EDM usually first to rupture. Test by independent elevation of little finger MCPJ with other digits flexed into palm.
- EDC (IV) and EDC (V) rupture next, then EDC (III) and finally(II). EIP unusual. Patient unable to elevate the MCPJs (beware alternative diagnosis of sagittal band rupture at MCPJ and, very rarely, PIN failure from compression by synovitis anterior to PRUJ)
  - *Sagittal band rupture*: patient cannot actively elevate proximal phalanx at MCPJ but can actively maintain extension once passively positioned.
  - *PIN palsy:* unable to elevate proximal phalanx actively and cannot maintain position of passively positioned. Tenodesis effect maintained (fingers automatically elevate if wrist passively flexed). Active wrist extension tilts int radial deviation.
- EPL ruptures independently of other extensors. Unable to elevate thumb MPJ backwards to the level of the palm (retroposition). Thumb IP extension partly preserved by intrinsic function of APB and adductor pollicis via extensor hood.

Tenosynovectomy

Dorsal midline approach. Extensor retinaculum elevated on 3/4 intercompartmental pillar. Tendon stripped of synovitis, Retinaculum split in H-fashion and half passed under tendons, half over (to protect tendons from erosion beneath yet avoid bowstringing). EPL left outside retinaculum.

Tendon rupture

- Direct repair not possible as tendons have lost substance and also retracted.
- Graft—suitable if recent rupture before muscle degraded. Donor-PL or ECRB/ECRL (if concomitant wrist fusion).
- Robust Pulvertaft weave to allow very early mobilization.

Transfer

- If EDM alone ruptured, leave but consider prophylactic ulnar head surgery before other tendons sequentially fail.
- EDC (V) and (IV): transfer EIP.
- EDC (V–III): adjacent hitch EDC (III) to EDC (II). Transfer EIP to EDC (IV), (V).
- EDC (II–V), EDM, EIP: Difficult problem, no ideal solution. Options:
  - tendon graft (if muscle still adequate);
  - FDS (III) to EDC (II,III) and FDS (IV) to EDC (IV), (V).
  - FCR prolonged with graft (synergistic transfer)

Ulnar head surgery

If tendons ruptured from DRUJ synovitis/instability then concomitant ulnar head surgery required. Options: Darrach's; matched hemi-resection; ulnar head replacement; Sauve–Kapandji.

Tendon lesions

If tendon ruptured by intratendinous nodule or synovial erosion then graft/transfer.

Radiolunate arthrodesis (Chamay)

Indications

Progressive ulnar translocation, volar subluxation or supination of carpus; relatively young patient; mid-carpal joint fairly mobile and preserved.

Technique

Dorsal incision. Denude joint surfaces. Local bone graft. Secure with memory staples or K-wires. Locking plate if good bone density. Often combined with ulnar head excision.

Outcome

Probably slows deterioration; good results for well-selected patients. Range of movement 80% normal. High patient satisfaction.

Radiocarpal fusion

See Chapter 15.

Indications

Pain, instability, deformity (e.g. non-correctible radial tilt with ulnar deviation of MCPJ), when joint-preserving procedure not suitable.

Techniques

Plate and screws: for osteoarthritic pattern, good bone stock.

Intramedullary Steinman pin. Via 3rd MC distal metaphysis (Mannerfelt technique) or via 2nd/3rd MC space (imparts some ulnar tilt useful for grip, avoids damage to metacarpal shaft or obstruction of MP replacement) Image intensification needed. If wrist spontaneously fusing in lower demand individuals then bone graft not needed. Needs prolonged plaster immobilization.

Often combined with Darrach's procedure if caput ulnae syndrome.

Wrist replacement

See Chapter 15. Patients generally prefer this to wrist fusion. Consider for lower demand patients with good bone stock. If one side fused then relatively stronger indication for replacement on the other side. Just a small arc of wrist movement greatly improves finger excursion and grip.

Ulnar head replacement

See Chapter 14. Role emerging. Preferable to Darrach's if instability a potential problem, Requires good bone stock, preserved sigmoid notch, competent dorsal DRUJ capsule and TFCC. Long-term results unknown. With soft sigmoid notch, risk of erosion.

Darrach's procedure

Indications

See Chapter 15. Caput ulnae syndrome, painful DRUJ synovitis, Vaughan–Jackson syndrome, Consider ulnar head replacement as an alternative wherever possible.

Sauve–Kapandji is an alternative (preserves buttress against ulnar translocation of carpus).

Procedure

Dorsal incision. Beware dorsal branch of ulnar nerve. Expose DRUJ capsule through floor of 5th compartment. Expose ulnar neck subperiosteally, preserving TFCC and ECU and radial cuff of DRUJ capsule. Divide neck. Remove head. Stabilize stump with strip of ECU or palmar capsule. Close dorsal capsule tightly, if fragile reinforce with retinaculum.

Concomitant procedures: radiolunate fusion, total wrist fusion, tendon reconstruction, wrist replacement.

Postoperative rehabilitation

- Sugar tong splint to maintain forearm in mid-rotation and wrist in 20° extension for up to 4 weeks
- Flexion and extension of the wrist is permitted 2 weeks after surgery
- Prevent pronation and supination for up to 6 weeks

Complications

Stump instability. Tendon rupture. Ulnar translocation of carpus. Cosmetic deformity. Stump instability is probably less important in low-demand rheumatoid patients with concomitant problems in the upper limb.

Sauve–Kapandji

Potential advantage over Darrach's
- Reduces possibility of ulnar translocation of carpus.
- Maintains contour of ulnar head (cosmetic)

Disadvantage
- Requires adequate bone stock.
- Fixation difficult in osteopaenic bone—wires or screw.
- Instability is a serious complication of this procedure although less likely in low demand rheumatoid.

Metacarpophalangeal joints

Features in RhA

Appearance

Commonly affected.

Early stages: swollen, painful, stiff.

Later stages: ulnar drift, subluxation of MCPJ, subluxation of extensor tendon ulnarwards, swan neck deformity, poor grip.

Function

Ulnar drift at index MCPJ causes reduced pinch grip. Accentuated by painful synovitis, weakened FDI, unstable thumb ulnar collateral ligament

Ulnar drift/extensor lag at ring and little MCP reduces opening span of hand. Power grip relatively well preserved especially if PIPJs still able to flex.

Radiology

- Early stages: erosions in the recess beneath the collateral ligaments. Best seen on Brewerton view (back of fingers on plate, MCPJ flexed 60°, beam from 30° ulnar).
- Later stages: erosion and destruction of head, palmar subluxation of P1, ulnar tilt of P1 on MC head.

Cause of ulnar drift

Multifactorial, progressive.

- Chronic synovitis of the metacarpophalangeal joints results in failure of the palmar plate and collateral ligaments.
- Powerful (cf extensor) flexor tendons pull proximal phalanx palmarwards, causing subluxation of the joint.
- Primary or secondary intrinsic muscle tightness pulls proximal phalanx palmarwards
- Joint erosion from synovitis causes incongruity and so loss of anatomical stability.
- Thumb pressure pushes index finger ulnarwards; weakened collateral ligaments and FDI (First Dorsal Intervenous) muscle reduces normal resistance to this force
- Radial deviation of wrist causes secondary MCPJ ulnar deviation (zig-zag mechanism)
- Ulnar drift becomes self-perpetuating with tightening of the ulnar intrinsic muscles and stretching of the radial intrinsics and radial collateral ligament
- Radial sagittal bands fail due to attenuation from joint synovitis, extensor tendon slips ulnarwards and palmarwards, further accentuating the deformity.

Classification

Nalebuff

Stage I synovial proliferation

Stage II recurrent synovitis without deformity

Stage III moderate articular failure, correctible deformity

Stage IV severe articular failure, fixed deformity

Treatment

Drugs

MCP synovitis usually responds to early and aggressive medial treatment to include the newer biological agents. The demand for surgery is now falling.

Cortisone injections

Readily administered. Suppress synovitis. Temporary.

Splintage

- Early ulnar drift may respond to splintage, worn at night:
  - To alleviate pain
  - Reduce inflammation
  - Prevent deformity
  - Promote functional independence
- Commonly used splints include:
  - Volar resting splint in position of function (worn at night)
  - Anti-claw splint for ulnar drift (worn during the day)
  - Early ulnar drift may respond to splintage, worn at night

MCP synovectomy

Indication

Failure of synovitis to respond to medical treatment (unusual), with painful joints and early changes on X-ray.

Procedure

Dorsal incision (longitudinal if one or two joints, transverse if more). Split extensor along natural cleavage. Excise synovium with scalpel and rongeurs. Close tendon securely. Early mobilization.

Rehabilitation

- Early oedema control
- Early gentle mobilization
- Maintain tendon glide, caution with vulnerable tendons

Sagittal band reconstruction and MCP realignment

Indication

Progressive but passively correctible ulnar drift of MCP and ulnar subluxation of extensor tendon with minor erosion on X-ray.

Procedure

Dorsal incision (longitudinal if one or two joints, transverse if more). Divide the attenuated sagittal band longitudinally along radial side of the extensor tendon, leaving adequate cuff for later repair. Release the tightened sagittal band along the ulnar side of the extensor tendon. Synovectomy. If joint destroyed consider silastic MP replacement. Release the tight ulnar collateral ligament from attachment to metacarpal neck. Release the attenuated radial collateral ligament from metacarpal neck, advance proximally and reattach with bone anchor or transosseous suture. Divide the tight ulnar intrinsic tendon as it runs alongside the joint. Consider attaching to the radial collateral insertion of the ulnar-adjacent digit ('crossed intrinsic transfer'). Double-breast the radial sagittal band, leave ulnar sagittal band open. If still unstable, augment with extensor tendon (split tendon longitudinally, divide radial half distally, pass under intermetacarpal ligament and reattach distally).

Rehabilitation
- Splintage:
  - Volar extension splint maintaining MCPs in extension, IPs free
  - Worn for 3–4 weeks continuously
  - Gradual weaning
- Exercise:
  - Whilst in the splint, range of motion should be maintained in all uninvolved joints
  - Weaning commenced at 3/4 weeks commencing with gentle active flexion, active extension and active assisted extension
  - Light ADL and gentle strengthening commenced at 6–8 weeks

MCP replacement
Implant choice
- *Anatomic surface replacement* (pyrocarbon, metal/polythene): for patients with well-aligned but destroyed and painful or stiff MCPJs and stable, robust soft tissues.
- *Silastic spacers:* for patients with destroyed joints and poorly aligned, tenuous soft tissues. Function as soft tissue spacers to hold the surgical soft tissue reconstruction in alignment. Slightly bend but also piston in and out of the medulla during movement.

Procedure (anatomical implants)
Incision longitudinal or transverse (for multiple replacements). Split tendon and capsule in midline. Proceed according to implant manual. Preserve collateral ligament insertion proximally and distally. Check alignment and size on image intensifier. Secure repair of dorsal capsule and extensor tendon to allow immediate mobilization.

Procedure (silastic implants)
Similar to soft tissue realignment (see above).

Rehabilitation
Differs according to implant.
- *Anatomical implants* should be mobilized early, just like a knee or hip replacement, as soft tissues are stable and the joint kinematics should be relatively normal.
- *Silastic implants:* The soft tissue reconstruction needs to be maintained as it heals despite the disordered kimematics of the hand.

Splints
- Static regime:
  - 2x splints (one with wrist in extension, MCPs flexion and IPs neutral: one with wrist in extension, MCPs and IPs in neutral)
  - Splints worn alternatively at night and for protection during the day

Exercises:
  - Splint removed during the day for hourly exercises:
  - MCP flexion with IP extension
  - MCP extension with IP flexion

- Active mass flexion
- Passive extension/flexion with active hold
- Intrinsic exercises
- Radial finger walking
- Active wrist flexion and extension
- Dynamic regime:

Splint:

- Dynamic extension splint to maintain MCPs in extension with radial pull to correct and prevent ulnar deviation
- Additional splint worn at night to maintain digits in extension and for protection
- Splints worn continuously for 4 weeks

Exercises:

- Active MCP flexion and IP extension
- Active MCP extension with IP flexion
- Active mass flexion
- Passive extension

At 4 weeks after surgery:

- Static regime:
  - Splints worn at night only
- Dynamic regime:
  - Splints worn for protection only
- Exercises:
  - MCP flexion and IP extension
  - MCP extension and IP flexion
  - Full composite flexion
  - Passive extension with active hold
  - Radial finger walking
  - Wrist flexion and extension
  - Pronation and supination
  - Light ADL commenced reinforcing joint protection techniques

At 6 weeks after surgery:

- Resistance increased

At 8 weeks after surgery

- Normal activities permitted following joint protection principles

Possible complications

- Scar tethering
- Extensor lag
- Oedema
- Ulnar deviation
- Pain
- Decreased ROM
- Decreased function (particularly if PIP ROM is poor)

Rheumatoid fingers

Many effects in rheumatoid. Some are multifactorial and codependent (e.g. arthritis of PIPJ with swan neck deformity).

Problems
- *Deformity*
  - Boutonnière
  - Swan neck
- *Tendon failure*
  - FDP rupture
  - FDS rupture
  - Mallet deformity
- *Joint failure*
  - Proximal interphalangeal joint
  - Distal interphalangeal joint

Boutonnière deformity
Cause
Synovitis or attrition causes central slip rupture as it attaches to base of middle phalanx. Unopposed flexion of the PIPJ. Lateral bands slip sideways and palmarwards, Now anterior to the axis of PIP joint rotation, aggravating the unopposed PIP flexion. The lateral bands still pass behind the axis of rotation of the DIPJ, but now relatively tighter, causing hyperextension of the DIPJ.

Classification

Type I   Mild passively correctible PIPJ (15–30°)
Type II   Moderate PIP deformity, correctible
Type III   PIP deformity not correctible

Treatment
- *Splintage:* For Type I. Splint PIP straight, DIP free (to allow excursion of lateral bands).
- *Acute rupture:* treat with static splint, holding PIP straight and DIP free, for 3 weeks. Then dynamic PIP extensions splint for further 3 weeks. Keep DIPJ moving passively and actively within the splint ('Lateral band exercises')
- See extensor tendon zone III & IV
Chronic correctible deformity: (Type I, Type II).
- If joint preserved and painless and if splintage has failed, extensor tenotomy (Eaton and Littler or Fowler) procedure: local anaesthetic, divide the extensor tendon 2/3 along the middle phalanx. Immediate mobilization. The distally conjoined lateral bands move proximally, the axilla centralizing and becoming an extensor of the PIPJ. The oblique retinacular ligament maintains extension of the DIPJ as a passive fixed constraint; (runs anterior to PIPJ axis, posterior to DIPJ axis) but the active hyperextension has been resolved by the extensor tenotomy.
- Reefing of central slip or V to Y proximal advancement, release of palmarly subluxed lateral bands. Splint as for acute rupture.
- Alternatives—various soft tissue reconstructions; none reliable.

Chronic fixed deformity: (Type III).
- soft tissue procedures unreliable. Leave alone if reasonable function or fuse PIPJ in optimal position for function. Joint replacement generally contraindicated unless good tendon balance across PIPJ (unusual).

Swan neck

Cause

Various causes in rheumatoid:
- Erosion of the PIPJ palmar plate by synovitis
- Rupture of FDS
- Intrinsic muscle tightness (spasm, ulnar drift, palmar subluxation of proximal phalanx on metacarpal head)

Classification

- *Type I* PIP joints flexible, independent of MP position (i.e. Bunnell's test negative). Due to palmar plate failure at PIPJ +/− failure of FDS
- *Type II* PIP joint flexibility dependent on MP position. Intrinsic muscle tightness. Bunnell's test: with MPJ passively extended, passive PIPJ flexion limited
- *Type III* PIPJ stiff regardless of MCP position. Due to contracture of joint
- *Type IV* Destruction of PIPJ.

Treatment

Depends on the primary cause, degree of deformity and passive correctibility.

Splintage: Figure-of-8 splint to hold the PIPJ in a few degrees of flexion. (Type I)

Palmar plate reconstruction: If passively correctible lax palmar plate is primary cause, Flexor sheath exposed in midline. A3 pulley opened at one edge. Slip of FDS exposed and divided proximally at level of mid-proximal phalanx. Attach proximal cut edge of FDS to scarified insertion of A2 pulley at about 30° PIP flexion. Temporary K-wire. Early DIP passive exercises. Early removal of wire and figure-of-8 splint (Type I).

Intrinsic muscle manipulation: Check whether intrinsics are tight (Bunnell test. Restricted passive flexion of PIPJ if MCPJ held extended). Sometimes, a swan neck deformity can be corrected by gentle manipulation then figure-of-8 splint (Type III).

Soft tissue release; dorsal capsule of PIP released, lateral bands mobilized longitudinally from central slip, lack of dorsal skin to heal by secondary intention (Type III).

Intrinsic muscle release: Dorsal incision over proximal phalanx. Either divide tendon alongside MCPJ or excise a triangle of lateral band along each side central component of extensor. Temporary K-wire across PIPJ. Early DIP passive exercises. Early removal of wire and figure-of-8 splint (Type III). Wound may need to be left open to heal by secondary intention (Type III).

Lateral band transfer: For correctible painless deformity without excessive hyperextension of PIP. Dorsal incision. Lateral bands freed from either side of central slip. One lateral band passed detached proximally, passed anterior through tunnel beneath attachment of A3 pulley and resutured to lateral band. Alternatively, keep lateral band intact and pass through a tunnel made in the lateral fascia. Figure-of-8 splint and active exercises post-operatively (Type I).

Joint Fusion: for painful PIPJ or failed soft tissue reconstruction (Type IV).

Flexor tendon synovitis

Common. Due to synovitis.

Problems
- Pain, stiffness. On examination, thickening of the flexor sheath, best felt by pinching from behind the digit (Saville's sign)
- Rupture: FDP, FDS or both
- Trigger finger
- Carpal tunnel syndrome
- Swan neck deformity.
- Attrition rupture over palmar aspect of carpus (FPL = Mannerfelt–Norman lesion)
- Rupture within flexor sheath (synovial erosion, ischaemia. Intra-tendinous lesion)

Treatment
Medical therapy

Synovitis: Cortisone injection. If fails, synovectomy

Rupture: if FDP alone then synovectomy (to protect FDS from future rupture) and fuse DIPJ If FDS alone then synovectomy but no tendon reconstruction. If both FDS and FDP then consider two-stage graft (high complication rate

Trigger finger: Cortisone injection. If fails then surgery. Do NOT release A1 pulley (can aggravate tendency to ulnar drift). Instead, synovectomy and excise one slip of FDS. 15% recurrence. May trigger in extension due to synovial thickening within the sheath.

Carpal tunnel syndrome: Cortisone injection. If fails, carpal tunnel release and flexor synovectomy.

Rheumatoid thumb

FPL rupture

Common. From synovitis within tendon sheath or from attrition rupture from front of radius or STT joint (Mannerfelt–Norman lesion) or from MPJ or IPJ. Leads to secondary hyperextension of IPJ.

Treatment

- *Leave:* if painless and tolerable function. Deterioration due to progressive hyperextension common.
- *Fusion:* Excise joint. Fix with intramedullary screw if bone stock allows. Otherwise, K-wires.
- *Two-stage graft.* Complex and only for high-demand individuals.
- *FDS (IV) transfer:* synergistic transfer.

Deformity

- **Type I (Boutonnière)**
  - Boutonnière: Most common. MCPJ synovitis attenuates EPB and displaces EPL. MCPJ then flexes and IPJ hyperextends.
  - Treatment depends on severity
  - Passively correctible—cortisone injection to MCPJ, splint. MPJ Synovectomy and extensor realignment—unreliable.
  - MCPJ fixed but IPJ passively correctible and CMCJ mobile—fuse MCPJ
  - MCPJ and IPJ fixed- fuse IPJ and either fuse or replace MCPJ
- **Type II (Boutonnière with CMCJ failure)**
  - Trapeziectomy and CMCJ stabilization, with MPJ and IPJ treated as above.
- **Type III (swan neck)**
  - CMCJ failure causes aduction contracture of the thumb base and then secondary MCPJ hyperextension.
  - Treatment depends on severity. Trapeziectomy with soft tissue reconstruction or fusion of MCPJ.
- **Type IV (gamekeeper's thumb)**
  - Synovitis attenuates ulnar collateral ligament. Pinch grip causes increasing deformity. Treat with ligament reconstruction (if bone and soft tissue quality allow) but usually MCPJ fusion.
- **Type V (swan neck with MCPJ and CMCJ preserved)**
  - Synovitis of MCPJ causes hyperextension with secondary passive flexion of IPJ. Treat with palmar plate advancement or, if soft tissues tenuous, MCP fusion.
- **Type VI (arthritis mutilans)**
  - Arthrodesis with interposition bone graft.

Scleroderma

Multi-system disorder
Diffuse scleroderma = systemic sclerosis, limited scleroderma = CREST syndrome.
CREST syndrome—Calcinosis, Raynaud's phenomenon, oEsophageal dysmotility, Sclerodactyly, Telangectasia.

Diagnosis

Features of sclerodactyly and Raynaud's syndrome along with evidence of inflammation (raised ESR) and antinuclear antibodies (ANA—particularly anti-centromere and anti-scl70). Pulmonary fibrosis and pulmonary artery hypertension may increase anaesthetic risk.

Hand involvement

- Raynaud's phenomenon
- Calcific deposits
- Fingertip ulceration
- PIP contractures +/− dorsal ulceration
- Sclerodactyly

Treatment

- Treatment is largely symptomatic although a number of immunosuppressive therapies are used (corticosteroids, penicillamine, mycophenolate mofetil). They are often ineffective. Iloprost is commonly used for severe Raynaud's.
- *Raynaud's phenomenon*: warm gloves, calcium channel blockers, ilioprost infusion. Refractory cases may respond to digital sympathectomy (stripping of the adventitia around the digital arteries in the distal palm). Botolinum toxin.
- *Contractures*: splinting; fusion (+ shortening if ulcerated)
- *Ulcers*: treat as for Raynaud's phenomenon. Occasionally amputation.
- *Calcific deposits*: excise if too troublesome (beware wound breakdown)

Psoriasis

Features

- Guttate or pustular rash
- 5% of those with psoriasis have joint involvement; 90% of which are small peripheral joints
- Nail pitting (onychodystrophy)
- Dactylitis (common cause)
- PIP and DIP erosive arthropathy ('pencil-in-cup')
- Auto-fusion of PIPJ and carpus
- Opera-glass hand
- Flexion contractures of PIPJ
- Acrolysis (spontaneous dissolution) of terminal phalanx

Diagnosis

- Rheumatoid factor negative
- HLA-B27, often positive and is a poor prognostic factor.
- Presents with features of inflammatory arthritis in one of five patterns of joint involvement:
  - DIP
  - Arthritis mutilans
  - RA-like
  - AS-like
  - Oligo-articular

Treatment

- *Medication:* similar approach to RA with methotrexate (first choice, sulfasalazine, gold (rarely). TNF inhibitors also effective.
- *Surgery:* PIP release; PIP replacement; PIP fusion; DIP fusion; interposition graft with fusion (for osteolysis/arthritis mutilans)

Dactylitis

Pain and swelling of one or more digits. Many causes.

- Psoriasis
- Sarcoidosis
- Tuberculosis
- Juvenile arthritis
- Leprosy
- Sickle cell
- Syphilis
- Osteoid osteoma

Systemic lupus erythematosus

Diagnosis

Autoimmune.

Women>men 10:1.

Antinuclear antibodies, anti-dsDNA antibodies and a number of ENAs (anti-RNP , anti-RO etc.)

Rash on cheeks (malar rash) and photosensitivity

Polyarthralgia (X-rays usually normal)

May have renal disease (glomerulonephritis) with hypertension and low albumin.

30% have associated thrombophilia (anti-phospholipid [Hughes] syndrome [APS]) with increased risk of peri-operative thrombosis.

Hand involvement

- Jaccoud's arthropathy (apparent deformity with no bone erosion on X-ray).
- Ligamentous laxity (especially ulnar drift of MCPJ) Raynaud's phenomenon, synovitis; swollen PIPJs; anterior subluxation of carpus (piano-key ulna).

Treatment

- *Medical:* broad, as many organ systems can be involved. Most commonly used are corticosteroids, hydroxychloroquine, immunosupressives (azathioprine, mycophenolate, mofetil, etc.). If APS is present then warfarin may be used. In most cases this should be converted to heparin prior to surgery rather than just stopping for a period.
- *Surgical:* soft tissue realignment of MCPJs (recurrence common); limited radiocarpal or intercarpal fusion; PIP and DIP fusion.

Juvenile rheumatoid arthritis

Features

Girls>boys.
Resolve entirely in about 25%, Significant consequences in 25% and mild consequences in about 50%.

Classification

- *Stills (25%):* systemic problems (rash, organomegaly, fever, muscle pain). Joint involvement.
- *Polyarticular (30%):* symmetrical large joint arthritis. Often preceded by dactylitis. Rheumatoid factor positive or negative. Antinuclear antibodies sometimes present.
- *Pauciarticular (45%):* asymmetric large joint arthropathy, 4 or fewer involved. Associated with iridocyclitis in females (slit lamp examination essential). In boys associated with HLA-B27 and spondylitis.

Treatment

Medical: similar approach to RA with adjustment of drug dose as needed. Symptomatic control with analgesia and anti-inflammatories and disease control with disease-modifying drugs such as methotrexate and sulphasalazine. Will resolve or greatly improve in most. Treat iridocyclitis to avoid blindness.

Hand Therapy: to maintain function, splintage in functional position (may auto-fuse).

Surgical: occasionally required. Fusion in functional position for painful or deformed joints—delay if possible until skeletal maturity.

Generalized ligamentous laxity

Causes

Benign joint hypermobility syndrome (common, end of normal spectrum)
Ehlers–Danlos
Other rare connective tissue disorders

Grading

Table 12.1 The 9-point Beighton scoring system for joint hypermobility scale.

The ability to		R	L
(1)	Passively dorsiflex the 5th metacarpophalangeal joint to $\geq 90°$	1	1
(2)	Oppose the thumb to the volar aspect of the ipsilateral forearm	1	1
(3)	Hyperextend the elbow to $\geq 10°$	1	1
(4)	Hyperextend the knee to $\geq 10°$	1	1
(5)	Place hands flat on the floor without bending the knees	1	
Maximum total			9

One point may be gained for each side for manoeuvres 1–4 so that the hypermobility score will have a maximum of 9 points if all are positive.
Reproduced from Grahame R et al. (2007) *J Rheumatology*, **27**(7), 1777–9, with permission.

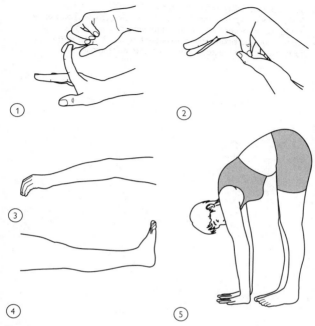

Fig. 12.1 Manoeuvres used in the Beighton scoring system for joint hypermobility.

Hand involvement
- Mid-carpal instability
- Thumb CMCJ and MCPJ instability
- Swan neck deformity
- Carpal supination
- DRUJ instability
- Rotatory instability of scaphoid

Treatment
- Adapt
- Splintage
- Surgery: soft tissue reconstructions tend to fail.
- *Thumb CMCJ*: FCR stabilization (half of FCR through drill hole across base of first metacarpal, returned around front of metacarpal base to attach to residual FCR). If fails than CMCJ fusion,
- *Thumb MCP*: soft tissue reconstruction likely to fail; fusion reliable with minimal effect on function.

- *Mid-carpal instability:* soft tissue reconstruction likely to fail. Arthroscopic capsular shrinkage with diathermy shows good early results. Four-corner fusion reduces movement significantly.
- *Carpal supination:* consider radiolunate fusion but other intercarpal laxity may not be treated or may become more apparent.

Diabetes and the hand

Diabetes can affect the hand in many ways; 40% of diabetics have hand problems, especially Type I and long duration. Abnormal glycosylation of collagen affects various tissues in the hand, explaining some of the effects.
- Type I: failed secretion of insulin, often early onset
- Type II: failed action of onset, usually later onset.

Trigger finger
- Far more common in diabetes
- Abnormal glycosylation of collagen probably affects the A1 pulley
- Injections less successful
- Release under local anaesthetic if does not respond to injection or time

Carpal tunnel syndrome
- More common in diabetes (40% increased risk). Alteration to the coactive tissue of the carpal tunnel; the diabetic neuropathic nerve is more susceptible to compression.
- May be confused with diabetic median mononeuropathy or diabetic diffuse peripheral neuropathy (often coexist).

Infection
- More prone to infection due to impaired immunity, reduced perfusion.
- Infection will destabilize diabetic control.

Wound healing
- Less likely to heal if poorly perfused, compounded by infection.

Dupuytren's disease
- Common in diabetics (20–30%)
- Tends to be mild and diffuse (palmar plaques) rather than digital contracture.
- Patients may have stiff joints and stiff tissues (diabetic cheiropathy) as well as a higher risk of complications. Therefore surgery may not be as reliable.

Peripheral vascular disease
- Microangiopathic (end capillaries, epineural vessels) and macroangiopathic (atherosclerosis)
- More common in diabetes
- Digital ischemia
- Infections
- Higher risk in surgery (wound healing, infection)

Diabetic cheiropathy
Aching and stiffness of the hand, diffuse waxy thickening, PIP contractures, nail changes. Compounded by stenosing tenovaginosis (trigger digit), plaques of Dupuytren's, neuropathy.
   Splinting and stretching limited value. No role for surgery.

Tendons

Anatomy and physiology

- Tendons consist of dense connective tissue which transmits muscle force to the skeleton.
- They comprise collagen fibrils (85% Type I collagen), arranged in parallel rows, which enable the tendons to withstand high tensile forces.
- Matrix of proteoglycans around the fibril. Few fibroblasts.
- The collagen fibrils are organized into **fascicles** surrounded by **endotenon**, which permits gliding between fibrils. A fine fibrous layer, the **epitenon**, covers the outer surface of the tendon which allows gliding beneath the sheath.
- Insertion into bone blends from tendon–fibrocartilage–ossifying fibrocartilage–bone.

Blood supply of tendons

A delicate balance exists between 2 nutritional sources:
- Blood supply
- Synovial diffusion

Blood supply to flexor tendons
- Vessels entering through the musculotendinous junction.
- Vessels entering the bone insertions of the tendon.
- Vessels enter the tendon at certain points through a mesotendon containing vinculae.

Blood supply to extensor tendons
- The extensor tendons are enclosed in sheath only where they travel through the extensor retinaculum, and are, for the most part, extra-synovial.
- Outside the sheaths the tendons are coated with a richly vascularized paratenon.

Synovial diffusion
- Nutrients and metabolites diffuse through the synovial fluid to and from the tendon.
- The flexor pulleys prevent bowstringing and provide a firm opposing surface to the avascular volar aspect of the tendon—this allows for contact lubrication and pumping of nutrients into the interstitium.

Tendon healing

Tendon healing

- After injury both the tendon itself (*intrinsic*) and all surrounding tissues (*extrinsic*) are involved in the healing process. There is no consensus about which process is more dominant.
- In non-stressed, immobilized tendons, extrinsic healing dominates; the proliferative phase is prolonged, and the strength of the repair is diminished.
- Mobilized, stressed repairs stimulate intrinsic healing; they develop fewer adhesions, achieve better excursion, and achieve earlier and greater strength of the repair.
- Tendons require long periods of time to regain their normal tensile strength following injury.

Phases of tendon healing

Phase 1—inflammatory phase

- Starts immediately after injury
- Repaired tendon undergoes proliferation of the cells on the outer edge of the tendon bundles during the 1st 4 days.
- By day 7 these cells begin to migrate into the substance of the tendon.
- Tensile strength of the repaired tendon diminishes in the 1st 2 weeks after injury due to softening of the tendon ends.
- Little collagen is laid down during this phase—thus end-to-end repairs are only held together by the strength of the suture.

Phase 2—fibroplasia

- By day 7 collagen synthesis is proceeding—initially the collagen fibres and the fibroblasts are orientated perpendicular to the long axis of the tendon—by day 10 the new collagen fibres begin to align parallel to the old longitudinal collagen bundles of the tendon stumps.
- Scar formation is rapid.
- From day 5–21 tensile strength increases as the collagen matures.

Phase 3—scar maturation.

- Collagen continues to *remodel* and increase its *tensile strength* for 3–4 months
- Increased repair strength allows application of greater force and stress to the repaired tendon.
- Scar remodelling can be characterized by a balance between collagen production and collagen lysis.

Effects of movement on tendon healing

- Early mobilization and stress is beneficial.
- Controlled passive mobilization during the first few weeks of healing stimulates an intrinsic healing response, which improves tendon glide and strength.
- A mobilized tendon is twice as strong as an immobilized tendon at 3 weeks.
- Immobilized tendons have even less tensile strength during the inflammatory phase of repair.

Control of adhesions

- Few adhesions would occur if tendons only healed intrinsically.
- Healing occurs en bloc, without differentiation into pre-injury tissue planes.
- Greater tissue damage causes a greater likelihood of adhesions, with subsequent restriction of tendon glide.
- If a tendon becomes ischaemic, fibrovascular tissue around the site of injury increases.
- Weak healing is needed between tendon and surrounding tissues to limit fixed adhesions.
- The aim when treating adhesions is not to break them—but instead to gradually lengthen the adhesion to allow a greater glide.

Factors affecting tendon healing

- Mechanism of injury:
  - Energy of injury
  - Distribution of energy within tendon
- Contamination
- Rehabilitation
- Anatomical location:
  - Zone of injury
- Age
- Tobacco smoking
- Nutritional status
- Systemic morbidity:
  - Diabetes
  - Inflammatory arthritis
  - Anaemia
  - Immunosuppressive drugs
  - Chronic illness
  - Digital ischaemia
- Tensile strength of repaired tendons:
  - Type and tensile strength of suture material
  - Type of repair
  - Single/multiple strand
  - Surface area grasped by suture
  - Quality of surgical technique
- Size of tendon
- Delay to repair
- Associated vessel and nerve damage

Flexor tendon anatomy

Anatomy

Long flexor (extrinsic) muscles

There are 6 long flexor muscles on the anterior aspect of the forearm:

Wrist flexors:
- Flexor carpi radialis
- Flexor carpi ulnaris
- Palmaris longus

Digital flexors:
- Flexor digitorum superficialis
- Flexor digitorum profundus
- Flexor pollicis longus

Short (intrinsic) flexor muscles
- Lumbrical muscles (flex MCPJs)

Superficial tendons

1. Flexor carpi ulnaris
Origin: humeral head: from the medial epicondyle of the humerus by the common tendon; ulnar head: arises from the medial margin of the olecranon of the ulna and the upper 2/3rds of the dorsal border of the ulna by an aponeurosis
Insertion: into the pisiform and via ligaments into the hamate and 5th metacarpal
Action: flexion and ulnar deviation of the wrist
Nerve:: ulnar nerve

2. Flexor carpi radialis
Origin: medial epicondyle of the humerus
Insertion: anterior side of the base of the 2nd metacarpal
Action: flexion and radial deviation of the wrist
Nerve: median nerve

3. Palmaris longus
Origin: medial epicondyle of the humerus
Insertion: palmar aponeurosis
Action: weak wrist flexion
Nerve: median nerve

Intermediate tendons

4. Flexor digitorum superficialis
Origin: humeral head: medial epicondyle of the humerus, medial margin of the coronoid process of the ulna; radial head: anterior surface of shaft of radius
Insertion: each tendon divides into two slips, which insert into the middle phalanx
Action: flexes PIPJ of finger
Nerve: median nerve (C7, C8, T1)

Deep tendons

5. Flexor pollicis longus

Origin: middle of anterior shaft of radius, interosseous membrane, medial epicondyle of the humerus and often the coronoid process of ulna
Insertion: palmar aspect of base of the distal phalanx of the thumb
Action: flexes IPJ of thumb
Nerve: anterior interosseous branch of median nerve (C8, T1)

6. Flexor digitorum profundus

Origin: upper ¾ of the medial and anterior aspects of the ulna and from the anterior aspect of the interosseous membrane
Insertion: palmar aspects of the bases of the distal phalanges. tendon to the index finger is separate, the other three have a common tendon which separates in the palm
Action: flexes DIPJ of finger
Nerve: index and middle fingers—median nerve; ring and little fingers—ulnar nerve

Examination of FDP and FDS

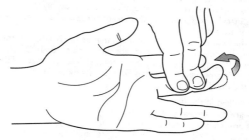

Fig. 13.1 Test to check integrity of FDP.

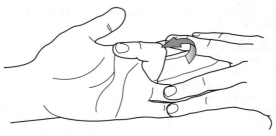

Fig. 13.2 Test to check integrity of FDS.

- Because FDP (III, IV, V) has a common muscle belly in the forearm, if the fingers are held straight at the tip, the flexor moment of FDP on the PIPJ is neutralized. FDS is now the only available PIP flexor and can be tested.
- This does not work for the index finger because FDP index has an independent muscle belly.
- To test the index finger FDS (II), the subject is asked to bend the PIP without bending the tip (producing a 'buttonhole'-shape against the thumb with DIP extended). If this cannot be achieved, so that only an 'OK' ring is made between thumb and index (i.e. tip flexed) then FDS may not be intact.

Flexor tendon sheath and pulley systems of the fingers

- The FDP and FDS tendons both enter the flexor tendon sheath in the palm.
- The index, middle and ring fingers enter the sheath at the level of metacarpal neck.
- The flexor sheath is composed of both synovial and retinacular components, and is sealed at both ends. The sheath provides nutrition, protection and ensures that the tendon glides smoothly.
- The retinacular component of the sheath consists of a series of annular and cruciate pulleys.
- Once the flexor tendons have entered the flexor sheath, FDS splits into two forming radial and ulnar slips that wrap around FDP at the chiasma of Camper. The slips conjoin again to insert dorsal to FDP on to the middle phalanx, permitting FDP to pass more distally to insert on to the distal phalanx.

Annular pulleys in the fingers
- There are five annular pulleys (A1–A5)
- These are thick, reinforced structures
- They keep the flexor tendons in close proximity to the digit when put under tension during flexion
- Odd numbers arise from the palmar plates of the small joints of the digits:
  - A5 pulley over DIPJ
  - A3 pulley over PIPJ
  - A1 pulley over MCPJ
- Even numbers arise from the periosteum of the middle and distal phalanges:
  - A4 over middle phalanx
  - A2 over proximal phalanx
- A2 and A4 are the most important pulleys and should be preserved where possible to prevent bowstringing.

Cruciate pulleys in the fingers
- There are three cruciate pulleys (C1–C3) in the fingers
- These are thin and flexible
- Permit full flexion of the digit

Flexor tendon sheath and pulley systems of the thumb

- The thumb has two annular pulleys that are located over the MP joint (A1) and the IP joint (A2) and one oblique pulley centred over the proximal phalanx.

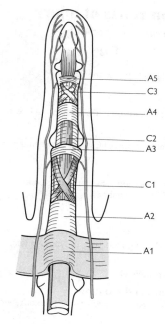

Fig. 13.3 Flexor pulley system (palmar view).

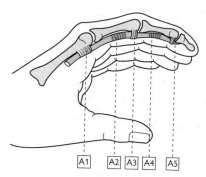

Fig. 13.4 Flexor pulley system (side view).

Flexor tendon zones of injury

The zones differ in the fingers and the thumb.

Flexor tendon zones in the fingers

Zone 1
- Distal to the insertion of FDS into the P2.
- Contains only FDP.

Zone 2
- From the origin of the flexor tendon sheath to the insertion of the FDS into the P2.
- Contains FDS and FDP.
- FDP passes through the chiasm of Camper between the two slips of FDS.

Zone 3
- Distal to the carpal tunnel and proximal to the tendon sheath.
- Contains FDS and FDP and lumbrical.

Zone 4
- The carpal tunnel
- Contains FDS (4), FDP (4), FPL, median nerve.
- Tendons are covered by a double layer of synovial membrane.

Zone 5
- Proximal to the carpal tunnel.

Flexor tendon zones in the thumb

Five zones; simpler than the fingers, as only one flexor tendon (FPL).

Zone 1
- Distal, at the insertion of FPL

Zone 2
- From the neck of the 1st metacarpal to the neck of the proximal phalanx.
- Contains flexor tendon sheath of the thumb.

Zone 3
- The area under the thenar muscles.

Zone 4
- The carpal tunnel.
- Thenar muscles also lie over part of zone 4.

Zone 5
- Proximal to the carpal tunnel.

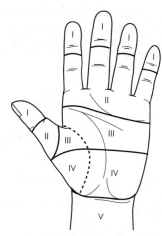

Fig. 13.5 Flexor tendon zones.

Flexor tendon suture techniques

- The most effective method of returning strength and excursion to repaired flexor tendons is to use strong, gap-resistant suture techniques, followed by frequent application of controlled movement/loading.

Ideal characteristics of a flexor tendon suture repair

- Easy suture placement
- Secure knots
- Smooth opposition of tendon ends with no bulge
- Minimal gapping potential
- Minimal compromise of tendon vascularity
- Strong enough to tolerate early active movement postoperative therapy regimens

Core sutures

- There are many types of core sutures. The most widely used is the modified Kessler suture.
  - This can be used as a four-strand repair by inserting two parallel modified Kessler core sutures.
- The strength of the flexor tendon repair is proportional to the number of strands of suture which pass across the repair site.
  - Four-strand techniques are approximately twice as strong as two-strand.
  - Six-strand techniques approximately three times as strong as two-strand.
  - Stronger suture equals stronger repair

Estimated repair strength of core sutures (no epitendinous suture) in grams

Type of repair	0 weeks	1 week	3 weeks	6 weeks
Two-strand	1800	1350	1350	2160
Four-strand	3600	2700	2700	4320
Six-strand	5400	4000	4000	6480

Epitendinous sutures

- Use of an epitendinous suture reduces gapping between the tendon ends, and increases the strength of the core repair by approximately 40% (or 700g).
- This improved strength is maintained during the healing period.
- Strongest epitendinous suture techniques:
  - Silfverskiöld cross stitch
  - Running lock stitch
  - Horizontal mattress are the strongest

Types of tendon suture material

- Use non-absorbable sutures.
- Curved, atraumatic needles cause less damage to the tendons than cutting needles.

Core sutures

- 3/0 and 4/0 braided polyester.
  - They must be inserted carefully, as they do not 'run' through the tendon easily because of the braiding.
- 3/0 and 4/0 polypropylene.
  - Runs through the tendon without resistance, and so is easy to insert.
  - The elasticity may lead to early gapping.

Epitendinous sutures

- 5/0 or 6/0 polypropylene or braided polyester.

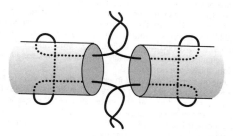

Fig. 13.6 Modified Kessler–Tajima suture.

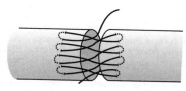

Fig. 13.7 Cross-stitch epitendinous repair technique (Silfverskiöld).

Flexor tendon repair

Open tendon injury

- Flexor tendons are most frequently divided by open sharp or crush injuries.
- Sharp injury over the course of a flexor tendon should usually be explored:
  - A partial division (undiagnosed) may appear to function normally when examined, and then rupture later if the patient continues to use the hand.
- A careful history should be taken about the exact mechanism of the injury. This will give useful information about the likely damage, and the requirements for surgery:
  - Hand posture during injury
  - Nature of wounding (e.g. knife, glass, metal, etc.).
- Flexor tendon injuries with the finger in extension usually have a division of one or both NVBs (and may require revascularization).
- FDS and FDP division with intact digital nerve sensibility usually means the injury was sustained with the digit in extreme flexion:
  - The digital nerves sublux laterally and dorsally in strong finger flexion, and so are not divided.
- Flexor tendon division sustained in extreme digital flexion (e.g. a defensive injury sustained when trying to grip an assailant's knife blade), when the tendon is at its shortest, will result in maximal tendon retraction, and the repair will be more difficult.
  - The tendon is likely to have retracted along the tendon sheath (and therefore will be difficult to retrieve).
  - The tendon repair will have to be performed with the finger in maximal flexion (difficult to operate between the pulleys).

Partial flexor tendon lacerations

- There is still contention about the treatment of partial division of flexor tendons.
- Insertion of a core suture into a partially divided flexor tendon may weaken it and increase bulk (thus reducing glide).
- Consider repairing flexor tendons with a division of 60% or more.
- Small lacerations can be tidied up by shaving off irregularities to allow improved glide.
- It is sometimes preferable to complete a tendon division, and perform a neat end-to-end repair, than to try and repair a significant partial division, which bulges, and does not glide well in the flexor tendon sheath.

Surgical techniques for flexor tendon repair

Skin incisions

- Extension of the wound requires thought and experience.
- Avoid long, narrow-based flaps.
- Use combinations of mid-lateral and Bruner-type incisions as required.
- Avoid a zig and a zag across the full span of a phalangeal bone—the tip of this flap will die, exposing your tendon repair.

Management of flexor tendon sheath
- Try to preserve all pulleys whenever possible.
- The A2 and A4 pulleys must always be preserved to prevent bowstringing. Try also to preserve the A3 pulley.
- A transverse or L-shaped window may be incised in the tendon sheath between the annular pulleys for access to the flexor tendons:
  - This can often be closed after repair using a fine (6/0) suture, as long as the tendon repair glides underneath it.
  - If the tendon repair sticks, leave the tendon sheath window open.

Tendon retrieval
- Handle the tendon minimally, and try to avoid unnecessary crush during retrieval.
- When the tendons have been retrieved, secure them using a hypodermic needle to minimize handling, and allow tension-free repairs.
- Avoid opening the whole palm to retrieve a tendon divided by a laceration in the finger.
- 'Milk' the tendon from proximal to distal, using the thumb. It may then appear in the flexor tendon sheath in the finger, or become retrievable.
- Try to retrieve the tendon using a fine artery clip, or tendon-passing forceps, passed down the flexor tendon sheath.
  - Repeated clumsy attempts to do this blindly will damage the synovial lining of the flexor tendon sheath, or mash the distal end of the cut tendon.
- It is important to ensure that the FDP passes through the chiasm of the FDS in the correct anatomical orientation to achieve proper tendon glide.
- If you cannot retrieve the FDS and/or FDP tendons up the flexor tendon sheath, make a small transverse incision in one of the palmar creases to find them.
- Alternatively, pass a fine umbilical catheter (from distal to proximal) down the flexor tendon sheath. Identify the catheter and tendon through a proximal incision (feel it first to position the incision). Suture the tendon to the catheter, and pull the catheter distally to retrieve the tendon. This has the advantage of ensuring that the FDP passes though the chiasm of the FDS slips in the correct orientation.

Repair of flexor tendons in each zone
Zone 1
- Only FDP divided (by definition of the zone).
- Preserve the A4 pulley.
- The DIPJ may need to be flexed to expose the distal end of the FDP.
  - Make a window between the C3–A5 pulley complex if necessary.
- The FDP usually retracts to the level of the PIPJ or proximal phalanx.
- The FDP can be exposed by making a transverse incision in the flexor tendon sheath at the C1–A3 or A3–C2 cruciate/annular pulley junction (on either side of the A3 pulley).
- Retrieve the FDP preserving the A4 pulley/flexor tendon sheath:
  - The needle of a core suture is passed through the laceration in the tendon sheath from distal to proximal (within the tendon sheath).

- This is easier if the needle is reversed, so the 'suture' end is advanced, rather than the sharp point of the needle.
- A core suture(s) is inserted in the tendon.
- The needle is passed back distally within the tendon sheath to the proposed site of repair.
- The tendon can then be pulled distally using the core suture.
- This allows preservation of the tendon sheath and minimizes handling of the tendon.
- If the FDP has retracted more proximally, the tunnel is longer than the suture needle, and the needle cannot be passed all the way along the tendon sheath. In this case, make several transverse incisions on either side of the A3 pulley, so the suture needle can be passed out, and then back into the tendon sheath, allowing it to progress distally.
- Once the FDP has been retrieved, transfix it transversely with an 23G hypodermic needle to hold it in position.
- It is usually easier to insert the back wall of the epitendinous suture before completing and tightening the core suture, as there is not much space within the flexor tendon sheath.
- The core suture can then be inserted into the distal FDP, tensioned correctly (remove the hypodermic and check the tenodesis and the glide in the flexor tendon sheath), and then tied (tension-free—replace the hypodermic first).
- The front wall of the epitendinous repair can then be completed.
- It is important to test the proper glide of the repair in the tendon sheath. If it is catching on the A3 or A4 pulley, the pulley can be 'vented' by making a 1–2mm nick in the leading edge. This should be done cautiously, and should not be used to accommodate a bad, very bulky repair (better to re-do it).

Zone 2

- Expose the flexor tendon sheath, preserving the NVBs.
- If the digital arteries and/or nerves are divided, mobilize them sufficiently for repair.
- Look for the tendon ends. Milk them from proximal to distal, and flex the DIPJ and PIPJ to find the distal ends.
- Make transverse or L-shaped incisions in the tendon sheath to retrieve the tendons, preserving the A3, as well as A2 and A4 pulleys.
- Deliver the tendons out of the tendon sheath through the windows, and transfix using a hypodermic needle.
- It maybe necessary to insert the sutures into the tendon ends at different levels in the tendon sheath if they have retracted. The sutures are then passed along the flexor tendon sheath using the technique described above.
- The repair is finished off with completion of the core suture and insertion of the epitendinous suture. It is often easier to insert the back wall of the epitendinous suture before completing the core suture when working within the flexor tendon sheath.

Zone 3

- Good prognosis after direct repair. Associated damage to neurovascular bundles and common digital vessels.

Zone 4
- Flexor tendons enclosed in synovial sheaths.
- May be associated injury to median nerve.
- The transverse carpal ligament is usually not repaired. Bowstringing of the tendons out of the carpal tunnel is possible if the wrist is splinted in extreme flexion.

Zone 5 proximal to the carpal tunnel
- Technically straightforward.
- Extend transverse lacerations using broad based flaps with gentle curved incisions.
  - Do not use sharp, triangular, zig-zag incisions across the full width of the wrist. These may not be well-vascularized, and die, exposing the tendon repairs.
  - If you need to extend the wound into the carpal tunnel, consider going from the middle of the transverse wrist laceration, rather then either end. This keeps the flaps broad-based, and therefore safe.
- Important to identify proximal and distal tendon ends correctly in multiple injuries.
- Associated injury of the median nerve and ulnar nerve should be repaired using an operating microscope at this level. The small nutrient artery can be used for correct orientation.
- FDS:
  - middle and ring finger FDS lie volar (i.e. superficial) to index and little finger FDS.
- FDP:
  - index FDP usually separate.
  - Middle, ring and little FDP converge to conjoined tendon by zone 5.
- Associated injury of the radial or ulnar artery should be repaired to maintain the vascularity of the hand. A small interposition vein graft may be required.

FPL repair
- The principles for flexor tendon repair described above should be followed.
- There is a higher rupture rate after FPL repair (due to poor vascularity), and a multi-strand repair is recommended.
- The oblique pulley should be preserved to prevent bowstringing.
  - Remember that the oblique pulley runs from ulnar/proximal (where it merges with A1 pulley) to radial/distal (as it merges with A2 pulley)
- The FPL is often difficult to retrieve when it has retracted beyond the thumb:
  - Consider using the umbilical catheter method of retrieval described above rather than extensive exploratory incisions.
  - Look for the proximal FPL in the wrist by the FCR tendon (rather than in the palm).

Flexor tendon repair in children

- As with all children's hand surgery, this should only be performed by specialist hand surgeons who operate on children regularly.
  - If you do not operate on children's hands regularly, refer the patient to someone who does.
- The surgery for flexor tendon repair in children is the same as for adults, except the structures are smaller. Loupe magnification is essential. The difference is in the **rehabilitation** after the injury.
  - Tendon repairs will heal quicker than in adults.
  - Children under 7 or 8 are unlikely to be able to comply with hand therapy, and participation should not be expected.
- Use absorbable sutures for skin closure.
- The hand should be placed in a dorsal splint to take tension off the flexor tendon repairs (10–30° of wrist flexion, MCPJs at 60°), and then wrapped up as a 'boxing glove' to prevent them from trying to use it.
  - The cast should be applied above the elbow, as young children can often wriggle out of short forearm casts. This is tolerated surprisingly well.
  - If the transverse carpal ligament has been divided (try to avoid this), place the wrist in neutral, and flex the MCPJs to 90° to prevent the flexor tendons bowstringing out of the carpal tunnel.
  - This allows the fingers to flex and extend within a shorter than normal range of movement.
  - The cast can be left undisturbed for 4–6 weeks, depending on the age of the child and family circumstances.
  - A general anaesthetic change of dressing may be required for young children.

Splints

- The repairs should be protected using a dorsal splint **beyond the level of the fingertips**, applied with the dressings in the operating theatre.
- The dressings over the front of the fingers should be **as light and loose as possible**; otherwise active flexion against resistance of dressings will increase risk of rupture.
- The wrist should not be put into extreme flexion, but either neutral or a little extension, depending on the nature of the repairs. Increased wrist flexion increases the force needed to flex the fingers
- The MCPJs should be flexed at approximately 60° (rather than >90°).
  - Remember that the force (or moment) required to initiate flexion **increases** with MCPJ flexion (the tendon is shorter), which then puts more force through the repair, and is more likely to rupture it.
- The patient should be seen by the hand therapists to start postoperative exercises according to local protocols.

Complications of flexor tendon repair
- Rupture of repair
- Wound infection
- Skin loss/wound breakdown leading to exposed tendons
- Adhesions leading to loss of movement
- Inability to flex fully (secondary to splinting by oedema)
- Bowstringing, secondary to pulley failure
- Tight in extension:
  - Repair too tight
  - Therapists have not moved in extension early enough

Closed flexor tendon rupture

Closed spontaneous tendon rupture of FDS or FDP is less common than open injury; seen in the finger, palm, wrist, and in the forearm at the musculotendinous junction.

Causes of closed flexor tendon rupture

- Sport (FDP rupture)
- Chronic tenosynovitis (e.g. rheumatoid arthritis)
- Partial tendon laceration
- Attrition rupture over bony prominence (e.g. STT OA, ulnar head OA)
- Gout
- Rheumatoid

Closed FDP rupture

- The commonest closed rupture is avulsion of the insertion of the FDP tendon.
    - Classic mechanism is rugby player grabbing another player's jersey in DIPJ flexion, while the fingertip is forced into extension.
    - A fragment of bone may also be avulsed with the tendon insertion.
    - Usually affects the ring finger (? Inherent weakness or mechanics of grip).
- It is often not diagnosed acutely .
    - The symptoms are relatively minor (pain, bruising, swelling).
    - The patient can still flex the PIPJ and MCPJ.
    - A bony fragment is not always seen on the X-ray.
- Classification of closed FDP rupture by *Leddy and Packer*.
    - *Type 1:* the FDP retracts into the palm. Repair within 7 days otherwise contracture develops.
    - *Type 2:* the tendon retracts to the level of the PIPJ, held by a small bony fragment at the A3 pulley, or vinculum. Most common. Repair up to 4 weeks usually successful.
    - *Type 3:* large distal fragment at mouth of A4 pulley. Repair up to 2–3 months can be successful.
- The patient must be consented for reconstructive options (if the tendon cannot be repaired directly) *before* initial exploration. These include:
    - Insertion of a silastic tendon spacer (as the first part of a 2-stage tendon reconstruction 📖 p. 414). Results are unpredictable for 2-stage reconstruction in this condition.
    - DIPJ arthrodesis.
    - No further reconstruction.

Surgical technique for closed FDP rupture

- Expose the flexor tendon sheath distally using Bruner or mid-lateral incisions.
- Confirm the FDP tendon has avulsed:
    - Staining and haematoma,
    - Distal end of the FDP within the flexor tendon sheath.
    - Open the flexor tendon sheath between the A4 and A5 pulley, and you will see that the FDP is not attached to the base of the P3.

- Retrieve the FDP tendon (📖 p. 405), and secure (tension-free) using a hypodermic needle to transfix the tendon.

Reattachment of the FDP tendon

- There are several methods to reattach the FDP tendon to its insertion at the base of the P3.

Pull-out suture method

- Drill parallel holes obliquely from the base of the P3 though the nail plate on the dorsum using broken off hypodermic needles in a K-wire driver.
- Insert a multiple-pass core suture into the distal and of the FDP tendon and cut off the suture needle.
- Pass the suture ends through the hypodermic needles and tie them over a button, or sponge on the dorsum of the nail plate.
- Remove the pull-out suture at 6–8 weeks after surgery, according to the patient's wound-healing status (leave longer in elderly, diabetics, smokers, etc.).
- **Advantage:**
  - Technically straightforward.
- **Disadvantages:**
  - Can deform nail plate.
  - Vulnerable to infection.
  - Prone to interference from patient, junior medical staff, nurses.
  - Tendon can still become detached after removal of pull-out suture, especially when there is poor wound healing.

Internal fixation to P3

- Drill a transverse hole through the base of the P3 (at 90° to the area of the FDP insertion) using a hypodermic needle (either drill with broken-off needle in K-wire driver, or drill with K-wire and then pass needle through hole).
- Insert a multiple pass core suture into the distal end of the FDP tendon and cut off the suture needle
- Pass the suture ends through the hypodermic needle in drill hole, remove needle, pull tight and tie, reattaching FDP to bone.
- **Disadvantage:**
  - Technically more difficult than pull-out suture.
- **Advantages:**
  - Hidden from interference.
  - More difficult for tendon to become detached (unless suture snaps, or knot fails).

Bone anchors

- Small bone anchors can be used to reinsert the FDP tendon into the distal phalanx.
- This must be done with great care, as there is very little bone stock, and accurate insertion is essential. Pull out strength may be inadequate.

Flexor tenolysis

Surgical release of flexor tendon adhesions.

Indications

- Flexor tendon adhesions which prevent unhindered tendon glide.

Timing of flexor tenolysis

- Probably no earlier than 3 months after injury or previous surgery to allow soft tissues to settle, and reduce risk of rupture.
- Leave it longer in children, who may 'grow out' of tendon adhesions with time.

Planning and informed consent

- Flexor tenolysis requires intensive rehabilitation to obtain a successful outcome.
- Some surgeons prefer to perform tenolysis under a regional anaesthetic block to allow the patient demonstrate their ability to move the tendon. This has the disadvantage of limiting the operative time because of tourniquet pain.
- If tenolysis is not possible during surgical exploration, 2-stage reconstruction (+/– pulley reconstruction) may be necessary, and this must be discussed/agreed before surgery.
- There is a risk of tendon rupture after surgery.
- There may be a skin shortage from scar contracture. Consider how you will deal with this in your pre-operative planning and consent.
  - Skin grafts need to be immobilized, and the hand must be moved following tenolysis, so a local flap may be a better option.
- Release of stiff joints in addition to tenolysis makes rehabilitation difficult. Surgery in two stages should be considered.
- If the pulley system is not intact, consider 2-stage flexor tendon reconstruction.

Technique

- Design incisions around old scars, forming Bruner zig-zags.
- Consider incorporating scar revisions (e.g. Z-plasty) if required.
- Find the level at which the tendons are stuck.
- Deflate the tourniquet before skin closure and check haemostasis.
- Close the skin carefully to ensure uncomplicated primary healing to facilitate postoperative hand therapy.

Division of adhesions within the flexor tendon sheath

- Expose the flexor tendon sheath, preserving the NVBs.
- Make transverse incisions in the flexor tendon sheath, between the annular pulleys.
- Try to divide tendon adhesions using sharp dissection with a scalpel (change blades frequently) or Beaver blade.
- A loop of strong suture material (eg 2/0 polypropylene) can be passed under the tendons inside the tendon sheath, from proximal to distal, or vice versa. This is used as a 'cheesewire' to divide adhesions, especially under the annular pulleys where access is limited.

- A fine periosteal elevator or dental probe may be useful to slide along the inside of the flexor tendon sheath.

Postoperative management

- Start supervised early active movement with the hand therapists on the same day, or day after surgery.
- A regional brachial plexus anaesthetic block allows hand therapy to start without pain.

Complications

- Haematoma
- Wound breakdown
- Infection
- Tendon rupture:
  - Early
  - Late
- Further tendon adhesions from lack of postoperative movement.

Flexor tendon reconstruction

Options

Fingers

Zones 1 and 2

- 2-stage tendon grafting.

Zone 3, 4 and 5

- 2-stage tendon graft (especially when there is extensive scarring)
- 1-stage interposition graft
- FDS tendon transfer
- End-to-side FDP transfer

Thumb

- The principles are the same as for the fingers.
- There is only one flexor tendon, so 'buddying' of FDP to FDS is not possible.
- The FDS to the ring or middle finger may be transferred.
  - The will reach to Zone 1 to reconstruct FPL.
  - The FDS can be used instead of a tendon graft as a 2-stage procedure.

One-stage flexor tendon reconstruction

- Occasionally considered in the first 3 weeks of injury, if no scarring, no infection, clean wounds, full passive movement, no swelling.
- Prone to adhesions, so two-stage grafting is usually preferred.

Two-stage flexor tendon reconstruction

Patient selection for two-stage tendon grafting

- This surgery is difficult, even for experienced hand surgeons.
- Indications for 2-stage tendon grafting decrease with experience!
- There is no point doing this surgery for educationally challenged, poorly motivated, non-compliant patients. It will not work, and they may be worse off than if they had not had it in the first place.
- The indication for 2-stage grafting of FDP in the presence of a functioning FDS is particularly debatable. Loss of only a few degrees of PIP flexion due to postoperative stiffness will outweigh any gain in DIP flexion with regard to total active flexion. Most likely indication is ring or little finger when full DIP flexion is essential (e.g. musicians).

Indications for two-stage tendon reconstruction

- Missed FDP division or closed rupture.
- Tendon adhesions unsuitable for tenolysis
- Reconstruction in Zones 1 and 2 (i.e. within flexor tendon sheath).
- Flexor tendon division with underlying fracture and defect in flexor tendon sheath (usually sticks).
- Flexor tendon division and requirement for pulley reconstruction
  - You can't reconstruct a flexor tendon and pulley at the same time—they will stick.
- Congenital absence (📖 see Chapter 16 p. 521)

Always consider leaving alone; amputation or DIP fusion may for many patients be better surgical options (quicker and more reliable restoration of function).

Outline of two-stage tendon grafting
Stage 1
- Exploration of the native tendon (+/– attempt at tenolysis).
- Excision of native FDP.
- Pulley reconstruction if required.
- Insertion of a silastic (silicone) tendon spacer (oval) or tendon rod (cylindrical) into the remaining flexor tendon sheath.
  - Smooth scar 'capsule' forms around the silicone, which acts as a new tendon sheath, allowing glide of the tendon graft.
- The tendon spacer is sutured distally (and not proximally) so that it pistons forward and backwards during passive flexion and extension of the digit.
- Commence hand therapy to regain full passive ROM.
- Range of movement:
  - The patient must get the maximum passive ROM before progressing to Stage 2.
  - In the best case, you will only get actively **after** Stage 2 tendon grafting, what you have passively **before** tendon grafting (and sometimes, a little less).
- Stage 2 is performed when the patient has regained a full passive ROM in the digit. This is usually 4 to 6 months after Stage 1.

Stage 2
- The tendon spacer is removed from the new tendon sheath.
- A tendon graft is inserted into the new tendon sheath.
  - This is secured distally with a technique similar to that for FDP reattachment (🕮 see p. 400).
  - Secured proximally with a three pass Pulvertaft weave (🕮 see Fig. 13.8).
  - There are a number of possible donor sources of tendon grafts (see below).
- Controlled active movement is started immediately after surgery, and the repair is protected for 3 months.

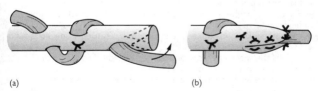

(a)   (b)

Fig. 13.8 Pulvertaft weave.

Informed consent points for two-stage tendon grafting.
- The outline of the surgery (see above) must be discussed in detail.
  - It is a good idea to get the patient to talk to one of your hand therapists to give them a more detailed overview of the treatment course.
- It is unlikely to be as good as a normal finger.

- The digit will take 2–3 weeks to heal after Stage 1, and you will then need hand therapy to regain the passive ROM.
- The source of tendon graft (and likely donor site scars and morbidity—especially for toe extensors) must be discussed.
- Stage 2 is likely to be performed 4–6 months after Stage 1. A longer (indefinite) gap between Stage 1 and Stage 2 is possible as long as the tendon spacer does not extrude.
- You will need up to 3 months of hand therapy after Stage 2.; you will need to wear a protective splint for 6–8 weeks, and you will not be able to do manual work during this time.

Sources of tendon graft

This should be discussed pre-operatively as part of the informed consent.

Palmaris longus (PL)

- PL is present in approximately 85% of the population.
- Test for palmaris:
  - Touch thumb to little finger.
  - Flex wrist against resistance.
  - Palmaris lies on ulnar side of FCR.
  - Ensure you are not palpating the median nerve, which is also on the ulnar side of the FCR, but deeper, and not attached to the palmar fascia.
- Harvest of palmaris graft:
  - Make a short transverse incision over the PL at the distal wrist crease.
  - Dissect under the PL with scissors.
  - Use a sharp tendon stripper, and divide the PL at the musculotendinous junction.
  - Alternatively, pass the tips of a pair of scissors under the PL tendon at the wrist. Flex the wrist, and pull up on the scissors to tension the PL. Feel the PL proximally, and cut at the musculotendinous junction using a number 11 scalpel blade through a small stab incision.

Plantaris

- Plantaris is present in approximately 80% of the population.
- Plantaris is long, and can be used for two fingertip to palm, or one fingertip to wrist, graft.
- Its presence/absence can be identified pre-operatively using ultrasound.
- Harvest of plantaris:
  - Feel the space just anterior and medial to the Achilles tendon.
  - Make a 5cm incision over this space.
  - Find the Achilles tendon, and then find the plantaris tendon just anterior to it.
  - Dissect the plantaris proximally, using the blunt end of a cat's paw retractor to lift the skin up. This makes subsequent stripping easier.
  - Divide the plantaris tendon distally.
  - Slide a tendon stripper over the plantaris tendon and hold the tendon distally with an artery clip.
  - Slide the tendon stripper distally, applying tension with the clip, and using a semi-circular oscillating movement. Advance to the proximal calf, and cut at the musculotendinous junction with the sharp edge of the tendon stripper.

Toe extensor
- The extensor digitorum tendons from the 2nd, 3rd and 4th toes may be used to provide long tendon grafts.
- Individual tendons may fuse distal to the ankle.
- Harvest:
  - Make small transverse incision over the extensor digitorum, just proximal to the webspace.
  - Find the tendon and strip to the ankle using a tendon stripper.
  - Make a further transverse incision and withdraw the tendon.
  - Use the tendon stripper to harvest up to the musculotendinous junction in the calf.
  - Avoid longitudinal incisions up the dorsum of the foot.

Pulley reconstruction
- You cannot reconstruct a tendon and a pulley(s) at the same time. This has to be done as a 2-stage procedure.

Donor material
- Discarded tendons (FDS, FDP, FPL).
  - When multiple pulley reconstruction is required, the long flexors may be taken via a small incision in the wrist to provide adequate length of graft.
- Tendon graft (PL, plantaris, toe extensors)
- Extensor retinaculum

Techniques of pulley reconstruction
Suture to pulley remnant
- If there is a reasonable cuff of pulley remaining, the graft can be sutured directly to this from side-to-side, or as an interweave.

Drill holes in bone
- Drill small holes in the phalanx for suture placement when there is no rim of pulley.

Slip of FDS
- If the distal insertion is intact, FDS slips can be sutured to the rim of the A2 pulley, or attached using a drill hole for the suture.

Encircling technique
- A loop of graft is used to encircle the phalanx, over and over. This provides a very strong reconstruction, but is a little bulky.
  - A2 pulley: place the loop **under** the extensor mechanism, and use a double loop.
  - A4 pulley: place the loop **over** the extensor mechanism.
  - This can be a little tricky, and a small vascular aneurysm needle is useful. Be careful not to encircle the NVB.
  - Approximately 6–8cm of graft is required to encircle the phalanx once. For a double loop to reconstruct the A2 pulley 10mm in length, 12–16cm of tendon graft is required.

Tendon transfer to reconstruct flexor tendons
- The principles of tendon transfer are discussed in the relevant section in Chapter 11.
- FDS to the ring and middle fingers can be used to reconstruct FPL (see above).

Extensor tendon anatomy

Extrinsic (long) extensor muscles

- The extensor muscles lie in the extensor compartment, on the radial/posterior aspect of the forearm.
- All the extensor tendons pass under the extensor retinaculum, a fibrous 'dorsal pulley'.
- Innervated by the radial and posterior interosseous nerves

Wrist extensors

Extensor carpi radialis longus (ECRL)
Origin: lateral humerus, above the lateral epicondyle.
Insertion: base of the second metacarpal
Action: radial deviation (and wrist extension)
Innervation: radial nerve

Extensor carpi radialis brevis (ECRB)
Origin: lateral epicondyle
Insertion: base of 3rd metacarpal
Action: wrist extension (and radial deviation)
Innervation: radial nerve or posterior interosseous nerve

Extensor carpi ulnaris (ECU)
Origin: proximal ulna
Insertion: base of 5th metacarpal
Action: ulnar deviation and wrist extension
Innervation: posterior interosseous nerve

Finger extensors

Extensor digitorum communis (EDC)
Origin: lateral epicondyle of humerus
Insertion: extensor mechanism of fingers
Action: extension of MCPJs
Innervation : posterior interosseous nerve

- There may be multiple slips of EDC (especially to the ring finger).
- EDC tendons are linked by slips (juncturae tendinae) distal to the extensor retinaculum.
- The EDC to the little finger may be absent in up to 50%, when it is replaced by a junctura tendinum from the ring finger to the extensor mechanism of the little finger.
- The additional finger extensors (extensor indicis proprius [EIP] and EDM) lie on the ulnar side of the EDC.

Extensor indicis proprius (EIP)
Origin: ulna and interosseous membrane
Insertion: extensor mechanism of index finger, ulnar to EDC
Action: independent extension of index finger
Innervation: posterior interosseous nerve

Extensor digiti minimi (EDM)/Extensor digiti quinti (EDQ)
Origin: proximal ulna
Insertion: extensor mechanism of little finger, ulnar to EDC.

Action: independent extension of little finger
Innervation: posterior interosseous nerve

Thumb abduction/extension

Abductor pollicis longus (APL)
Origin: ulna and interosseous membrane
Insertion: base of 1st metacarpal
Action: abduction of 1st metacarpal
Innervation: posterior interosseous nerve
• Usually has more than one tendon

Extensor pollicis brevis (EPB)
Origin: radius and interosseous membrane
Insertion: into proximal phalanx of thumb via saggital bands
Action: extension of proximal phalanx with abduction of 1st metacarpal
Innervation: posterior interosseous nerve

Extensor pollicis longus (EPL)
Origin: ulna and interosseous membrane
Insertion: distal phalanx of thumb
Action: extension of distal phalanx, retropulsion of 1st metacarpal
Innervation : posterior interosseous nerve

Extensor retinaculum

• Runs from ulnar head and neck to the volar/radial edge of radial styloid.
• Average width 5cm, measured over the 4th compartment.
• The space under the extensor retinaculum is divided into 6 compartments by vertical septa.
  • There are 5 fibro-osseous compartments
  • There is 1 purely fibrous compartment (5th compartment containing EDM).

Extensor compartments (from radial to ulnar)	Tendons
1	APL, EPB
2	ECRL, ECRB
3 Ulnar to Lister's tubercle	EPL
4	EDC, EIP
5 Overlying DRUJ	EDM
6	ECU

Extensor mechanism of the fingers

Summary

- The extensor mechanism is a complex, subtle system, which extends 3 joints (MCPJ, PIPJ, DIPJ), and flexes one joint (MCPJ).
- The finger extrinsic system originates in the forearm, is radially innervated, and has 4 insertions (the dorsal capsule of the MCPJ and the dorsal base of the 3 phalanges).
- The finger intrinsic system consists of the seven interosseous, and four lumbrical muscles, which pass volar to the axis of the MCPJ, and dorsal to the axes of the IPJs.
- The intrinsic muscles divide and insert into components of the extrinsic extensor tendon to form the extensor mechanism.
- The extrinsic extensors extend the MCPJ, PIPJ and DIPJ.
- The intrinsics flex the MCPJ, and extend the PIPJ and DIPJ.

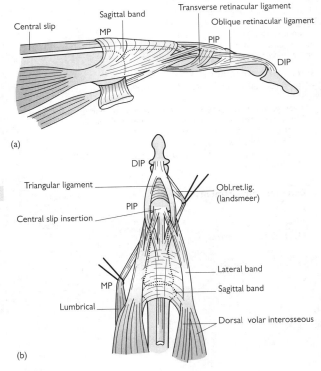

(a)

(b)

Fig. 13.9 Extensor mechanism.

Anatomy

- The extensor tendon at the level of the MCPJ is held in place by a combination of the tendons of the intrinsic muscles and the sagittal bands (transverse lamina) to centralize the tendon over the joint.
- The sagittal band arises from the volar plate and the intermetacarpal ligaments at the metacarpal neck.
- The extensor mechanism over the proximal part of the finger consists of a cross-hatched fibres which 'concertina', to allow the lateral bands to move volarwards in flexion, and return to the dorsum in extension.
- The intrinsic tendons (the lumbricals, palmar and dorsal interossei) join the extensor tendon, merging to form the extensor hood, at the proximal to mid-portion of the proximal phalanx.
- At the MCPJ, the intrinsic tendons are **palmar** to the joint's axis of rotation.
- At the PIPJ, the intrinsic tendons are **dorsal** to the axis of rotation.
- At the PIPJ, the extensor mechanism divides into three slips, which must be in balance for effective function.
  - The single **central slip** attaches to the central dorsum of the base of the P2.
  - The central slip extends the P2 at the PIPJ.
  - The two **lateral bands** pass on either side of the PIPJ, and continue distally to insert into the dorsal base of the P3.
  - The lateral bands extend the P3 across the DIPJ.
- The transverse retinacular ligaments maintain the position of the extensor mechanism at the level of the PIPJ.

Extensor tendon zones of injury

Zone	Finger	Thumb
I	DIPJ	IPJ
II	P2	P1
III	PIPJ	MCPJ
IV	P1	Metacarpal
V	MCPJ	CMCJ/radial styloid
VI	Metacarpal	
VII	Extenso retinaculum	
VIII	Distal forearm	
IX	Mid and proximal forearm	

- Original classification of Zones I to VIII by Kleinert and Verdan.
- Additional zone (IX) required to include muscles in middle and proximal forearm.

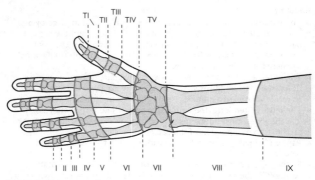

Fig. 13.10 Extensor tendon zones.

Extensor tendon repair

The repair of extensor tendon injuries depends on the zone and type of injury.

Mallet finger (zone I, DIPJ)

- Loss of continuity of the combined lateral band insertion into the distal phalanx results in a loss of extension of the distal phalanx, and is known as a 'mallet finger'.
- Full passive extension is usually present.
- Unopposed action of the central slip on the P2 +/− laxity at the PIPJ may cause hyperextension at the PIPJ leading to a swan neck deformity.

Mechanism of mallet injury

Closed (common)
- Sudden forced flexion of extended digit
- Sports, occupation or domestic activities.
- Causes rupture of extensor mechanism insertion into dorsum of P3, with or without fragment of bone.

Open
- Sharp injury
- Crush injury

Incidence

- Sex and age incidence vary geographically.
- Males greater than females:
  - Higher in adolescent/young males
  - Higher in middle-aged women
- Commoner on ulnar side of hand in both sexes.

Classification of mallet finger

Type 1
- Closed injury, +/− avulsion fracture
- Commonest injury

Type 2
- Open division of tendon at, or proximal to DIPJ

Type 3
- Associated loss of skin or tendon

Type 4A
- Transepiphyseal plate injury

Type 4B
- Hyperflexion injury
- 20–50% fracture of the articular surface

Type 4C
- Hyperextension injury
- >50% fracture of articular surface
- Volar subluxation of P3

Non-operative treatment of closed (Type 1) mallet finger
- The majority of Type 1 Mallet fingers can be treated non-operatively by application of a splint
- No bone fragment:
  - 8 weeks continuously
  - 4 weeks more at night
- Bone fragment:
  - 6 weeks continuously
- The patient is advised to only remove the splint for washing, maintaining the DIPJ in extension.

The goals of therapy
- To promote healing of the tendon
- To maximize function
- To maximize ROM
- To maintain full ROM of uninvolved joints
- To prevent development of a swan neck deformity

Types of splint
- Aluminium with foam which can be cut to size
  - Ensure no sharp edges
- Pre-moulded plastic (Stack)
- Custom-made moulded thermoplastic

Splint application
- A dorsal splint permits freedom of the PIP joint and allows fingertip sensation.
  - A volar splint compromises both.
- The DIPJ should be immobilized at 0° or slight hyperextension.
  - Extreme hyperextension can compromise circulation.
  - Slight flexion can result in an extension lag.
- Splint position and skin integrity should be monitored on a regular basis.
- Proper splint application should be taught.

After 6 weeks (fracture), after 8 weeks (no fracture)
- Begin gentle active flexion exercises.
- Week 1 no more than 20–25° active flexion of DIP joint.
- Week 2 if no lag, DIPJ can be flexed to 35°.
- If DIP joint is very tight in extension the oblique retinacular ligaments might need to be stretched.
- If an extension lag occurs, a period of re-splinting may be indicated (and exercises delayed).
- Splinting between exercises is recommended during the first 2 weeks of mobilization, with a night splint for 4 weeks.
- Desensitization of a painful fingertip may be necessary.
- Exercises should gradually proceed to resistive grasp and pinch.
- Flexion should be increased if extension is maintained.
- If PIPJ develops a slight posture of hyperextension, splint at 30–45° flexion with the DIP joint in extension.

Complications of splint immobilization
- Maceration/skin necrosis.
- Maceration/necrosis of the nail bed.

- Tape allergy.
- DIP joint extension lag.

Operative treatment of closed (Type 1) mallet finger

- Open repair techniques are described, but do not give superior results to non-operative treatment. High complication rate.
- K-wire immobilization (bury the wire, and place obliquely [not longitudinally] to avoid pain at the fingertip) is occasionally indicated for patients who cannot use a splint because of their occupation, or for social or psychological reasons.

Type 2 mallet finger (open division of tendon at, or proximal to DIPJ)

- Acute injuries are treated by surgical repair of the extensor mechanism, followed by immobilization for 8 weeks, using a splint or buried K-wire.

Type 3 mallet finger (associated loss of skin or tendon)

- This requires reconstruction of the soft tissue defect(s).
  - 📖 Extensor tendon reconstruction p. 434.
  - 📖 Local flaps to the dorsum of the finger p. 221.

Type 4 mallet finger with fracture

Type 4A transepiphyseal plate injury

- The extensor mechanism is attached to the basal epiphysis.
- Can be corrected by closed reduction.
- Splint in extension for 4 weeks, then check X-ray to monitor fracture healing and reduction.

Type 4B

- Hyperflexion injury
- 20–50% fracture of the articular surface
- Can be treated by splinting, K-wires, or ORIF.
  - Be careful not to shatter the small bony fragment with drills or screws.

Type 4C

- Hyperextension injury
- >50% fracture of articular surface
- Volar subluxation of P3 from the proximal fragment (which is in the correct anatomical position, held in place by the extensor tendon attachment, and the joint capsule).
  - The distal fragment has subluxed volarwards **off** this.
- Can be treated by splinting, K-wires, or ORIF.
- *Ishiguro* K-wire technique is useful when there is volar subluxation of the main fragment of the P3.
  - Flex DIPJ.
  - Insert K-wire through dorsum of P2 1–2mm dorsal and proximal to the fracture fragment. This wire blocks extension of the DIPJ.
  - Pull the P3 distally and extend to reduce it.
  - Insert an axial K-wire through the P3 across the DIPJ.
  - Apply a protective splint.
  - Remove the K wires at 4–6 weeks.

Mallet thumb (zone T I, IPJ)

- Closed mallet thumb is treated by splint for 6–8 weeks.
- Open mallet thumb injuries can be treated by suture of the tendon.
- The mobilization protocol is the same as for Type 1 mallet finger.

Finger P2 (zone II) and thumb P1 injury (Zone T II)

Finger middle phalanx

- Usually following open sharp or crush injury (rather than closed rupture as in zone I).
- Often incomplete division of tendon due to its width over the middle phalanx.
- Division less than 50% may be treated without repair of the tendon.
- Repair using a running over-and-over suture or Silverskiöld-type cross-stitch.
  - The tendon is too thin (0.5mm) to use a core suture.

Postoperative therapy
- Splint DIPJ in full extension for 6 weeks.
- Allow active flexion of PIPJ during this time.

Thumb proximal phalanx

- Laceration of the EPL over the proximal phalanx may be sutured, either as above, or sometimes using a core suture with a Silverskiöld-type cross stitch.

Postoperative therapy
- Splint the IPJ in full extension for 6 weeks.
- Allowing active flexion of the MCPJ.

Finger boutonniere lesion (zone III, PIPJ)

The boutonnière deformity

- The finger is held with the PIPJ flexed and the DIPJ hyperextended.
- This is due to a dorsal disruption of the extensor mechanism at the PIPJ, and is initially a dynamic imbalance of the extensor system.
- A fixed deformity can develop when left untreated.

Acute boutonnière deformity

- Division of the central slip into the base of the middle phalanx with volar subluxation of the lateral bands results in the boutonnière deformity:
  - Loss of extension at the PIPJ, with unopposed action of FDS.
  - Volar migration of lateral bands due to attenuation of transverse retinacular ligament, so that lateral bands lie volar to the axis of the PIPJ.
  - Pull of intrinsics directed (around PIPJ) to distal joint, leading to hyperextension at the DIPJ.
  - The dorsum of the PIPJ appears to 'buttonhole' (hence *Boutonnière*) through the middle of the lateral bands of the extensor tendon).
  - Some patients can maintain full active PIPJ extension when the joint is placed at 0°. Once the joint flexes enough for the lateral bands

to displace volarly, active extension is lost as the lateral bands pass volar to the axis of the PIPJ.

Causes
- Closed avulsion of central slip.
- Closed avulsion of central slip with avulsion fracture.
- Laceration of central slip.
- Volar dislocation of PIPJ with avulsion of central slip insertion into P2.

Pseudoboutonnière deformity
- Usually follows hyperextension injury of the PIPJ.
- PIPJ flexion contracture leads to contraction of oblique retinacular ligament and therefore loss of flexion of DIPJ.

Treatment of closed acute boutonnière injury
- Splint PIPJ in extension, leaving DIPJ free.
- Allow active flexion of DIPJ, and tighten strap across dorsum of PIPJ to bring it into full extension.
- Flexion of DIPJ brings the lateral bands into their anatomical position, dorsal to the axis of the PIPJ.
- Splint until PIPJ is fully extended, and DIPJ can be flexed fully:
  - This may take several weeks, and requires regular supervision by Hand Therapists.
- Mobilization at the PIPJ starts when full passive extension of the PIPJ and full active flexion of the DIPJ are achieved.
- Week 1 Start PIPJ flexion/extension in 30° ROM with MCPJ in neutral.
- Week 2 If no extensor lag, then increase ROM to 40–50°
- Week 3 Increase ROM by 20° each week.

Treatment of open acute boutonnière injury
- The laceration may be repaired directly.
- In untidy injuries, with loss of tendon substance, an alternate method must be used to reconstruct the central slip.

Direct repair
- Adequate stump of central slip—direct suture, with core suture and cross-stitch on dorsal surface of tendon.
- Inadequate stump of central slip—use transverse drill hole in the base of the P2, or micro bone anchor.

Free tendon graft
- This can be done immediately, or as a delayed procedure (as long as there is a full passive ROM and the soft tissue cover on the dorsum of the P1 and PIPJ is suitable).
- A piece of split PL (or other suitable graft) is passed through a transverse drill hole in the base of the P2, and the ends crossed over in a figure-of-8.
- The free ends of the grafts are woven through the lateral edges of the extensor mechanism.
- The PIPJ is protected in extension for approximately 2 weeks, followed by gentle short range active mobilization, progressing to full flexion over the next 6 weeks.

Distally based central slip flap
- Use a portion of the proximal central slip turned over to reconstruct central slip defect.
- Close the defect in the proximal central slip.

Split lateral band reconstruction
- Dissect the lateral bands from their lateral attachments to the oblique retinacular ligaments.
- Split the lateral band longitudinally for 2cm.
- Suture the medial part in the midline, leaving the lateral parts to function as lateral bands.

Thumb injury (zone T III, MCPJ)
- This involves EPL and/or EPB.
- The extensors are usually large enough to permit use of a core suture with a dorsal cross-stitch.

Finger P1 injury (zone IV)
- Be careful to avoid length imbalance between the central slip and lateral band components of the extensor mechanism.
- Start early short arc movement to avoid adhesions.

Partial lacerations
- Repaired using cross-stitch or epitendinous suture.
- Mobilize early to avoid adhesions.

Complete lacerations
- Repair using core suture with cross-stitch or epitendinous suture.

Thumb injury (zone T IV, metacarpal)
- EPL and EPB are well defined oval tendons.
- See *Thumb injury (zone III, MCPJ)* above.

Finger injury (zone V, MCPJ)
Punch injury (fight bite)
- 📖 Chapter 10 Infection bites.
- The MCPJ is injured by a punch injury, often to the mouth of the opponent. The patient may be reluctant to admit to the cause of the injury.
- This results in a laceration from a tooth, which penetrates the extensor tendon and the joint capsule, and is contaminated by oral flora.
- These injuries often present late, only when infection has developed.
- Septic arthritis can develop within 48 hours of the injury.
- The punch injury is sustained with the hand clenched into a fist, with the MCPJ flexed maximally.
    - The wound track goes through skin, extensor tendon, joint capsule and synovium into the joint.
    - There may be an defect of the articular cartilage, a fracture, or a foreign body (e.g. a fragment of tooth) in the metacarpal head.

Investigations
- Obtain an X-ray to look for fractures or foreign body.

- Blood tests
- Send a wound swab for microbiology culture.
- Monitor white cell count and C-reactive protein, especially when infected.

Surgical treatment of zone V punch injury
- Check that tetanus immunization is in date.
- Start IV antibiotics.
- Explore the wound in the operating theatre.
  - When the hand is explored with the MCPJ in extension, the relative position of the skin, tendon, and joint capsule changes (as they overlap).
  - It is easy to miss the hole in the joint capsule.
- Excise the skin edges of the wound with a 1–2mm margin.
- Extend the wound, proximally and distally.
- There is usually a visible laceration in the extensor tendon, which can be extended. If not, the extensor tendon should be split longitudinally for access to the MCPJ.
- There may be a visible defect in the capsule of the MCPJ. **When there is a clear history of a punch injury, the joint should be opened longitudinally and washed out (even if there is no visible puncture wound).**
- The wound should **not** be closed primarily.
- If the joint is infected, the patient should return to the operating theatre for further washout of the joint, until it is clean.
  - Repeat microbiology swabs.
- Significant tendon injuries should be repaired as a delayed procedure, when the wound is clean.
- Small splits in the extensor tendon can be left to heal without surgery.

Laceration to extensor hood
- The thick tendon of the extensor hood can be repaired using a core suture with cross-stitch.

Open sagittal band injury
- Laceration of the sagittal band is uncommon as their position protects them from injury.
- The sagittal bands should be repaired, or the main extensor tendon will sublux laterally, with discomfort and loss of extension.

Closed sagittal band injury
- Closed rupture (partial or complete) of the radial sagittal band with ulnar subluxation of the extensor tendon can occur in the non-rheumatoid patient following trauma (forced flexion or extension).
- This results in discomfort, with 'clicking' of the tendon during flexion of the MCPJs, and extensor lag.

Acute treatment of closed sagittal band injury
- For injuries less than 2 weeks old.
- Splint the MCPJ in 10–20° of flexion for 6 weeks.
- Leave the IPJs free.

Delayed treatment of closed sagittal band injury
- Some form of reconstruction is required to stabilize and centralize the extensor tendon. These include:
  - Direct repair of the radial sagittal band.
  - Use of a junctura tendinum.
  - Use of a slip of EDC, passed under the intermetacarpal ligament and back to EDC.
  - Use of a free tendon graft.
  - Little finger—transfer of the EDM for extensor subluxation with abduction of the little finger at the MCPJ.
- Limited release of the ulnar sagittal band may be necessary for rebalancing.

Thumb injury (zone T V, CMCJ)
- EPB and APL (2–4 tendon slips) may be injured in zone V.
- EPL is included in zone VII (wrist).
- These tendons can be repaired using a core and epitendinous suture as described previously.
- The superficial branch of the radial nerve (SBRN) may be injured.
  - This should be repaired, as neuroma or neuropathic pain is disabling.

Finger injury (zone VI, metacarpal)
- Division of extensor tendons in zone VI have a better prognosis than in Zones II to V.
- These can be repaired using a core and epitendinous suture as described previously.

Wrist injury (Zone VII)
Open injury
- Suture of the tendons at this level is similar to that described for Zones V and VI.
- Sorting out the correct tendon ends when there are multiple divisions (usually the case) can be difficult. Be systematic, and if necessary, use sutures for labelling.

Management of the extensor retinaculum
- Extensor injuries at the wrist involve the extensor retinaculum.
- Lacerations to the retinaculum must sometimes be extended for access (proximally and distally).
- Try to preserve part of the retinaculum in each compartment to avoid bowstringing.

Closed rupture
- EPL, EDC, EIP, EDM and ECU may rupture following distal radial or ulnar fractures.
  - Immediate
  - Delayed attrition rupture over a bony spur.
- ECU may dislocate ulnarwards, with the supination, palmar flexion and ulnar deviation following a Colles' fracture.

EPL reconstruction
- The EIP can be used to reconstruct the EPL.
- The transfer should be made subcutaneously, and not under the extensor retinaculum, for smooth glide and a straight line of pull.
- The EIP should be routed around the **radial** side of Lister's tubercle.

Surgical technique for EIP to EPL transfer
- Make a 1cm transverse incision on the ulnar side of the 2nd MCPJ to find the EIP (this is on the ulnar side, and deep to the EDC II).
- Palpate and mark Lister's tubercle.
- Make a 1cm transverse incision over the mid-point of the 2nd metacarpals and tension the EIP with scissors.
- Make a 2cm transverse incision over the 4th compartment at the proximal edge of the extensor retinaculum (ulnar to Lister's tubercle) and find the EIP again.
- Tension the EIP in the 4th compartment, and divide distally at the level of the MCPJ. Flip the tendon back. It may be necessary to divide juncturae tendinae, through the mid-metacarpal incision.
- Make 1cm transverse incision just proximal to the thumb MCPJ, and find the distal end of the EPL.
- Make a straight line subcutaneous tunnel from the 4th compartment incision to the thumb incision.
  - Easy with McIndoe-type dissecting scissors.
- Use tendon passing forceps to pass the EIP through the tunnel.
- Weave the EIP to the EPL, with the wrist and thumb in extension.
- Splint in 30° of wrist extension and thumb extension at MCPJ and IPJ for 10–14 days, and then start gentle short arc active movement.

Distal forearm injury (Zone VIII)
- Tendon repairs are the same as above.
- Lacerations at the level of the musculotendinous junction can be sutured if there is some tendinous substance proximally.
- Side-to-side suture, or tendon transfer (acute or delayed) can be performed when it is not possible to obtain good suture purchase in the muscle belly.

Proximal forearm injury (Zone IX)
- Wrist extensors, EDC, EDM arise from the lateral epicondyle.
- Thumb extensors, APL and EIP arise from the proximal forearm.
- Loss of function following an injury may be from;
  - Transection of muscle
  - Nerve injury
  - A combination of both.
- The internal injury may be more extensive than the skin laceration implies.

Muscle
- Muscle bellies are difficult to repair.
  - It is sometimes possible to oppose cut edges with a suture through the epimysium.
  - Avoid large suture 'bites' through muscle, which may cause ischaemia and necrosis.

Radial nerve

- The radial nerve gives branches to brachialis, brachioradialis and ECRL in the distal upper arm.
- It then divides into a motor and a sensory branch.
  - The posterior interosseous nerve (motor) innervates ECRB and supinator. It then passes between the 2 heads of supinator into the extensor compartment to supply ECU, EDC, EDM, APL, EPL, EPB, EIP.
  - The superficial branch of the radial nerve (sensory) continues distally under the brachioradialis, emerging from its distal third across the anatomical snuffbox.
- Division of the motor branches must be sought during exploration, and repaired where possible.
- Reconstruct lost nerve function by secondary nerve surgery, or tendon transfer.

Extensor tendon reconstruction

Reconstruction of extrinsic extensor tendon reconstruction in the forearm, wrist and dorsum of hand

General principles

- The commonest injury is a composite loss of skin, tendon (and sometimes bone, or associated fractures) on the dorsum of the hand, usually after a road traffic accident.
- Immediate reconstruction of tendon loss in Zones III to VII, especially when there is dorsal composite loss requiring complex soft tissue reconstruction, can produce delayed recovery and poor results because of oedema and tendon adhesions.
- It is often better to reconstruct the soft tissue envelope, and commence therapy to regain a full passive range of movement, and then perform a delayed extensor tendon reconstruction.
- The cut proximal tendon end should be sutured out to length in the defect at the time of soft tissue reconstruction, to prevent shortening and contracture of the muscle belly (which compromises function of delayed reconstruction using an interposition tendon graft).
- Silicone tendon spacers may be used through reconstructive flaps to recreate a tunnel for extensor tendon reconstruction using free graft or tendon transfer.
  - The requirement for a smooth, gliding tunnel is not as important for extensors (compared with flexors).
  - Tendon grafts or transfers can be performed successfully (without tendon spacers) as long as the soft tissue cover is adequate. This means a flap, rather than scar or tight skin graft

Free tendon graft

- In the presence of a proximal functioning musculotendinous unit, and an intact distal extensor mechanism, free tendon grafts can be used for reconstruction of the defect.
- It is difficult to reconstruct the large defects of the extensor mechanism distal to the central slip insertion.
- Fixation should be strong at either end (weaves and bone anchors) to permit early mobilization and avoid adhesions.
- PL, plantaris, toe extensors and extensor retinaculum may be used.

Tendon transfer

- The tendon transfers for the extrinsic extensor muscles are similar to those described for radial nerve injury.
- If the tendons are not long enough to reach the recipient site, they can be elongated using intercalated tendon graft.

Injured tendon	Tendon transfer
EPL	EIP
	PL
APL	Brachioradialis
EDC	Side-to-side to adjacent EDC
	EIP
	FCU or FCR
EDM	EIP
ECRL or ECRB	PT

Composite microvascular flap reconstruction

- Skin, fascia and tendon may be reconstructed in a single stage by microvascular free tissue transfer.
- A composite flap from the dorsum of the foot (skin, fascia and toe extensor tendons) is supplied by the dorsalis pedis vessels.

Advantage

- Promotes primary healing of defect.
- Allows immediate mobilization.

Disadvantage

- Poor donor site—tight, insensate skin graft on dorsum of foot may cause difficulties with footwear.
- Can be difficult to orientate vascular pedicle, skin and tendon components correctly relative to recipient site.

Extensor deformity

Chronic mallet finger

See mallet finger Zone I and mallet thumb Zone TI pp. 424–427 for treatment of acute mallet finger injuries. For a thorough understanding of the chronic mallet deformity, this section should be read **before** the section below.

Presentation
- A chronic mallet finger presents as absence of extension at the DIPJ.
- Patients present late for several reasons:
  - Pain in the joint.
  - Deformity of the flexed fingertip, which catches on things.
  - Appearance.

Examination
- Examine the PIPJ—loss of extension at DIPJ may be due to swan neck of the PIPJ, with dorsal displacement of lateral bands, and consequent loss of extension at the DIPJ.

Types of late mallet deformity
- Passively correctable deformity (+/– fracture).
- Fixed deformity (+/– fracture).
- Established secondary osteoarthritis.

Treatment of late mallet deformity
Extensor tendon (+/– small avulsion flake only), no significant fracture, no OA, no swan neck
- Tighten extensor tendon;
  - Either 'reef' technique
  - Or resect scar, with end-to-end repair.
- Insert K-wire across DIPJ for 4–6 weeks.
- Immobilize using splint for 6–8 weeks.

Swan neck, passively correctable, no fracture of the P3, no OA of DIPJ or PIPJ
- Oblique retinacular ligament reconstruction with free tendon graft (Thompson).

Displaced Type 4C or 4D fracture
- Arthrodesis of DIPJ if symptomatic.

Established secondary osteoarthritis
- Arthrodesis of DIPJ if symptomatic.

Chronic boutonnière lesion

Acute boutonnière deformity is covered in finger boutonnière lesion (Zone III, PIPJ) p. 427.

Causes
- Untreated injury to central slip of extensor mechanism.
  - Closed avulsion of central slip.
  - Closed avulsion of central slip with avulsion fracture.
  - Laceration of central slip.
  - Volar dislocation of PIPJ with avulsion of central slip insertion into P2.

- Attrition rupture of central slip.
  - Osteoarthritis
  - Rheumatoid, or other inflammatory arthritis.

Mechanism of the chronic boutonnière deformity

- An untreated acute boutonnière will develop into a fixed deformity:
  - The central slip (if present) continues to lengthen.
  - The dorsal transverse retinacular ligaments continue to lengthen.
  - The volar transverse retinacular ligaments tighten.
  - The lateral bands become fixed **volar** to the PIPJ axis, and shorten.
  - The oblique retinacular ligaments thicken and shorten.
  - Secondary joint changes develop.
- Both the flexors and extensor mechanism flex the PIPJ:
  - FDS and FDP flex the PIPJ.
  - The extensor mechanism also flexes the PIPJ, as the lateral bands are now volar to the PIPJ axis.

Classification of the chronic boutonnière deformity

- There are three stages:

Stage 1
- Dynamic imbalance.
- Passively supple.
- Lateral bands subluxed volarwards, but not adherent.

Stage 2
- Cannot be corrected passively.
- Thickened, shortened lateral bands.
- No secondary joint changes.

Stage 3
- Stage 2 with secondary joint changes.

Treatment of the chronic boutonnière deformity

- The best treatment is to recognize the problem and prevent the development of a chronic boutonnière.
- Many respond to intensive therapy, which will often produce a better result than surgery.
- Surgery is difficult, although possible.

Non-operative

Therapy is by a combination of exercises and splinting.
There are two important exercises;
- Active assisted PIPJ extension stretches tight volar structures.
  - This causes the lateral bands to move dorsally, and puts the lateral bands and oblique retinacular ligaments under tension.
  - This will increase the tenodesis effect across the DIPJ into hyperextension.
- Forced flexion at the DIPJ while the PIPJ is held at 0° (or as near to 0° as the joint will allow).
  - This stretches the lateral bands and oblique retinacular ligaments to their normal length, to allow normal flexion at the DIPJ.
- Splints. Use a combination of active and static splints during the day, and static splints at night.

Operative
- Surgeons should be aware that even careful surgery may fail, and progressive attenuation may compromise a good early result.
- Consider the following when planning surgery:
  - These procedures are difficult and should only be attempted by experienced (not occasional) hand surgeons.
  - Many patients with a boutonnière deformity have good function, especially in flexion, with good grip. Ensure you do not downgrade their function by surgery.
  - Passively correctable, chronic boutonnière deformities usually respond to non-operative treatment.
  - The patient must be compliant with several months of hand therapy.
  - If the joint is stiff, this must be released as a first stage. The extensor mechanism may rebalance following joint release, obviating the need for a secondary boutonnière correction procedure.
  - If there is established OA, perform extensor rebalancing with an arthroplasty, or an arthrodesis.

Extensor tenotomy (Eaton and Littler) (Fig. 13.11)
- Dorsal midline incision over PIPJ.
- Divide the extensor mechanism transversely.
  - Over the middle and proximal third of the middle phalanx
  - Distal to the dorsal transverse retinacular ligaments
- Do not divide the oblique retinacular ligaments.
- The lateral bands retract proximally so the crux between them centralizes, acting as a central slip. The intact oblique retinacular ligament maintains extension of the DIP as a fixed tether in front of the axis of the PIPJ and behind the axis of the DIPJ.
- This can be augmented by the *Littler* split lateral band technique if the central slip insertion into the base of the P2 is attenuated.
  - The lateral bands are rolled dorsally, and sutured to the central slip insertion.
- Splint PIPJ straight, and allow active flexion of DIPJ.

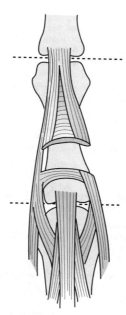

Fig. 13.11. Eaton–Littler tenotomy.

Free tendon graft
If the central slip and lateral bands are inadequate, use the free tendon graft technique described above.

Swan neck

- This is hyperextension at the PIPJ with flexion at the DIPJ.
- Initially this is an imbalance, which occurs during full active finger extension.
- The dynamic imbalance can progress to a fixed deformity with joint changes.

Causes of swan neck deformity

- Volar plate laxity at PIPJ.
- Spasticity.
  - Stroke
  - Cerebral palsy
- Rheumatoid arthritis
- Fractures of P2 healed in hyperextension.
- Mallet deformity of DIPJ with laxity of volar plate at PIPJ.

Non-operative treatment
- The swan neck deformity does not respond well to non-operative splinting techniques. The volar late laxity persists, along with PIPJ and DIPJ imbalance, to maintain the deformity.
- Splinting may help to correct PIPJ contractures or intrinsic tightness

Operative treatment
- Consider the whole hand when planning a swan neck correction; where there is a cause in addition to isolated volar plate laxity (see list above) this should be corrected.

Spasticity
- Treat the neurological condition if possible.
- Consider anti-spasm drugs (e.g. baclofen) and *Botulinum* toxin
- Tendon transfers.
- Arthrodesis of the PIPJ.

Rheumatoid arthritis
- Correct tendon imbalance or flexion contracture at MCPJ before treating swan neck.

Fracture of P2 in hyperextension
- Osteotomy to correct length and alignment allows rebalance of the extensor mechanism.

Mallet finger
- Correction of the mallet deformity will correct the PIPJ extensor tone and the swan neck deformity.

Volar plate laxity at PIPJ
- Surgical correction involves rebalancing of the extensor mechanism, with correction of volar plate laxity at the PIPJ.
- Significant joint changes must be treated to regain passive ROM before specific correction of the swan neck deformity.
- There are two main techniques for reconstruction:
  - Oblique retinacular ligament reconstruction
  - FDS tenodesis at the PIPJ

Oblique retinacular ligament reconstruction using lateral band (Littler)
- Ulnar dorsolateral approach.
- Detach ulnar lateral band proximally at level of MCPJ. Leave attached distally.
- Re-route the distally attached lateral band volar to Cleland's ligaments:
  - Dorsal to DIPJ
  - Volar to PIPJ
- Tension proximally to flex PIPJ at 20° and position DIPJ at 0°.
- Secure the lateral band proximally using one of the following methods:
  - Pass through a small window in the flexor tendon sheath at the level of the A2 pulley, and suture to itself
  - Use a drill hole in the proximal part of the P1.
  - Use a micro bone anchor in the proximal part of the P1.

Oblique retinacular ligament reconstruction with free tendon graft (Thompson)

- Use the same exposure as for the lateral band technique.
- Use PL (or other free graft) instead of the lateral band.
- Secure distally through the P3.
- Pass the graft from distal surface of P3, around P2 on the volar aspect of the PIPJ (deep to the NVBs), to the opposite side of the proximal P1.
- Secure proximally into P1.

FDS tenodesis (Littler)

- Uses a slip of FDS to make a 'check-rein' for the PIPJ to prevent hyperextension.
- It does not rebalance the extensor mechanism at the DIPJ (and may not correct the extensor lag at the DIPJ) so best for isolated palmar plate laxity.
- Use Bruner zig-zag incisions over the P1 and P2.
- Make a window in the flexor tendon sheath at the distal edge of the A2 pulley.
- Retract a slip of FDS, and divide it as proximally as you can (so it is distally based).
- Pass the slip of FDS through a volar-to-dorsal drill hole in the P1 and tension to flex PIPJ at 20°.
- Alternatively, pass the slip around the A2 pulley (proximal to distal) and suture to itself.

Postoperative care

- Splint for 4 weeks (+/− K-wire across PIPJ).
- Start gentle short arc active movement with dorsal splint to block full extension.
- Increase range over next 6 weeks
- Joint will be flexed at 5–10° at PIPJ because of tenodesis effect of correction—do not try to extend to 0°.

Complications

- Stretching or rupture of tenodesis with recurrence of swan neck deformity.
- Tenodesis too tight producing PIPJ flexion deformity (and potentially boutonnière).
- Loss of joint mobility due to scarring around flexor tendons (especially after FDS tenodesis).

Tendon pulley rupture

A2 rupture

Open injury

- Associated with burst fracture and damage to flexor tendon sheath, and sometimes tendon laceration.
- When there is a fracture, rupture of the pulley mechanism and flexor tendon sheath, and division of the tendon, it may be better to insert a silastic tendon spacer during the initial surgery. These injuries stick, and are very difficult to rehabilitate.

Closed pulley rupture

- Seen in elite rock climbers, gymnasts.
- Usually A2 pulley, occasionally A4.
- Ring and middle fingers most frequently affected

Investigation of closed pulley rupture

- X-ray to exclude fracture
- USS to image pulley system
- MRI:
  - T1 sequence can image dehiscence of tendon from bone
  - T2 sequence demonstrates tenosynovitis.

Treatment of closed pulley rupture

- Mostly conservative by hand therapists
- Non-steroidal anti-inflamatories
- Short period of rest +/− immobilization
- Taping:
  - 1.5cm tape over A2 pulley provides protection up to force of 500 Newtons
- Graduated return to easy activities, using taping and protection with pulley rings for 6–8 weeks.
- Return to full activities in 3 months, with taping for protection for further 6 months.
- Surgical reconstruction
  - for failed conservative treatment
  - delayed presentation
  - wrap extensor retinaculum graft, synorial ride towards tendon, around proximal phayarx
  - rehabilitate with tape and graduated return to activity

Attrition rupture

- Unreduced fractures and fixation plates
  - EPL over distal radius
  - EDC/EIP over distal radius
  - EDC/EDM over distal ulna
  - FPL over distal radius
- OA ulnar head (Vaughan–Jackson syndrome)
- OA radiocarpal joint or STT joint (Mannerfelt lesion)

Rehabilitation of flexor tendon repairs

Therapist must have a clear understanding of:
- Physiology
- Biomechanics
- Tendon and soft tissue healing
- Operative procedure performed
- Surgeons preferences
- Anatomy including the level of injury

Aim
- Preserve joint mobility
- Encourage development of strong tendon
- Tendon glides freely
- Normal tendon function—without hindrance

Factors affecting outcome
- Experience of therapist
- Quality of splints
- Surgical expertise (careful handling/careful repair/type of suture/sheath closure—may stop triggering)
- Patient's age
- General health of patient
- Patients rate and quality of scar formation
- Patient motivation
- Socio-economic factors

Flexor tendon excursion
- As a tendon glides it encounters a certain amount of normal resistance from surrounding tissues.

Normal excursion
- MCPJ produces no relative motions of the tendons within the sheath.
- DIP joint motion produces excursion of the FDP through FDS of 1mm for 10° of flexion.
- PIP joint produces excursion of FDP and FDS of 1.3mm for 10° of flexion.

Excursion after injury
For the first few weeks after repair, resistance is increased by:
- post-traumatic oedema
- post-surgical oedema
- lacerated tissues
- extra bulk of sutures
- bulk of scar formation

Care must be taken to allow for this increased resistance.

Postoperatively, excursion decreases:
- DIPJ: 10° flexion produces 0.3mm excursion of FDP through FDS
- PIP J: 10° flexion produces 1.2mm excursion of FDP and FDS

Treatment options
- Initial immobilization
- Early controlled mobilization
- Early active mobilization

Immobilization

For non-compliant patients and children. Complete immobilization of tendon repair for 3–4 weeks, before beginning active and passive mobilization. Dorsal blocking splint (DBS). A palmar splint provides resistance which would encourage tendon rupture.

Splint
Wrist: debatable. 10–30° flexion; neutral or slight extension (to reduce power generated in flexing fingers)
MCPJ: 60° flexion
PIPJ/DIPJ: extended

Advantages
- Decreases the risk of gap formation
- Reduces risk of inadvertent early extension causing rupture
- Minimizes therapist input

Disadvantages
- Healing is slowed by the absence of tension as a stimulus
- Slower return of strength
- Higher risk of adhesion formation

Early controlled mobilization

Implies passive mobilization of the flexor tendon within the first few days either manually or by dynamic flexion traction. About 4 weeks after the repair active motion can begin.

Advantages
- Inhibits restrictive adhesion formation,
- Promotes intrinsic healing and synovial diffusion
- Produces a stronger repair.

Regime options
- Kleinert
- Duran and Houser
- Modified Duran

1. Kleinert method
- Developed for zone 2 injuries
- Dynamic passive flexion using rubber bands
- Active extension

Splint
DBS with dynamic traction
Wrist: 45° flexion
MCPs: 40° flexion
PIPJ/DIPJ: neutral

Modifications
- Standard Kleinert splint does not flex DIP joint, therefore dynamic traction is now directed through a palmar pulley.
- Some believe that to achieve a better glide the IP joints should be strapped into extension at night.
- Some also believe that traction should be applied to all fingers.

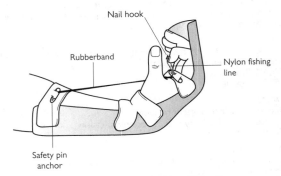

Nail hook

Rubberband

Nylon fishing line

Safety pin anchor

Fig. 13.12 Dynamic splinting for flexor tendon injury (Kleinert).

Exercises
- 0–4 weeks
  - Extension to the splint—20 repetitions hourly
  - Passive flexion with the rubber band
- 4–6 weeks:
  - Active flexion commenced.
- 6–8 weeks:
  - Resisted exercise begins.

2. Duran and Houser method
Controlled passive mobilization, originally for zone 2 and 3 repairs.
- Based on the principle that restrictive tendon adhesions can be prevented by passively moving the tendon through 3–5mm of excursion.
- Passive flexion and extension of the DIP joint with MCPs and PIPS in flexion moves an FDP repair distally away from an FDS repair.
- Passive motion of PIP joint with MCP and DIP joints held in flexion moves both repairs away from the injury site and from any surrounding tissues, to which adhesions may have occurred.

Splint
DBS with rubber bands
Wrist: 20° flexion
MCPs: relaxed position of flexion
PIPJ/DIPJ: allowing full IP extension

Exercise:
- 0–4 weeks
  - MCP and PIP joints held in flexion—DIP joint is passively extended
  - DIP and MCP joints held in flexion—PIP joint is passively extended

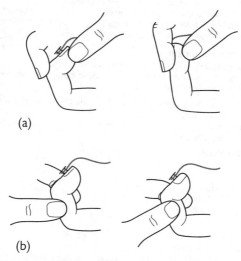

(a)

(b)

Fig. 13.13 Duran and Houser method of flexor tendon rehabilitation. (a) passive extension and flexion of the DIP joint with MCP and PIP flexion, (b) passive flexion and extension of the PIP joint with MCP and DIP flexion.

These exercises should be carried out twice daily, 6–8 repetitions for 4.5 weeks:
- 4.5 weeks:
  - Splint is removed and a wristband applied with rubber bands still attached, allowing for tenodesis exercises to be conducted.
- 7.5–8 weeks:
  - Resisted flexion starts.

3. Modified Duran
Uses active extension without rubber band resistance, which reduces the risk of flexion contracture.

Splint
DBS
Wrist: 30 flexion
MCPs: 40° flexion
PIPJ/DIPJ: strapped into extension between exercises and at night

Exercise
- Straps removed 1–2 hourly.
- Passive flexion.
- Active extension 5–20 repetitions.
- Exercises conducted 4–6 times daily.
- Wrist flexion is accompanied by finger extension.
- Passive mobilizations are still conducted.
- At the end of 3–4 weeks the protocols are very similar.
- Gentle active motion can be commenced.

Early active mobilization
- Mobilization of the repaired tendon within 48 hours.
- Active contraction of the involved flexor, within carefully prescribed limits.
- Used on recently injured tendons.

Various protocols have been devised and modified but have primarily been based on the following 2 regimes:
- Belfast regime
- Active hold/place hold

4. Belfast method
Splint
DBS
Wrist: 20° flexion
MCPs: 80–90° flexion
PIPJ/DIPJ: allowing full extension

Exercise
- 0–4 weeks:
  - Zone 3 injuries initiated 24 hours after repair
  - Zone 2 48 hours after repair to allow for postop oedema to subside.
  - 2 repetitions 4 hourly:
  - Full passive flexion
  - Full active flexion
  - Active extension
- 4–6 weeks:
  - Splint discontinued if tendon glide poor—5 weeks for most patients
  - 3 weeks after the splint has been discontinued residual flexion contractures can be dealt with.
  - Protected passive IP extension (MCPs held in flexion)
  - Continuation of existing exercises—with introduction of graded resistance
- Heavier use of hand at 8 weeks—full function by 12 weeks.

Active hold/place hold mobilization
Proponents attempt to quantify the amount of force/muscle tension of the flexors during passive and active mobilization and also against resistance.

For their EAM regime Strickland (1993)[1] and Cannon (1993)[2] concluded forces of 500g for FDP and 1500g for light grip—FDS is 15% that of FDP. Their protocol assumes that some margin must be allowed for oedema—they also rely on tensile strength of 2150 to 4300g during the 1st 3 weeks after repair (using a 4-strand suture).

This regime is classified as an 'active hold' protocol—digits are passively placed into flexion and the patient then maintains the flexion with gently muscle contraction.

Regime
- 0–4 weeks:
  - 2 splints provided:
  - 1. DBS:
  - Wrist: 20° flexion
  - MCPs: 50° flexion
  - PIPJ/DIPJ: neutral
  - 2. Exercise splint:
  - Hinged wrist that allows:
  - Full wrist flexion but limited extension to 30°
  - Full digit flexion and full IP extension
  - MP extension limited to 60°
- Exercise:
  - 15 repetitions hourly of:
  - PROM to PIP, DIP and entire digit
  - 25 repetitions of: place and hold digit flexion in tenodesis splint.

The patient actively extends the wrist and allows the digits to passively flex, maintaining digit flexion for 5 seconds. The patient then relaxes the wrist into flexion allowing the digits to extend.
- 4 weeks–7/8 weeks:
  - Tenodesis splint is discontinued, but DBS is used, except for tenodesis exercises.
  - Tenodesis exercises every 2 hours, plus active wrist and digit flexion and extension, avoiding simultaneous wrist and digit extension.
- 5–6 weeks
  - Blocking exercises/hook fists added, for tendon gliding.
- 7–8 weeks:
  - Splint discontinued
  - Progressive resistance commenced
  - No restrictions by 14 weeks.

1. Strickland JW (1993) Flexor tendon repair. Indiana method. *Indiana Hand Center Newsletter* **1**:1.
2. Cannon NM (1993) Post flexor tendon repair: motion protocol. *Indiana Hand Center Newsletter* **1**:13–18.

Strengthening flexor tendons

Gentle strengthening through light ADL is generally commenced at week 6/7

Resistance to FDS should begin early, as FDS does not pull through strongly in the full fist unless resisted.

Resistance can start with:
- Light prehension
- Isometric strengthening
- Sustained grasp activities
- Light ADL

Progressing AROM

Decision to progress is usually dependent upon the quality of the glide, which is measured through assessment/palpation and observation.

Rehabilitation of extensor tendon repairs

Treatment goals

- Prevent complete extensor tendon rupture
- Reduce swelling and pain
- Prevent lateral band subluxation
- Prevent oblique retinacular ligament contracture
- Restore active and passive ROM of MCP, PIP and DIP joint
- Maintain ROM of uninvolved joints
- Return to previous level of function

Boutonnière

Conservative management

- 6 weeks of dynamic PIP extension splintage (i.e. Capener)
- 3 weeks static immobilization of PIP (i.e. gutter splint or cylinder POP) joint followed by a further 3 weeks of dynamic PIP extension splintage.

Short arc motion regime

- Splints:
  - Dorsal-based thermoplastic splint maintaining PIP and DIP extension worn between exercises.
  - Exercise splint: volar splint moulded to permit 30° active PIP joint flexion and 25° of DIP joint flexion.
- Exercises:
  - Performed hourly.
  - Wrist held in 30° of flexion and the MCP joint in neutral or slight flexion.
  - With exercise splint in place the patient actively flexes the IP joints within the confines of the splint and actively extends to neutral.
  - 20 repetitions.
  - With the dorsal splint *in situ* the distal strap is removed and active DIP joint flexion is performed to maintain excursion of the lateral bands and the oblique retinacular ligament.
  - Composite flexion is permitted at the end of week 5.
  - Resisted ADL avoided until week 10.
- If no extensor lag develops then range of movement can be increased.
- Splintage is terminated after 6 weeks.

Surgical management:

- Primary repair
- 3 weeks static splintage followed by dynamic PIP joint extension splintage for a further 3 weeks

Complications

- Extension lag
- Hyperextension of DIP joint
- Persistent boutonniere deformity
- PIP joint oedema
- Joint stiffness
- Intrinsic tightness
- Tethering

Zones V– VII

Controversy over rehabilitation of the extensor tendons:
- immobilization.
- controlled early mobilization.

Immobilization
- Usually lasting 3–4 weeks, until scar-remodelling phase is established.
- Priorities:
  - Wound care
  - Oedema control
  - Proper postop immobilization to protect the repair
- Splinting:
  - Wrist: 30–45° extension
  - MCPJ: slight flexion
  - IPJ: neutral
- 0–4 weeks:
  - Total immobilization
- 4–6 weeks:
  - Splinting between exercise
- 6–8 weeks:
  - At night time only

For isolated injuries of EIP, EDM and EPL only the affected joint/digit needs to be immobilized. For EDC the therapist must consider the juncturae tendinum. If the repair is proximal to the interconnecting tendon all fingers should be splinted. However, if it is distal those fingers injured and the adjacent fingers should be splinted.

Exercise
- Active mobilization begins at 4 weeks:
  - Begin gently with the wrist in extension
  - Active and active assisted MCP extension
  - IPS—with wrist and MCPS held in extension
  - Composite flexion with wrist held in extension
  - Hook fist
- 6 weeks:
  - Full fist making
  - EDC gliding (starting in gentle fist and extending MCPS whilst maintaining IP flexion)
  - Light ADL commenced
  - Combined wrist and finger flexion
- 7–8 weeks:
  - Gentle passive flexion
  - Resisted extension

Controlled early mobilization
1. Dynamic extension splint (DES)
- Static splint for 2 weeks
- DES for 4 weeks (complicated to make)
  - Wrist 30° extension
  - MCPs neutral
  - IPs free

- Permits active flexion and passive extension
- Prevents stiffness and adhesions
- Light ADL commenced at 4 weeks
- 4–8 weeks graded activity
- 8–12 weeks strengthening

2. Early active mobilization
- Palmar splint:
  - Wrist: 30–45° extension
  - MCPs: 0–50° flexion
  - IPs: extended
- 1st day postop: controlled active mobilization begun.
  - Two exercises are taught:
  - Combined IP and MCP extension
  - MCP extension with IP joint flexion
  - 4 × 6-hourly
- 5 weeks on:
  - Splint discarded during the day but continued at night for 2 weeks more
  - Gentle flexion MCPs and IP joints, steadily increased to full flexion and power grip
  - Light ADL commenced at 4 weeks
  - 4–8 weeks graded activity
  - 8–12 weeks strengthening
- Results: 92% excellent/good results by week 6 compared with DES.

Benefits:
- Easier to use
- Easier to design
- Cheaper to make
- Low-cost maintenance

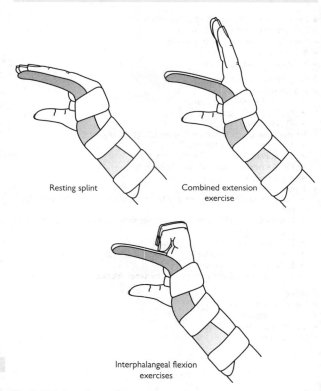

Resting splint

Combined extension exercise

Interphalangeal flexion exercises

Fig. 13.14 Splint and exercise for extensor tendon injury.

Extensor injuries to the thumb

Zone TI
Splint IPJ 8 weeks in slight hyperextension.

Zone TII
Hand-based splint immobilizing MCPJ and IPJ joint straight. AROM initiated at 3 weeks starting with 25–30° flexion and gently increasing ROM over next 3 weeks. Splint protection for 6 weeks.

Zone TIII & TIV
Thumb MCPJ: 0° and slight abduction
Wrist: 30° extension

Zone TV
Dense adhesions frequently limit excursion of EPL at the retinacular level

Improper immobilization will create stiff MCPJ, 1st webspace contracture and poor tendon glide.

Extensor excursion

Tendon migration necessary to maintain functional glide and to stimulate cellular activity may be in the range of 3–5mm.

Early active and passive motion allowing 5mm of excursion is successful with extensor tendon repairs in zone V–VII and TIV–TV and 4mm of active excursion in zone III–IV.

EPL

Excursions for EPL vary in the literature from 25–60mm. Calculating the excursion is further complicated by the oblique course the takes at Lister's tubercle and by the different movements at the CMC joint.

Work-related upper limb disorders (WRULD)

Introduction

The Health and Safety Executive (HSE) in 2006/07:

- estimated that 426 000 people in the UK believed that they were suffering from a musculoskeletal condition affecting mainly the upper limbs or the neck, with symptoms apparent during their current or past work.
- This equates to approximately 3.5 million working days that are lost each year,
- Each person taking an estimated 13.4 days off work .

WRULD can form a significant proportion of referrals to a hand clinic and given the ambiguity that surrounds the definition it is essential that the correct diagnosis is made.

Sometimes work factors are important. There generally has to be a combination of factors

- Load
- Unaccustomed use
- Frequency
- Abnormal posture

Definition

WRULD

Useful term which, without intrinsic implication of blame, is applied to conditions which are apparent at work. Alternative terms should be avoided.

Repetitive strain injury (RSI)

This is a misnomer. It is accusative and presumptive of causation. There is no clear definition of 'overuse' and no good evidence that 'overuse' is always harmful. Human tissues are designed to respond to use, not to degrade with use—that is why athletes train. Human structures do not, in general, alter their length with load (the mechanical definition of strain). The term 'injury' implies that the patient has been harmed by a negligent act of omission or commission by an employer; there is rarely a good case for such harm.

Simply because symptoms are apparent at work does not mean that work caused them. If a postman has a stone in his shoe then his work will expose pain from that stone. His work did not put the stone there. If a patient dies in bed, the bed did not kill him; he just happened to be in bed when a medical event occurred.

The use of the diagnosis 'RSI' can lead to a trail of social and psychological suffering underpinned by an unfounded or weak medicolegal premise. Furthermore, it is all too easy to use a fatuous term like RSI and thus deny the patient the chance of a clear diagnosis of a treatable condition.

Cumulative trauma disorder (CTD)

Equally devoid of logical support as a diagnosis.

Occupational overuse syndrome

Rather less perjorative but still implies causation without justification.

New definitions

An alternative newer term is Work-Relevant Upper Limb Symptoms which is not accusatory or presumptive of cause nor implies pathology yet acknowledges the influence of symptoms on working ability.

Classification

Since WRULD is a vague term, it is essential to make a clear distinction between conditions that have a specific and recognized medical diagnosis, and the more vague/diffuse group of conditions, which lack a clear diagnosis.

Type I

Localized, well-defined conditions with established pathologies and aetiology:
- Carpal tunnel syndrome
- Tendonitis
- De Quervain's
- Tennis elbow
- Tenosynovitis
- Trigger finger
- Ganglion
- Frozen shoulder
- Raynaud's syndrome

There is little, if any, evidence, to suggest that work causes any of the above conditions.

Type II

Diffuse group of conditions characterized by a variety of symptoms:
- Ache
- Pain
- Cramps
- Numbness
- Tingling
- Heaviness
- Tightness

Symptoms vary in location, intensity and nature. Diagnosis is extremely difficult as the conditions largely escape clinical tests and sophisticated medical investigations.

Cause

The actual cause of Type II WRULD is still unknown, however several theories if not risk factors have been identified:

Static muscle loading

Muscular activity that focuses on maintaining a certain position with little or no movement. Static work has been shown to impede blood flow. When muscles contract they compress the blood vessels which feed them. If static activity is maintained for a significant period of time blood supply is reduced and waste products accumulate. This results in muscle fatigue and discomfort (which is usually transient).

Unaccustomed repetitive use

Repetition of certain activities causing overuse of specific muscles may result in tissue failure. Fatigue may initially occur and where activity is not changed then aches, pains and injury may result. An example is the pain we feel in muscles after running too far or too fast. Another example is peritendonitis crepitans or de Quervain's in which a period of unaccustomed use such as rowing or trimming a hedge can cause inflammation of the tenosynovium in the 2nd and 1st dorsal compartments respectively.

Stress
Stress at work and other psychological factors may play a role in the onset of WRULD. Stress can cause increased muscle tension; perhaps this can sensitize the nervous system and increases the perception of pain.

Common work stress:
- Workload
- Job insecurity
- Lack of job description
- No recognition
- Poor working relationships
- Demands to work harder, more intensely or for longer

The psychological aspects are complex but very relevant. Unhappy working conditions and a conviction that a patient has been injured, compounded by a medico-legal claim, may alter the way in which an individual can cope with their experience of the aches and pains of normal life.

Ergonomic
- Poor posture
- Repetitive tasks
- Work environment:
  - Noise
  - Temperature
  - Workstation set-up
- Muscle loading/contact stresses

Malingering
True malinguering is rare but in some patients there are likely to be aspects of secondary gain for *social reasons* (e.g. to change work, extra help at work or home), *psychological* reasons (sympathy) and *financial* reasons (compensation claims). Characterized by delayed recovery, exaggerated symptoms, unlikely patterns of symptoms and physical signs.

Incidence

Gender
The HSE (2006/07) reported that males had a higher prevalence than women.

Age
55–64 years for males.
55–59 for women.

Occupation
- HSE (2006/07) report that the incidence of musculoskeletal disorders is statistically significantly greater in:
  - skilled construction and building trades
  - skilled agricultural trades, health and social welfare
  - transport and mobile machine drivers and operators.

- However, these occupations may require the use of the arms and thus expose symptoms that other workers would not realize they are prone to. Causation is not implied.
- It can be argued there is a 'survivor effect' such that those who have symptoms may change jobs, and so the prevalence of WRULD may be potentially even higher in certain occupations since a proportion will have left that occupation because of symptoms, leaving 'survivors' less prone to such symptoms.

Diagnosis

To date there are no standardized objective diagnostic tools to confirm a diagnosis of type II WRULD. Diagnosis typically is based on exclusions or the basis that the condition is exposed during or following a repetitive task and is relieved by rest.

Management

The application of unhelpful terms like RSI can do nothing but harm. The superimposition of (often unjustified) blame, conflict with employer, legal wrangling will not help patients to cope; they are more likely to cope if they understand that work is exposing the symptoms and that they can be controlled. If not, then the patient should be encouraged to find a more suitable job.

Unfortunately many patients suffering with WRULD do no seek medical intervention until their symptoms start to significantly interfere with their social or work life. Early intervention typically produces the quickest and most favourable results and is often a combination of several treatment modalities. Treatment should be tailored to individual requirements in terms of their clinical presentation.

Rehabilitation

Unfortunately there is no single treatment approach. Keller et al. (1998)[1] recommends three-phase programme to pace the treatment:

Phase 1—symptom control
- Educational
- Postural retraining
- Body movement awareness
- Ergonomics

1. Keller et al. (1998) Resetitive strain injury in computer keyboard users. *J Hand Therapy* **11**: 9–26.

- Pain management techniques (thermal modalities, soft tissue massage)
- Joint mobilization
- Gentle stretching
- Nerve gliding
- Home exercise programme

Phase 2—strengthening (commenced once symptom control achieved)
- Strengthening programme to rebalance muscles
- Improve joint function
- Improve soft tissue extensibility
- Improve muscle tone
- Improve nerve mobility

Phase 3—conditioning
- Maintaining changes
- Application of principles at work

Ergonomics
Ergonomic principles include:
- Fitting the person to the job, and
- Fitting the job to the person
- Good posture
- Taking regular breaks
- Work pacing
- Changes in job tasks

A work place assessment will highlight the abilities of the patient and the demands placed on them in work, including work activities/load and work-station set up.

Key workstation ergonomics
- Workplace organization:
  - Sufficient desk area to position keyboard and mouse
  - Place items used regularly within easiest reach
  - Work pacing
- Chair:
  - Ensure the chair is comfortable
  - Thighs need to be horizontal
  - Ensure support is given to the lower back
  - Ensure feet are flat on the floor
  - Change sitting position regularly
- Keyboard and mouse:
  - Position keyboard to ensure arms are relaxed and forearms are horizontal
  - Shoulder relaxed
  - Wrists in neutral/slight extension
  - Allow hands to glide over the keyboard
  - Place mouse close to keyboard
- Display:
  - Position to minimize glare/reflections
  - Top of the screen should be just below eye level
  - Maintain a comfortable viewing position, about 20–24inches
  - Keep head upright

- Adjust contrast and brightness according to room changes
- Palm rest:
  - Do not use whilst keying but between periods of keying
- Keyboard support:
  - Maintain wrist in neutral
- Footrest:
  - Keep feet supported
  - Should tilt front to back
- Lumbar support:
  - Provides additional support

Prognosis in WRULD

The majority of patients with WRULD make a good recovery if treated as soon as symptoms commence; it probably helps if terms like RSI are avoided. However, some patients may develop symptoms that take longer to resolve or may be left with debilitating symptoms, which may require lifestyle changes.

It is characteristic of 'injured' tissues to heal—patients must be reassured about this. There is no biological reason why long-term damage has been caused.

The presence of litigation is a very poor prognostic factor.

Miscellaneous tendon disorders

Saddle syndrome

- Rare condition.
- Follows crush injury to hand or can be spontaneous.
- Painful excursion between the intrinsic muscles and the intermetacarpal ligament (between the metacarpal necks).

Treatment

- Intrinsic stretching
- Ultrasound
- Cortisone injection
- Surgical release

Congenital anomalies

- Common, rarely cause symptoms of pain or functional impairment.
- Asymptomatic anomalies may cause confusion in the interpretation of the physical examination.

Palmaris longus

- Absent in about 15%
- Implicated in carpal tunnel syndrome as it is absent in only 3% of patients with this condition
- Useful as a tendon transfer or free tendon graft

Flexor pollicis longus

- *Lindburg–Comstock anomaly*: a tendinous slip or tenosynovial adhesion connecting the flexor pollicis longus tendon to the flexor digitorum profundus tendon of the index finger.
- Found in 25% of cadavers.
- Causes pain by restricting independent movement of the index and thumb.
- Pathognomonic sign is coincidental flexion of the index finger when the thumb is flexed actively; pain in the wrist if flexion of the index is blocked as the thumb is flexed.
- Usually only problematic in musicians.
- Surgical division of the connection is usually curative.

Flexor digitorum superficialis

- FDS of index, middle, and ring fingers have individual muscle bellies and can act independently.
- The little flexor digitorum superficialis tendon:
  - may be linked to the flexor digitorum superficialis of the ring finger, leading to uncertainty when interpreting physical signs after lacerations of the little finger
  - 60% of little fingers have an independent FDS
  - 20% of the little flexor FDS is linked to the ring FDS
  - 20% have no discernible function of the little FDS
  - Cadaver dissections suggest that the FDS tendon is generally present but may be linked to the little FDP tendon
  - Linkage of the ring and little FDS tendons can be shown by the standard and modified flexor digitorum superficialis tests: the little

finger cannot be flexed actively at the proximal interphalangeal joint whilst the other digits are held extended.

Abductor pollicis longus
- Considerable variation in the number of tendon slips and their insertion.
- Slips may attach to:
  - APB
  - Trapezium
  - Base of the thumb metacarpal.
- The tendon may fuse with the tendon of extensor pollicis brevis.

Extensor pollicis brevis
- 30–60% of wrists, the extensor pollicis brevis tendon runs in a subcompartment of the first extensor compartment
- Symptoms of de Quervain's syndrome may persist if a subcompartment is overlooked at the time of release

Extensor digitorum communis
- Many variations
- Variations account for the variable deficit that results from rupture or laceration of the extensor digiti minimi.
- Rupture of extensor digitorum minimi, which may herald rupture of extensor digitorum communis tendons in rheumatoid arthritis, may pass unnoticed unless independent extension of the little finger is tested.

Tenosynovitis and tendonitis

Terminology

Tendonitis
Inflammation of the tendon or tendon insertion.

Tenosynovitis
Inflammation of the tendon lining.

Presentation
- Recognizable and reproducible physical signs:
  - Swelling
  - Tenderness
  - Crepitus along the line of the tendon or sheath
  - Specific tenderness at a tendon insertion or along its course
  - Pain on resisted active contraction
  - Pain on passive stretching.
- Characteristic pathological changes on histology.
- In the absence of these features, and especially in the context of pain in the workplace, it is inappropriate to assign these diagnoses.
- Terms such as forearm pain or non-specific arm pain should be used when the symptoms and signs are poorly localized.

Types of tenosynovitis
There are many causes.
- Acute gout
- Sarcoidosis
- Amyloid
- Calcium pyrophosphate deposition
- Unaccustomed overuse
- Rheumatoid disease
- Infection:
  - Pyogenic
  - Fungal
  - Mycobacterium
- Retained foreign body:
  - Foreign material within the tendon sheath may incite an inflammatory response in the absence of infection.
  - The thorns of the blackthorn tree (*Prunus spinosa*) and Pyrocantha species are particularly liable to cause a subacute aseptic inflammation of joint or tendon sheath.

de Quervain's syndrome

Anatomy
First dorsal compartment of the wrist, containing the tendons of APL and APB.

Aetiology
- The cause is unknown.
- Occurs spontaneously
- More often in females than males,
- May arise during or just after pregnancy.

Clinical features

- Pain during use of the thumb
- Loss of ulnar deviation of the wrist
- Triggering of the abductor pollicis longus tendon seen occasionally
- Pain on resisted active extension of the thumb
- Swelling and tenderness over the first compartment
- Positive Finkelstein's test:
  - Reproduction of pain by 'grasping the patient's thumb and quickly abducting the hand ulnarward'
  - Another test, originally described by Eichhoff but often attributed erroneously to Finkelstein, deviates the wrist ulnarward while the thumb is held in the palm beneath the flexed fingers
- Differential diagnosis includes:
  - intersection syndrome
  - arthritis of the trapeziometacarpal, scaphotrapezial, or radioscaphoid joints.

Management

- Rest, analgesics, splintage
- Steroid injection:
  - effective in at least 70%
  - avoid subcutaneous extravasation of long-acting steroid, which can produce an unsightly patch of atrophic skin and subcutaneous tissue.
- Operative release:
  - Transverse skin incision gives good exposure and a better scar than a longitudinal incision
  - Crucial to protect the superficial radial nerve; a neuroma can be very troublesome
  - Release of the retinaculum toward the dorsal edge of the compartment leaves a palmar ridge of retinacular tissue that may help to prevent the uncommon complication of palmar subluxation of the abductor pollicis longus tendon on wrist flexion
  - Explore for any subcompartments (30–60% of first dorsal compartments have a septum that separates APL from EPB).

Intersection syndrome

Alternative names

- Cross-over syndrome
- Peritendinitis crepitans

Aetiology

- Tenosynovitis of the radial wrist extensor tendons in the second extensor compartment. Swelling cannot distend the firm roof of the compartment and thus presents just proximal to it, where the abductor pollicis longus and extensor pollicis brevis tendons cross over.
- Originally thought to be bursitis or tendinitis due to friction between the abductor pollicis longus and extensor pollicis brevis muscle bellies and the radial wrist extensor tendons.
- Probably the only tendon disorder for which a consistent association with overuse has been demonstrated.

Clinical features
- Pain, swelling, and, in severe cases, crepitus where the abductor pollicis longus and extensor pollicis brevis muscle bellies run obliquely across the longitudinally orientated second dorsal compartment (about 5cm proximal to the radial styloid)
- Proximal to the site affected in de Quervain's syndrome.

Treatment
- Rest
- Splintage
- Steroid injection
- Operative release of the second extensor compartment

Flexor carpi radialis

Anatomy
- FCR tendon passes in front of the wrist through a fibro-osseous tunnel lined with synovium
- Runs past the ulnar side of the tubercle of the scaphoid
- Along a groove in the medial face of the trapezium
- Inserts onto the base of the second metacarpal

Clinical features
- Spontaneous pain related to FCR tendon may arise spontaneously.
- Typically in females of late middle age (in whom it may be associated with scaphotrapezial osteoarthritis).
- Occasionally be associated with activities requiring strenuous flexion of the wrist.
- Pain localized to the tendon at the wrist, aggravated by resisted flexion of the wrist.
- Tenderness and swelling of the tendon sheath.
- The differential diagnosis includes:
  - de Quervain's syndrome
  - palmar wrist ganglion
  - scaphotrapezial osteoarthritis.

Treatment
- Rest, splintage, analgesics
- Steroid injection of the sheath
- Operative release of the sheath is occasionally required

Other tendons
- Several other tendons, including:
  - EPL ('drummer's thumb')
  - EPB
  - EIP
  - FCU
  - ECU
- Diagnosis is made from the findings of pain, swelling, local tenderness, and pain on active resisted tendon action.
- The management follows the lines described above.

Trigger finger and thumb

Trigger finger and trigger thumb in adults
Cause
- Nodular thickening of the flexor tendon, accompanied by stenosis of the first annular (A1) pulley of the tendon sheath at the level of the metacarpophalangeal joint.
- Much more common in diabetes, rheumatoid.
- Rare associations: mucopolysaccharidoses, amyloidosis.

Clinical features
- Most common in middle-aged females. Usually spontaneous.
- Ring finger, middle finger, and thumb most frequently affected.
- Clicking or locking of the interphalangeal joints of the fingers or the thumb during flexion and extension.
- Often most troublesome on waking.
- Although locking appears to affect the PIPJ, the pathology is more proximal at the level of the MCPJ
- Tenderness over the tendon sheath at the level of the MCP
- Thumb occasionally locks in extension.
- Persistent locking of the finger may lead to a fixed flexion contracture at the PIPJ.

Treatment
- Mild triggering may resolve spontaneously.
- Splintage of the interphalangeal joints in extension at night improves locking on waking and may suffice in mild cases.
- Steroid injection of the tendon sheath cures about 70%:
  - less likely to be effective in diabetes.
- Surgical release of the A1 pulley: 95%+ success.
- Percutaneous needle release equally effective, safe, shortens recovery.
- Long-standing cases with persistent PIP contracture and tendon thickening: resection of the ulnar slip of FDS.
- Release of the A1 pulley is contraindicated in rheumatoid (may exacerbate a tendency to ulnar drift). Synovectomy and resection of one slip of FDS is preferred.

Trigger thumb in children
See p. 545.

Trigger finger in children
See p. 545.

Trigger wrist

Cause
- Thickening of the flexor tendons or synovium impedes gliding at the wrist.
- Occasionally discrete mass or extensor tendon pathology.

Clinical features
- On flexion of the fingers, crunching is felt just proximal to the carpal tunnel. The fingers may lock in flexion or clunk as the hand is opened.
- Associated with median nerve compression.

Treatment
- Ultrasound scan or MRI to exclude space occupying lesion or demonstrate tenosynovitis
- Surgical release

Ulnar corner

Anatomy

Anatomy of stability

Bone

Ulnar head—270° cartilage, articulates with sigmoid notch of distal radius. Variable concavity of sigmoid notch = variable contribution to stability and variable exposure to ulnar corner symptoms after distal radius malunion.

TFCC

Triangular fibrocartilage complex. Primary stabilizer of DRUJ. Components: central disc (avascular, aneural); ulnar collateral ligament; anterior radius–ulnar ligament; posterior radius–ulnar ligament; meniscal homologue; underside of ECU sheath; ulnalunate ligament; ulnatriquetral ligament.

Ligaments

Ulna-otriquetral ligament and ulna-olunate ligament: anterior wall of ulnocarpal joint, blend perpendicularly proximally into the anterior radioulnar ligament (i.e. part of TFCC).

Others

Interosseous membrane: radius proximal to ulna distal.
Muscles: several muscles cross from radius to ulnar or vv.
DRUJ capsule: minor stabilizer. Contraction after injury limits rotation.
PRUJ capsule and annular ligament.
NB deletion of ulnar head will destabilize the quadrilateral forearm joint; avoid unless no other option.

Anatomy of rotation

Ulna is main load-bearing bone of the forearm, radius suspended by interosseous membrane, PRUJ—capsule and annular ligament, DRUJ—capsule and TFCC. Radius rotates around ulna—ulna remains fixed.

Ulnar head translates and rotates against sigmoid notch. Variability—planar notch—more translation (and less prone to symptoms of dorsal malunion of distal radius).

More supination with elbow flexed, more pronation with elbow extended.
Radius relatively long in supination, relatively short in pronation.

Muscles

Biceps (musculocutaneous nerve) powerful supinator in flexion
Supinator (radial nerve) more powerful in extension
Pronator quadratus (anterior interosseous nerve)
Pronator teres (median nerve) more powerful in extension

Kinetics

Ulnar head trasnmits load transversely to sigmoid notch, especially in miid-rotation.

Distal surface of ulna articulates with underside of lunate, lunatetriquetrum and triquetrum, via the central part of the TFCC. Load spread by TFCC.

About 80% of load transmitted across radiocarpal joint, 20% across ulnocarpal joint.

Decreasing variance by 2.5mm decreases ulnocarpal load to 5%; increasing by 2.5mm increases ulnocarpal load to 40%.

Pronation increases ulnocarpal load to about 35% (as ulna relatively long in pronation since radius obliquely crosses forearm).

Ulnar deviation increases ulnocarpal load to about 25 to 30%.

Causes of ulnar corner pain

Tendon

ECU tendonitis
ECU instability
FCU tendonitis

Bone

Hook of hamate fracture

Joint

- Mid-carpal instability
- Lunate-triquetrum instability
- Radiocarpal joint:
  - Ulnar translation of carpus
- Distal radioulnar joint:
  - Osteoarthritis
  - Rheumatoid arthritis
  - Instability
- Ulnocarpal joint:
  - TFCC perforation
  - Ulnocarpal instability
  - Ulnocarpal impaction
  - Styloid-carpal impaction
- TFCC:
  - Perforation
  - Tear
  - Crystal deposition
- Pisotriquetral joint
  - Arthritis
  - Instability
  - Ganglion
- Fifth and fourth carpometacarpal—Hamate arthritis
- Lunate—Hamate arthritis

Nerve

- Ulnar nerve—Guyon's canal
- Cubital tunnel syndrome
- Cervical radiculopathy
- Neuroma dorsal branch of ulnar nerve

Vascular

- Hypothenar hammer syndrome

Tendon

ECU tendonitis

Can occur spontaneously or following unaccustomed use. Occasionally due to previous ulnar styloid fracture or more likely surgical fixation.

Symptoms and signs

Pain aggravated by grip and ulnar deviation in dorso-ulnar corner. On palpation: swelling, tenderness and crepitus over ECU.

Treatment

Rest, NSAID, cortisone injection. Surgery rarely needed. Remove metalwork from ulnar styloid. Release and z-widening of ECU sheath with synovectomy.

ECU instability

Anatomy

The ECU tendon runs in a fibro-osseous tunnel over the dorso-ulnar corner of the ulnar head. The sheath is complex at this site, forming an important component of the TFCC and contributor to the stability of the ulnar head. As the forearm rotates, the ECU tendon translates (dorso-radialwards on supination, palmar—ulnarwards on pronation). ECU becomes an ulnar abductor of the forearm in pronation with no extension moment. In supination it is an extensor with no ulnar—deviation moment.

Pathology

The ECU sheath can become incompetent, occasionally due to attenuation or attrition (e.g. rheumatoid) or after sudden trauma. Most commonly seen in racquet sports. On rotation, the ECU subluxates out of the 6th compartment. Pathological if this is accompanied by a painful clunk, with ECU palpably snagging over the back of the ulnar head.

Symptoms and signs

Clunking over the back of the ulnar head on rotation. The ECU can be felt to snap across the back of the ulnar head and edge of the ulnar styloid, especially on ulnar deviation with the forearm supinated. Compare with normal side to judge the normal tendon movement in that patient. Subluxation may be bilateral and asymptomatic.

Consider TFCC tear, LTIL instability, mid-carpal instability or DRUJ instability as differential diagnoses.

Dynamic ultrasound useful to confirm diagnosis.

Treatment

- If mild symptoms rest, modification of racquet technique, strapping.
- Acute injury, with tenderness, swelling and demonstrable instability over the ECU sheath may respond to above elbow splint in pronation, wrist in slight extension and radial deviation for 4 weeks.
- Chronic instability (the usual presentation) requires surgery for intrusive symptoms. Spinner and Kaplan operation. Dorsal incision, extensor retinaculum identified and divided in 'H' fashion, transverse piece of retinaculum detached ulnarwards then passed under ECU tendon and back radialwards on itself, secured with non-absorbable sutures. Above elbow cast in mid-rotation for 5 weeks then rehabilitation.

Alternative is anatomical reconstruction and reattachment of ECU sub-sheath onto ulnar groove with suture anchors.

FCU tendonitis

Most common tendonitis. Can occur spontaneously or following unaccustomed use.

Symptoms and signs

Pain on flexion and ulnar deviation. Swelling, Tender and crepitus over FCU, pain on resisted contraction. X-ray may show calcific deposits.

Treatment

Rest, NSAID, splint, cortisone injection. Surgery rarely needed—synovectomy, removal of calcific deposit.

Hook of hamate non-union

Caused by blow on ulnar side of palm, usually impact from golf club or tennis racquet. Pain on grip in ulnar side of palm.. Tender over hamate hook (1cm distal and radial to pisiform). Resisted flexion of little and ring finger tip causes pain (hook of hamate is a pulley drawing FDP (IV) and FDP (V) radialwards).

Investigation

Plain X-rays do not show this injury very well; occasionally demonstrated on a 'carpal tunnel skyline' view. CT scan is investigation of choice.

Treatment

Excision gives excellent relief (carpal tunnel incision, subperiosteal excision, avoid ulnar artery superficially and deep motor branch of ulnar nerve). Bone grafting and screw fixation technically complex with unnecessary potential complications for no potential gain.

Luno-triquetral instability

Background

Anatomy and kinematics

U-shaped luno-triquetral interosseous ligament (LTIL). Thickest anteriorly (cf scapholunatre which is thickest posteriorly). If ruptured, the lunate and scaphoid flex as no longer held in neutral by the tension of the LTIL. A static VISI *in vitro* requires rupture of the dorsal radio-triquetral and dorsal radiocarpal ligament.

Cause

Degenerative
Fall on ulnar corner of outstretched hand.
Does not lead to a progressive arthritis (cf. SLIL instability)

Clinical features

Symptoms

Ulnar corner pain and clunk. Aggravated by grip, ulnar deviation and rotation

Signs

Localized tenderness over LTL. Sagging/supination of ulnar corner. Lunate–triquetrum shear test positive (thumb of one hand on front of pisiform, index on back of triquetrum; thumb of other hand over front of lunate, index over back of lunate; shear in antero-posterior plane; painful movement more than other side is positive).

Investigation

True lateral X-ray: VISI 10 degrees or more of palmar tilt of lunate. Decreased scapholunate angle.
Arthrogram (MRI preferable, otherwise CT or fluoroscopic); contrast passing across lunotriquetral space. Not particularlty sensitive or specific.
Arthroscopy: Definitive diagnosis. Quantification of laxity. Assessment of other pathology e.g. ulno-carpal impaction.

Treatment

Conservative treatment

Pain relief, modification of activity, splintage.

Surgical treatment

Literature on techniques and outcomes is limited.
If diagnosed in first few weeks at most, arthroscopic debridement and percutaneous pinning or ligament repair (volar approach) and pinning.
- *Ligament reconstruction* (slip of ECU through bone tunnels).
- *Luno-triquetral fusion* (joint excision, distal radius cancellous graft, cannulated compression screw). Range of movement about 85%, grip strength 75%, non-union 20–25%. 50% still have pain.
- *Ulnar shortening osteotomy*: will tighten the extrinsic ligaments and reduce symptomatic instability. Especially indicated if associated ulno-carpal impaction.

Ulnar translation of carpus

Rare condition. Failure of the radiocarpal ligaments (rheumatoid, trauma, Madelung's) can lead to progressive ulnar translation of the carpus. Can occur after Darrach's or over-aggressive radial styloidectomy. Increased load on the ulnar head. Treatment includes early repair of ligaments (but rarely diagnosed early). Later, consider radio-lunate fusion or radial tilting osteotomy if symptoms very intrusive.

Distal radioulnar joint

Arthritis

Aetiology
- Spontaneous
- Intra-articular fracture
- Instability
- Incongruity from malunited distal radius fracture
- previous ulnar shortening

Clinical features
Pain in DRUJ, worse on rotation. Crepitus and tenderness. Occasionally rupture of EDM and EDC V, IV. (Vaughn–Jackson syndrome over the sharp osteophytic head.

Treatment
- Cortisone injection
- NSAIDs
- Ulnar head replacement
- Ulnar head deletion (Darrach's or Sauve–Kapandji). *NOT recommended in OA patients with working demands as poor results and risk of instability.*
- Extensor tendon reconstruction.

Instability

Aetiology
- Ligamentous laxity (rheumatoid, connective tissue disorders).
- Traumatic rupture of the anterior or dorsal limbs of TFCC.
- Traumatic avulsion of TFCC from fovea.
- Displaced or un-united unstable ulnar styloid basal fracture.
- Malunion of radius (distal radius, shaft) with secondary incongruity of sigmoid notch.
- Previous ulnar head deletion.
- Essex–Lopresti injury (radial head fracture with dissociation of interosseous membrane.
- Radius fracture with DRUJ dislocation (Galeazzi)

Clinical features
Symptoms: Clunking with or without pain in DRUJ on rotation and grip.
Signs: prominent ulnar head sometimes at rest, sometimes only on stressing (with palm tilted ulnarwards to relax secondary constraint from ulnocarpal ligaments).

Investigation
Plain X-ray: ulnar styloid fracture. Radius malunion
CT scan: transverse cuts to assess sigmoid notch in pronation and supination
MRI arthrogram: TFCC injury
Examination under anaesthesia with fluoroscopy and arthroscopy.

Treatment

Acute injury: reduce joint (open if needed). Accurate reduction and stable fixation of any associated bone injury (ulnar styloid base, radius). Hold position (above elbow plaster, transfix DRUJ with wires if unstable). Palmar dislocation of head reduces in pronation, dorsal dislocation of head in supination,

Non-operative treatment: Brace usually not sufficient.

Restorative surgery: treat primary cause when possible:
* Avulsed TFCC: reattach TFCC to fovea with bone anchors or drill holes, open repair probably more robust than arthroscopic.
* Ulnar head deletion: ulnar head replacement.
* Malunion of radius: radius osteotomy.

Indirect reconstruction: when primary cause cannot be restored.
* Tendon graft with drill holes through fovea and across radius to anatomically reproduce palmar and dorsal limbs of TFCC. *This is the most robust and reliable procedure if restorative treatment fails.*
* Ulnar shortening osteotomy to tighten ulnar corner soft tissues.
* Reinforce dorsal capsule and dorsal limb of TFCC with extensor retinaculum.
* Advancement of pronator quadratus (Johnson).
* Re-routing of FCU or ECU (various patterns described).
* Deepening of sigmoid notch.
* Radius–ulna fusion. *Last resort as greatly impedes function.* No ideal position of rotation.

Stiffness of the DRUJ

Loss of rotation substantially compromises hand function. Investigation and treatment depends on cause.

Malunion of distal radius

Some sigmoid notches are deeper than others. The deeper the notch, the greater loss of rotation for a given tilt of the distal radius in sagittal plane. Flat notches compensate well for dorsal malunion, deep notches do not. CT scan to demonstrate incongruity—transverse cuts in different positions of rotation. Corrective radius osteotomy usually restores rotation.

DRUJ arthritis

An incongruous ulnar head after malunion or with osteoarthritis will lose rotation. See above.

Capsular contracture

Following trauma (e.g. distal radius fracture with DRUJ dislocation) the capsule contracts. Usually supination is reduced. If the radius is proven to be normally aligned then capsular release can be very effective (anterior DRUJ capsule exposed between FCU and FDS avoiding retraction on ulnar nerve; capsule divided longitudinally under image intensification, anterior limb of TFCC preserved; supination splint and therapy post-operatively).
⚠ **Do not delete the ulnar head unless anatomical reconstruction not possible and patient has intrusive symptoms or low functional demands.**

Ulno–carpal joint

Traumatic TFCC tears: classification

Clinical features

Symptoms: fall on outstretched hand. Ulnar corner pain, worse on grip, rotation and ulnar tilt. Sometimes clicking and locking. Sometimes instability described

Signs: tender over ulnar head. Pain on passive ulno–carpal compression. DRUJ instability (type B, C, D).

Diagnosis

Plain X-ray: Associated fracture. OA from prolonged instabilit. Positive ulnar variance—predisposes to central perforation

MRI arthrography; not entirely specific or sensitive

Wrist arthroscopy. Direct visualization of central perforation and tears. Loss of trampoline effect in peripheral avulsion.

Treatment

Type 1A: NSAID, rest, injection. Arthroscopy = 85% satisfactory.

Type 1B: treatment: early diagnosis—reduce and above elbow plaster 6 weeks. Later diagnosis: reattach, open probably more secure than arthroscopic

Type 1C: literature sparse. Plaster.

Type 1D: debride flap if unstable. ? role for open or arthroscopic repair.

TFCC perforation and ulnocarpal impaction: classification

Central portion of TFCC is avascular. Prone to perforation as asymptomatic natural aging process (60% of cadavers). More likely in those with long ulnar (positive ulnar variance). May also be perforated after trauma.

Palmer Type 2 Degenerative TFCC Tear	
A	TFCC wear
B	TFCC wear
	+lunate and/or ulnar chondromalacia
C	TFCC perforation
	+lunate and/or ulnar chondromalacia
D	TFCC peforation
	+lunate and/or ulnar chondromalacia
	+ lunotriquetral ligament perforation
E	TFCC perforation
	+lunate and/or ulnar chondromalacia
	+ lunotriquetral ligament perforation
	+ulnocarpal arthritis

Clinical features

Symptoms: Ulnar corner pain, worse on grip, rotation and ulnar tilt. Sometimes previous trauma, sometimes spontaneous. Sometimes clicking and locking.

Signs: Tender over ulnar head. Pain on passive ulno–carpal compression.

Investigation

Plain X-ray: positive ulnar variance in most (not all). The wrist should be in neutral rotation, elbow flexed 90°, shoulder abducted 90°. The ulna lengthens relative to the radius in full pronation as the radius crosses over the ulna, this obliquity losing relative length. In advanced cases, secondary sclerotic or cystic changes to surfaces of lunate and triquetrum which abut the ulnar head.

MRI arthrogram: demonstrates the tear and also any signal change in lunate and triquetrum secondary to pressure.

Arthroscopy: gold standard test.

Treatment

Rest. NSAIDs. Cortisone injection often effective for small perforations with minimal secondary changes, Can repeat.

Arthoscopy: to confirm diagnosis. Trim irregular edge of central perforation. Consider supplementary surgery for ulno–carpal abutment.

Abutment operations

- Arthroscopic wafer operation: dome of ulnar removed through the perforated TFCC with burr. Suitable for up to 4mm positive variance.
- Open wafer operation (Feldon): rarely indicated if arthroscopic skills available.
- Ulnar shortening osteotomy: for greater degrees of positive variance whuch cannot be managed by arthroscopic wafer excision. NB reverse oblique sigmoid notch contraindicates ulnar shortening osteotomy.
- Ulnar *head deletion is contraindicated for ulnocarpal abutment.*

Ulno–carpal instability

Carpus supinates with the triquetrum and hamate sagging palmarwards from the ulnar head. The ulnar head appears prominent but is stable within the sigmoid notch. Caused by failure of the ulnar–lunate and ulna–triquetrum ligaments (trauma, rheumatoid, generalized laxity).

Treatment

Reconstruction of dorsal ulnar-sided capsule with reefing of dorsal radio-triquetral ligament and reinforced with strip of ECU tendon.

Radio–lunate fusion is an effective method as well. The carpus adapts well to this procedure. See Chapter 15, p. 489.

Pisotriquetral joint

Anatomy

Smallest carpal bone, only carpal bone attached to a tendon (embedded as sesamoid within FCU); only one articulation—triquetrum. Communicates with ulnocarpal joint in about 80%. Ossifies by age 8, rarely accessory bone (os pisiforme secondarium). Radial border—ulnar nerve. Complex ligament attachments to surrounding structures.

Arthritis

Cause

May occur spontaneously, usually after a previous fall on outstretched hand, landing on ulnar corner of palm (same mechanism for other ulnar corner injuries) or after long-term instability.

Symptoms and signs

Persisting pain on grip in flexion/ulnar deviation (e.g. cutting meat, holding iron). Pain with coarse crepitus on shearing the pisiform radialwards and dorsally against the underlying triquetrum with wrist slightly flexed. Spontaneous rupture of FDP(V). Secondary ulnar neuropathy common.

Investigation

X-ray: direct lateral will not show the joint. Specific lateral in 25° supination will provide a diagnostic skyline view of the piso-triquetral joint.
Carpal tunnel view: variable information.
CT scan: usually not needed if adequate plain X-ray acquired.

Treatment

Cortisone injection helpful in confirming diagnosis and alleviates symptoms for a while.
Surgical excision of pisiform gives excellent relief (zig-zag incision over distal FCU and pisiform, subperiosteal excision, avoid motor branch of ulnar nerve, repair FCU, splint 2 weeks).

Outcome

Excellent pain relief. No difference in power grip or wrist flexion.

Instability

Spontaneous or after trauma (direct fall or forced hyperextension).

Symptoms and signs

Pain and clunking on grip in flexion/ulnar deviation (e.g. cutting meat, holding iron). Painful with clunk on shearing the pisiform radialwards along the underlying triquetrum with wrist slightly flexed.

Investigation

X-ray: direct lateral will not show the joint. Specific lateral in 25° supination may show secondary arthritis but otherwise normal.
CT scan: can usefully suggest malalignment if clinical diagnosis not certain.

Treatment

Taping. Cortisone injection. Ligament repair—difficult. Surgical excision of pisiform successful.

Loose bodies

Rare—spontaneous or post-traumatic. Diagnosed by X-ray or CT. Excision.

Ganglion

A ganglion from the pisiform hamate region can cause pain in the ulnar corner of the palm. Associated with compression neuropathy of the ulnar nerve,

Diagnosis

- MRI scan or ultrasound
- Nerve conduction studies

Treatment

Surgical treatment (zig-zag incision over Guyon's canal, ulnar nerve trifurcation carefully exposed, ganglion removed.

Other causes of ulnar corner pain

Ulnar styloid impaction

Cause
- Long ulnar styloid abuts underside of triquetrum.
- Congenital
- After distal radius malunion
- Iatrogenic (hemiresection arthroplasty of ulnar head)

Clinical features
Ulnar corner pain, worse on ulnar deviation.

Investigation
X-rays in ulnar deviation.

Treatment
Rest, cortisone, subperiosteal excision of tip of styloid.

5th and 4th metacarpal–hamate arthritis

Post-traumatic condition with previous (often missed or improperly treated) fracture dislocation of the 5th CMCJ ('reversed Bennett's fracture') or fracture dislocation of both 4th and 5th CMCJ.

Symptoms and signs
Ulnar-sided pain, especially on grip (the 4th and 5th MCs flex on the hamate when gripping). Localized tenderness, painful crepitus on passive movement.

Treatment
Cortisone injection may extemporize.
Excision arthroplasty: if only 5th CMCJ involved (CT scan if any doubt) then fuse basal metaphysis of 5th MC to 4th MC using bone graft from distal radius held with wires or screws, then excise 5mm of base of 5th metacarpal. Plaster 6 weeks then X-ray. Excellent results as metacarpal flexion preserve in 4th CMCJ yet arthritic joint deleted.
Fusion: If both 4th and 5th CMCJs involved (CT scan if any doubt), then hamate–metacarpal fusion (distal radius graft; K-wires, memory staples or circular plate).

Lunate–hamate arthritis

Anatomy and pathology
- Type I lunate: 30%; does not articulate with hamate
- Type II lunate: 70%; articulates with hamate.

Rare pattern of arthritis, associated with Type II lunate and LT ligament instability.

Symptoms and signs
Ulnar-sided pain, worse on ulnar deviation. Point tenderness. Possible LT signs.

Treatment
Arthroscopy: to confirm diagnosis, exclude or confirm associated injuries, arthroscopic resection of proximal pole of hamate. Radial mid-carpal portal (scope); ulnar mid-carpal portal (burr). Remove 3mm.

Outcome

Usually good to excellent results, durable. Less reliable if associated pathology.

Neurogenic pain

Pain with neurogenic quality can affect the ulnar side of the wrist and hand. This would include compression neuropathy in Guyon's canal, cubital tunnel syndrome and a C8 cervical radiculopathy. Diagnose with careful history and examination (+/– neurophysiological studies and cervical spine MRI).

Other pathology in the ulnar corner (e.g. piso-triquetral OA, DRUJ instability) can cause secondary neurological symptoms from irritation of the ulnar nerve.

Neuroma

Cause

The dorsal sensory branch of the ulnar nerve leaves the main trunk 2–10cm proximal to the ulnar side of the ulnar styloid then passes dorso-ulnarwards, dividing into terminal branches over the back of the triquetrum. Vulnerable from a direct blow, penetrating trauma and especially surgery (ulnar shortening, ulnar styloid excision, 6R arthroscopic portal, reconstruction over dorsum of ulnar carpus).

Symptoms and signs

Neurogenic pain. Dystrophy (complex regional pain syndrome). Point tenderness with positive Tinel's sign at site of injury. Hypoaesthesia or dysaesthesia over dorsum of ulnar side of hand.

Treatment

Avoidance of the nerve by meticulous surgery! Like all neuromata, otherwise very difficult to treat.

Hypothenar hammer syndrome

Caused by repeated blows to ulnar side of palm, e.g. labouring, martial arts. Various structures vulnerable and can cause symptoms:
- Pisiform–triquetrum arthritis
- Neurogenic symptoms from ulnar nerve
- Ulnar artery aneurysm with cold intolerance or even microemboli in little and ring fingers

Investigation
- Duplex ultrasound and angiography if aneurysm suspected
- Nerve conduction studies
- CT scan to examine piso–triquetral joint and hook of Hamate
- MRI scan to examine ganglion

Treatment

Reconstruct with reversed vein graft. Treat associated pisiform or nerve symptoms by excision or neurolysis.

Surgical procedures

Wrist arthroscopy

Indications
Diagnostic: mechanical wrist pain of uncertain cause, localization of arthritis (e.g. to decide between proximal row carpectomy and 4-corner fusion), assessement of interosseous ligamentous instability. assessment of TFCC laxity

Therapeutic: debridement of TFCC perforation, localized or full synovectomy, removal of occult wrist ganglion, radial styloidectomy, removal of loose bodies, capsular shrinkage for laxity, guided reduction of fractures and ligamentous pinning; TFCC reattachment, ulnar head dome or total excision, removal of dorsal soft tissue or bone impingement, proximal row carpectomy; lavage of crystal arthropathy, lavage of sepsis; capsular release.

Technique
Distraction device, 2 fingers held with Chinese finger traps; distend radiocarpal joint with saline through 3–4 portal (synchronous inflation of midcarpal joint or DRUJ suggests interosseous ligament tear or TFCC perforation); small vertical skin incision, spread to capsule with fine-tipped clip; perforate capsule; insert scope (about 2.9mm); routine diagnostic procedure; surgical procedures and mid-carpal assessment via further portals.

Complications
- Rare (3% approx)
- Portal pain from neuroma
  - Dorsal branch of ulnar nerve (6r portal)
  - Superior radial nerve (1–2 portal)
- Infection
- Dystrophy
- Tendon rupture

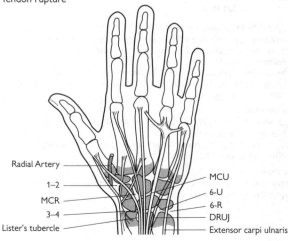

Radial Artery		MCU
1–2		6-U
MCR		6-R
3–4		DRUJ
Lister's tubercle		Extensor carpi ulnaris

Fig. 14.1 Arthroscopic portals.

Ulnar shortening

Indications

Ulnocarpal impaction; DRUJ laxity; Madelung's deformity; distal radius malunion with axial shortening but no tilt (easier than radial lengthening).

Technique

Tourniquet. Mid-lateral incision; meticulous avoidance of dorsal cutaneous branch of ulnar nerve; expose ulna between FCU and ECU; minimal periosteal stripping; double parallel osteotomy with cooled saw (cutting jig highly recommended); fixation with compression plate and lag screw.

Complications

- Delayed union
- Non-union
- Plate protrusion (about 30% need removal once healed)
- Dorsal cutaneous branch of ulnar nerve injury (numbness, neuroma, dystrophy)
- DRUJ arthritis (reduced contact area, increased pressure if reverse oblique DRUJ)

Ulnar head replacement

Indications

Unstable previous ulnar head deletion; primary treatment for ulnar head osteoarthritis or rheumatoid.

Implants

- *Silastic implants:* withdrawn due to synovitis and poor loading characteristics.
- *Anatomical implants:* head materials: ceramic (Herbert), metal (Avanta); pyrocarbon (Ascension); stem materials: metal with or without coating, impaction fit.
- *Other devices:* semi-constrained sigmoid notch/ulnar head (Scheker, for unstable arthritic DRUJ); spherical head (Fernandez, for unstable Sauve–Kapandji procedure)

Technique

Pre-operative templating; prophylactic antibiotics; tourniquet; dorso–ulnar incision; meticulous avoidance of dorsal cutaneous branch of ulnar nerve; expose DRUJ capsule through floor of EDM sheath; preserve ECU sheath; capsulotomy preserving radial cuff for later repair and preserving TFCC distally; divide neck at correct length; remove head; ream ulnar shaft; trial implants—check for length, width and stability; formal implants.

Complications

- Instability
- Infection
- ? Later sigmoid notch arthritis or erosion (long-term follow-up needed)

Results

No long-term results available, 2–5-year results suggest good early outcome with low complication rates in selected patients.

Resection arthroplasty

Indications

NB *Avoid deleting the ulnar head unless intrusive symptoms, low demand and no reconstructive alternative.*

- Ulnar head pathology (rheumatoid, osteoarthritis, un-united or malunited fracture, painful instability)
- Malunion distal radius with DRUJ incongruity
- Tendon rupture from synovitic DRUJ (rheumatoid) or osteophytic ulnar head (Vaughan–Jackson syndrome)
- Ulnocarpal impaction

Techniques

Approach similar to ulnar head replacement

Darrach's: excision of ulnar head; stabilized with anterior capsule (Blatt) or ECU tendon loop.

Matched ulna resection: curving of head preserving ulnar styloid to allow congruous rotation and minimize instability

Sauve–Kapandji: fusion of ulnar head to sigmoid notch; excile 7mm ulnar metaphysis to restore rotation

Baldwin's: excision of 1cm of ulnar distal metaphysis, ulnar head left in place

Outcome

Good results reported in selected patients especially low demand rheumatoid. Avoid in higher demand post-trauma patients (because of risk of stump instability).

Complications

- Ulnar stump instability (pain, weakness, cosmetic deformity, clunking) can be very problematic and difficult to solve (ulnar head replacement most promising).
- Stylo-carpal impingement (from matched ulnar resection, ulnar styloid impinging on triquetrum)
- Non-union (Sauve–Kapandji)
- Extensor tendon rupture from distal edge of ulnar shaft
- Infection, scar pain, dorsal branch of ulnar nerve neuroma

Wrist

Anatomy

Bones

Distal radius–lunate fossa (quadrangular/spherical), scaphoid fossa (triangular/spoon-shaped) sigmoid notch (articulates with ulnar seat in DRUJ, variable concavity).

Eight carpal bones—scaphoid, lunate, triquetrum, pisiform (sesamoid in FCU). hamate, capitate, trapezioid, trapezium.

Ossification

Radius physis—appears age 2, fuses age 16 to 18

Other bones develop ossification centres in clockwise order right-hand face down: capitate (1 month), Hamate (year 1); triquetrum (Year 2–3); lunate (year 4); scaphoid (year 4–6); trapezium (year 4–6); trapezioid (year 4–6); pisiform (year 8–10).

NB In an adolescent, the incompletely ossified scaphoid resembles scapholunate dissociation.

Anomalies

Scaphoid: bipartite (confused with fracture)
Lunate–triquetrum coalition (usually asymptomatic)
Os styloideum (accessory bone at tip of styloid)

Ligaments

The extrinsic ligaments are discrete consolidations of the capsule. Palmar stronger than dorsal.

Extrinsic carpal ligaments (dorsal)

Dorsal radiocarpal ligaments (radio–scaphoid, radio–triquetral). Rupture contributes to VISI.

Dorsal intercarpal ligament (triquetrum to scaphoid and trapezioid). Available as a donor for tenodesis against palmar rotation of scaphoid.

Extrinsic carpal ligaments (palmar)

Radio–scapho–capitate. Attaches to palmar edge of radial styloid. Fulcrum for scaphoid flexion. Divided then carefully repaired during palmar approach to scaphoid. Readily seen in arthroscopy. Beware removing attachment by enthusiastic radial styloidectomy.

Long radiolunate ligament. Restrains lunate from palmar dislocation.

Ligament of Testut (radio–scapho–lunate): synovial fold, no stabilizing function. Landmark for scapholunate ligament in wrist arthroscopy.

Short radiolunate ligament. From ulnar edge of distal radius to lunate, blends ulnarwards with the ulno lunate ligament.

Ulnocarpal ligament = ulno-capitate, ulno-lunate, ulno-triquetral. Blend into volar radiolunate ligament (i.e. anterior limb of TFCC). Ulno-triquetral ligament blends into subsheath of ECU (also part of TFCC).

Space of Poirier = gap between lunate and mid-carpal joint through which lunate can dislocate anteriorly.

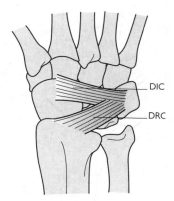

Fig. 15.1 Palmar ligaments.

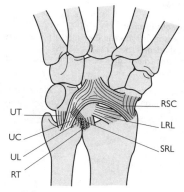

Fig. 15.2 RT Dorsal ligaments.

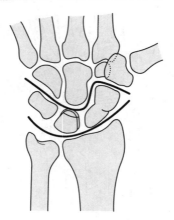

Fig. 15.3 Gilula's lines.

Intrinsic (interosseous ligaments)
Scapholunate interosseous ligament: C-shaped, thickest dorsally.
Lunotriquetral: C-shaped, thickest palmarwards.
Capitate–hamate, trapezium–capitate; trapezium–trapezioid.

Blood supply
Dorsal and palmar arches, supplied by radial artery, ulnar artery, anerior interosseous artery. Can be used as flaps to vascularize scaphoid and lunate.

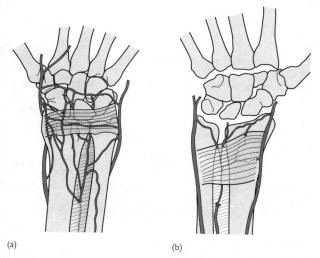

(a)   (b)

Fig. 15.4 Artorial supply to the wrist a) dorsal b) palmar.

Lunate

Volar and dorsal (80%); volar only (20%)
Three configurations of intraosseous vessels—I, X, Y

Scaphoid

80% via vessels from radial artery into dorsal ridge of scaphoid. 20% into volar scaphoid tubercle.

Radiological anatomy

Plain X-rays: taken with wrist in mid-rotation, elbow flexed 90°, shoulder abducted 90°.

Ulnar variance: varies with pronation (ulnar longer) and supination. Range −4 to + 4mm—compare other side.

Gilula's arcs: disturbed in mid-carpal instability, Kienbock's, dislocation,

Normal angles: radial tilt 22°, palmar tilt 11°; scapholunate angle 30–65°.

Carpal height: ratio distal edge capitate to proximal edge lunate/3rd metacarpal. Usually 0.54+/−0.03. Reduced in carpal collapse, e.g. Kienbock's disease. SLIL rupture.

Biomechanics

Kinetics
Study of forces acting apon an object and the resulting change in motion

Kinematics
Study of motion of objects without consideration of the forces acting apon them

Kinetics
About 80% of load transmitted across radiocarpal joint, 20% across ulno-carpal joint.

60% of radiocarpal load over scaphoid, 40% over lunate.

Decreasing variance by 2.5mm decreases ulnocarpal load to 5%; increasing by 2.5mm increases ulnocarpal load to 40%.

Pronation increases ulnocarpal load to about 35% (as ulna relatively long in pronation since radius obliquely crosses forearm).

Ulnar deviation increases ulnocarpal load to about 25 to 30%.

Kinematics
- Radiocarpal joint—ellipsoid biaxial joint
- Proximal carpal row: scaphoid, lunate, triquetrum. no tendon attachments so 'intercalated segment'. Movement of bones determined by force transmitted through the interosseous ligaments (scapholunate and lunotriquetral) and by the shape of the articular surfaces.
- Centre of rotation in head of capitate
- Distal carpal row: hamate, capitate, trapezioid, trapezium. Move very little in relation to each other.
- 4th and 5th CMCJ—movement between hamate and 4th and 5th metacarpals, called metacarpal descent. Cups the ulnar side of hand on grip. Variable range, around 30°.
- 3rd and 2nd CMCJ—minimal or no movement.
- Scaphoid—part of proximal and distal carpal row. Moves within proximal carpal row relative to lunate and radius; moves alongside capitate in distal carpal row.

Movements
- *Wrist flexion:* proximal row and distal row flex and ulnar deviate.
- *Wrist extension:* proximal row and distal row extend and radially deviate.
- *Radial deviation:* two movements. 1: proximal row flexes (to prevent scaphoid blocking flexion between radial styloid and trapezium); distal row slightly extends. 2: scaphoid slides ulnarwards, pushing lunate and triquetrum, Variable flexion and sliding between individuals—'column wrist' and 'row wrists'.
- *Ulnar deviation:* proximal row extends; distal row slightly flexes.
- *Radial–ulnar deviation:* 60% mid-carpal, 40% radiocarpal/ulnocarpal.
- *Flexion–extension:* variable descriptions, about 50% mid-carpal, 50% radiocarpal.

Range of movement
Normal: mean arc of flexion/extension 112–150°; Radial tilt 30°, ulnar tilt 45°.
Functional: 10° flexion to 30° extension.

Wrist pain

Many pathologies affect the wrist. Most can be diagnosed simply from history and careful examination, since the symptoms are often typical and the signs are usually very well-localized.

Ulnar—dorsal
- Ulnocarpal impaction
- TFCC perforation
- Lunotriquetral Instability
- Distal radioulnar joint arthritis
- Distal radioulnar joint instability
- ECU synovitis
- ECU instability
- Triquetrum impingement syndrome

Ulnar—palmar
- Pisotriquetral arthritis
- Pisohamate ganglion
- FCU synovitis
- Hook of hamate non-union

Dorsal—central
- Kienbock's disease
- Ganglion
- Dorsal synovial impingement
- EDC synovitis
- Radiocarpal and pan-carpal arthritis

Dorsal—radial
- Radiocarpal arthritis
- Scaphoid pathology
- CMC pain
- Scapholunate instability
- Tendonitis—EPL, ECRB, ECRL, cross-over syndrome

Palmar—radial
- De Quervain's synovitis
- STT osteoarthritis
- Radiocarpal arthritis
- Scapholunate pain
- FCR tendonitis

Palmar—central
- Flexor synovitis
- Median nerve irritation

Investigations for wrist disorders

Plain X-rays

Standard investigation for diagnosis of:
- Radiocarpal and mid-carpal arthritis
- Static wrist instability (e.g. fixed scapholunate diastasis)
- Established avascular necrosis (Preiser's, Kienbock's)
- Fractures, malunion, dislocation
- Ulnocarpal impaction and ulnar variance
- Opaque foreign body
- Calcification (gout, chondrocalcinosis)

Special X-rays

When certain conditions are suspected.
- 30° supinated lateral (for pisotriquetral OA)
- Carpal tunnel view (hook of Hamate fracture)
- Antero-posterior clench fist view (dynamic scapholunate instability)
- Scaphoid views (early diagnosis of fracture)
- Lateral tilt view (screw impingement in joint)

CT scan

Establishes cortical bone margins, therefore useful in:
- Confirming union of scaphoid and other fractures
- Planning osteotomy
- Planning fixation (scaphoid, distal radius)
- Localize osteoid osteoma
- Occult trauma (e.g. fracture hook of hamate, pisiform, capitate)
- Occult osteoarthritis (pisotriquetral, lunocapitate)
- Metalwork impingement after fixation
- Articular malalignment
- Confirm union (scaphoid)
- Bone fragmentation (Kienbock's)
- Bone tumours

Three-dimensional reconstruction can be helpful. Images may be degraded in presence of metalwork.

Ultrasound

- Ganglion
- Pigmented villonodular synovitis
- Tenosynovitis
- Tendon rupture
- Foreign body
- AV malformation

Isotope bone scan

Very *sensitive* (will demonstrate the existence of certain pathologies) but not too *specific* (may not localize the site or condition precisely).
- Infection
- Osteoid osteoma
- Undisclosed fractures (e.g. scaphoid)

Indications now very limited and generally superceded by MRI.

Arthrography (CT)

- Central perforation of the TFCC
- Tears of scapholunate and lunato-triquetral interosseous ligaments.
- Ganglion
- Larger chondral lesions
- Relatively low radiation—only 1.5x scaphoid X-ray

MRI scan

Special extremity coils speed up acquisition and reduce claustrophobia. Presence of loose metal elsewhere in the body is a contraindication. No one protocol will answer all possible diagnoses—the radiologist needs a clear question to answer so the correct sequence is used.

Some conditions very clearly demonstrated—ganglia, avascular necrosis, osteoid osteoma, ulnocarpal impaction, acute intrinsic/extrinsic ligament tears, acute fractures). Other conditions are not so clearly shown (osteoarthritis, cortical bone abnormalities, joint or fracture malalignment). The resolution of the scan may not detect the smallest tears of the TFCC and interosseous ligaments in the more chronic phase (once the initial oedema, which is very clearly seen on T2-weighted MRI) has resolved. *Arthrography* will enhance sensitivity.

Gadolinium-enhanced

To establish vascularity in scaphoid fractures (proximal pole ischaemia), reduced perfusion of lunate (Kienbock's disease) or scaphoid (Preiser's disease).

Dynamic MRI

Ulnocarpal abutment, interosseous ligament instablity.

DEXA scan

Indicated after a distal radius fracture in postmenopausal women. Findings of reduced bone density may be an indication for treatment.

Arthroscopy

📕 See p. 486.

Crystal arthropathy

Gout

Idiopathic or secondary (cyclosporine, psoriasis, haemolytic anaemia). Can cause sudden acute inflammation of the wrist. Easily mistaken for septic arthritis (severe rest pain, passive movement very painful, raised temperature, malaise). Features elsewhere include gouti tophi, arthropathy in first toe MTPJ. Tendon involvement.

Investigation

Urate levels: often normal.

Aspiration: urate crystals, needle-shaped, negatively birefringent under polarized microscopy.

Plain X-ray: tophi in soft tissues, punched out intra-articular erosions.

Treatment

If severe wrist inflammation, treat initially as infection with joint aspirate, then provisional antibiotics and joint wash-out. If crystals confirmed and bacteria excluded on aspirate then NSAIDs and splintage. Consider colchicine or intramuscular corticosteroid if symptoms too severe. Allopurinol for repeated attacks.

Pseudogout

Calcium pyrophosphate deposition in cartilage. Wrist is a common site. Episodic pain, usually less severe than gout.

Investigation

Plain X-rays: may show calcification of TFCC.

Aspiration: crystals (rod-shaped, weakly birefringent under polarized microscopy).

Treatment

Splint. NSAIDs. Intra-articular cortisone injection.

Carpal instability

Classification

Complex, several descriptions. Dobyn's:

Carpal instability dissociative (CID)

Occurs within the proximal carpal row due to failure of scapho-lunate interosseds ligament (SLIL) or lunotriquetral interosseous ligament (LTIL).

Carpal instability non-dissociative (CIND)

Occurs between rows, e.g. mid-carpal instability (between proximal and distal row) or ulnar translocation (between proximal carpal row and radius/ulna)

Carpal instability combined

Peri-lunate instability and other complex instabilities.

Taleisnik described static and dynamic instability:

Static instability

Seen on plain X-rays.

Dynamic instability

Provoked by stress, e.g. clenched fist AP view for SLIL dynamic instability. Also on dynamic MRI, videofluoroscopy, arthroscopy.

Adaptive instability

Alteration of usuial alignment secondary to another malalignment. E.g. flexion of distal row to compensate for a dorsal malunion of distal radius.

Intercalated segment instability

Intercalated segment

= the proximal carpal row, comprising scaphoid, lunate and triquetrum. Connected by SLIL and LTIL. No tendons attach, therefore movement determined by shape of articular surfaces and tension in the LTIL and SLIL.

Dorsal intercalated segment instability (DISI)

Failure of SLIL-scaphoid defaults into flexion; lunate narrower anteriorly than dorsally, so tends to fall into extension, dragging triquetrum with it via intact LTIL.

- *Lateral X-ray:* scapholunate angle increases above the normal of 30–60°. Radiolunate angle decreases.
- *Antero-posterior X-ray:* widening of scapholunate gap if static. May need stress views if dynamic.

Volar intercalated segment instability

Failure of LTIL-triquetrum defaults into flexion; scaphoid defaults into flexion, dragging lunate with it via intact SLIL. Capitate hyperextends, also pushing lunate into flexion. *In vitro* studies show that dorsal radiotriquetral and ulnotriquetral ligament, triquetrohamate ligament and LTIL must be sectioned to create a VISI.

- *Lateral X-ray:* scapholunate angle decreases below normal of 30–60°, radiolunate angle increases. Antero-posterior X-ray rarely shows a gap.

Lunotriquetral instability

📖 See Chapter 14 p. 478.

Scapholunate instability

Cause

Failure of SLIL. Usually traumatic. Sometimes seen in generalized ligamentous laxity and rheumatoid. Prone to degenerative failure (precursor to typical SLAC pattern of osteoarthritis), although actual risk and timescale unknown.

Acute trauma: fall on outstretched hand, extension, ulnar deviation and supination. Radial-sided wrist pain and swelling. Diagnosis often delayed as may not be clear radiographic signs, mistaken for an occult scaphoid fracture (similar mechanism of injury, symptoms and signs).

Symptomatic failure of SLIL accompanied by failure of other extrinsic ligamentous constraints.

STT arthritis: About 25% of those with STT arthritis have a DISI (in which case avoid distal pole scaphoid excision)

Clinical features

Symptoms

Acute: as above. Later: radial-sided pain, weakness of grip, clunking.

Signs

Tender over SLIL and scaphoid tubercle. Dorso-radial swelling. Positive scaphoid shift sign (Watson's test). Dorso-radial soft swellin if arthritis established.

Watson's scaphoid shift test

Examiner's fingers over back of carpus, thumb over scaphoid tubercle anteriorly with wrist in ulnar deviation. Wrist passively deviated radial-wards. Scaphoid should automatically flex. If SLIL failed, scaphoid cannot flex and will displace backwards with a painful clunk. As thumb releases, scaphoid reduces into scaphoid fossa with a clunk.

Investigation

Plain X-ray

May be normal, changes can develop over time as secondary restraints fail. Comparative views of other wrist helpful because of normal variation in angles and interosseous space.

Increased scapholunate gap ('Terry-Thomas sign', >4mm).

Scaphoid ring sign (flexed scaphoid looks round on postero-anterior view.) Anteroposterior view in full supination or clenched fist view may accentuate SLIL gap.

In later stages, osteoarthritic changes apparent (see scapho-lunate advanced collapse (SLAC) wrist, p. 504)

Videofluoroscopy

Demonstrates dynamic instability. Can be combined with intra-articula contrast but false positive rate.

MRI arthrogram

May demonstrate contrast passing through space (false positive rate increases with age). Signal changes around insertion of ligament into scaphoid (high false negative rate beyond initial injury).

Arthroscopy

📖 See p. 486. Gold standard. Allows direct visualization of ligament. Dynamic stress can be applied (Watson's test, direct manipulation with probe). Ligament structural injury best viewed from radiocarpal joint; instability best judged from mid-carpal joint.

25% of asymptomatic adults have some degree of SLIL tear.

Geissler classification:

Probable tear: from mid-carpal view, if probe can be rotated in the inrterosseous space. Confirmed tear: if probe or scope can be passed into radiocarpal joint.

Table 15.1 Arthroscopic classification of SLIL failure (Kozin)

Grade	Appearance
1	Attenuation of ligament
2	Step-off of interosseous space, slight gap less than probe width
3	Step-off, probe passes into space
4	Step-off. 2.7mm scope passes into space

Treatment

Acute (<8 weeks)

If diagnosed early (often missed as mistaken for sprain), immobilization in plaster 8 weeks if well-apposed lunate and scaphoid.

If displaced, direct repair. Open approach, ligament sparing capsulotomy, attach ligament to scaphoid (usually) or lunate (sometimes with bone-anchors or drill holes. Consider supplementary capsulodesis. Support with K-wires and plaster 8 weeks. Excellent outcome unusual.

Rupture, reducible, no degeneration

Direct repair no longer feasible beyond about 8 weeks as ligament retracts. Aim to either restore normal kinematics (probably impossible due to complexity of associated injuries) or at least prevent uncontrolled scaphoid flexion.

- *FCR tenodesis (Brunelli, several modifications):* Half of FCR passed through drill hole across scaphoid, passed across back of wrist, secured to dorsal ligament over triquetrum. Long-term results unknown. Grip about 80%, lose about 20° flexion. Usually some persisting pain and reduced function.
- *Bone-retinaculum-bone graft:* from extensor retinaculum attached into troughs in back of lunate and scaphoid.
- *Blatt capsulodesis:* rectangle of dorsal capsule tightened between radial half of dorsum of radius and scaphoid. Capsulodesis alone is usually successful for those with rotatory instability secondary to spontaneous laxity. Lose 20–30° flexion, 80% grip strength.

Rupture, irreducible, no degeneration

- Scaphoid-lunate fusion. Distal radius graft. Double-headed compression screw. Unreliable union, carpal kinematics disrupted. Poor range of movement.
- STT fusion. 📖 See p. 515.
- Scapho-capitate fusion. 📖 See p. 516.
- Four-corner fusion or PRC. 📖 See p. 515.

Rupture, degeneration (SLAC wrist)

An unstable scaphoid will alter joint forces and lead to degeneration—Scapho-Lunate Advanced Collapse (SLAC wrist). (📖 see p. 504.)

Mid-carpal instability

= carpal instability, non-dissociative. Instability between proximal and distal carpal row.

Cause

Occurs after trauma or spontaneously (ligamentous laxity). Can be dorsally instable, palmarly unstable or both. Can develop as an adaption to keep hand coaxial with forearm after a dorsal malunion of distal radius (adaptive instability).

Clinical features

Symptoms

Ulnar mid-carpal pain. Clunking and weakness. Sometimes history of trauma.

Signs

Palmar sag on ulnar side of wrist. As wrist in full pronation moved from radial to ulnar passively by examiner, clunk felt. Sometimes other signs of ligamentous laxity.

Investigation

Plain X-rays: usually normal. Sometimes VISI.

Videofluoroscopy: mid-carpal shift may be demonstrable. In ligamentous laxity, head of capitate subluxates out of the lunate.

Treatment

Acute injury

Rarely diagnosed: rest in splint 8 weeks.

Established instability

Non-operative: always try first. NSAIDs, splintage. Hand therapy (proprioceptive feedback, gyroscopic exerciser)

Four-corner fusion: hamate, capitate, lunate, triquetrum—most reliable. Range of movement only 60% normal, grip about 70% normal, about 50% still have pain. which can be very troublesome and worse than the original condition for some.

Ligament reconstruction: complex, variable patterns described, results uncertain.

Adaptive instability

Distal radius osteotomy.

Wrist osteoarthritis

Causes
- Spontaneous, idiopathic
- Infection
- Trauma:
  SNAC (scaphoid non-union advanced collapse)
  SLAC (scapholunate advanced collapse)
  Intra-articular fracture
- Avascular necrosis:
  Kienbock's
  Preiser's

Symptoms
- Pain, weakness, catching
- Occasional carpal tunnel syndrome

Signs
- Dorso-radial soft swelling (different from the firm central ganglion—cyst)
- Reduced range of movement, especially radial deviation and flexion
- Tenderness
- Instability (if previous scapholunate rupture)

SLAC wrist

Aetiology
Primary degenerative arthritis or following traumatic scapholunate ligament failure. Failure of SLIL—uncoordinated scaphoid flexion—abnormal radioscaphoid joint loading—proximal migration of capitate. Specific pattern of arthritis develops, progressing through the following stages.

Classification
Watson
Stage 1: radial styloid and distal scaphoid
Stage 2: entire radioscaphoid joint
Stage 3: capitate–lunate joint

Treatment
Simple: rest; splint; adapt activities; NSAIDs; cortisone injection
- *Stage 1:* arthroscopic debridement with arthroscopic radial styloidectomy and neurectomy, The instability continues and so only likely to extemporize. Success of additional ligament stabilization procedures uncertain.
- *Stage 2:* the spherical lunate–radius articulation is almost always preserved, however advanced the rest of the arthritis. This allows the option of movement-preserving surgery. Since scaphocapitate joint preserved, proximal low carpectomy or scaphoidectomy and four corner fusion.
- *Stage 3:* SFCF to preserve movement. PRC not an option as capitate head now arthritic.

SNAC wrist

An un-united scaphoid may stabilize in a congruous position with robust scar tissue in which case it may be asymptomatic. However, an unstable fracture will probably lead to arthritis eventually.

Similar progression to SLAC wrist but some differences.

Classification

Stage 1: radial styloid and distal scaphoid

Stage 2: scaphocapitate joint (proximal scaphoid and reciprocal radius spared cf. SLAC)

Stage 3: peri-scaphoid arthritis, lunate–capitate arthritis.

Treatment

Minimal surgery: arthroscopic debridement and arthroscopic radial styloidectomy, neurectomy, The non-union and instability continue and so symptoms likely to recur.

- *Excision of distal pole of scaphoid :* option for those with arthritis confined to the radial styloid–proximal pole. However, the residual proximal pole will remain unstable so outcome uncertain.
- *Motion-preserving surgery:* the lunate–radius articulation is almost always , and lunate–capitate joint usually, preserved, however advanced the rest of the arthritis. This allows the option of movement-preserving surgery (PRC or SFCF)

Radiocarpal arthritis

Usually associated wirth previous intra-articular fractures of the radius. Mid-carpal joint preserved.

Treatment

- Motion-preserving: radio–scapho–lunate fusion, with or without distal pole scaphoid excision
- Salvage: total wrist fusion
- Wrist replacement: for non-dominant wrist in older or low-demand patient

Hamate-lunate

Anatomy and pathology

Type I lunate: 30%; does not articulate with hamate
Type II lunate: 70%; articulates with hamate.

Rare pattern of arthritis, associated with Type II lunate and LT ligament instability.

Symptoms and signs

Ulnar-sided pain, worse on ulnar deviation. Point tenderness. Possible LT signs.

Treatment

Arthroscopy: to confirm diagnosis, exclude or confirm associated injuries, arthroscopic resection of proximal pole of hamate. Radial mid-carpal portal (scope); ulnar mid-carpal portal (burr). Remove 3mm.

Outcome

Usually good to excellent results, durable. Less reliable if associated pathology.

Swellings around the wrist

Dorsal ganglion

Symptoms
Sometimes cosmetic only, swelling over back of wrist. Can be painful especially after activity or on full flexion–extension.

Signs
Smooth swelling, overlies the dorsal mid-carpal joint. Sometimes no swelling to be seen ('occult wrist ganglion') but focal tenderness over the back of the mid-carpus. Underlying range of movement should be full, no crepitus and pain-free except at end of range. If not, consider underlying pathology, e.g. wrist osteoarthritis, interosseous, ligament tear.

Investigation
Not needed if obvious diagnosis
Ultrasound or MRI if occult wrist ganglion suspected

Treatment
- Leave alone. May just need reassurance if otherwise asymptomatic. Can spontaneously resolve.
- Aspiration. Typical gel, clear-coloured or straw-coloured fluid. Diagnosis confirmed, patient reassured and symptoms (usually temporarily) relieved. Recurrence in most patients.
- Cortisone injection. At the same time as aspiration. Unlikely to affect the success or recurrence rate, but may help if ganglion painful.
- Surgery. If occult, can be removed arthroscopically. Portals—3–4 and 6–R. Root of ganglion identified attached to dorsal capsule, removed with arthroscopc abrader or diathermy wand. Larger ganglia removed by open technique. Transverse incision, root excised, closure with subcuticular dissolvable suture. Recurrence up to 30%. Small risk of stiffness, dystrophy, wound falure.

Volar wrist ganglion

Less common than dorsal ganglion. Derived from FCR tendon sheath, STT joint or anterior radiocarpal capsule. Can be asymptomatic, but may be painful if underlying FCR tendonitis or STT arthritis.

Treatment
- Leave
- Aspirate (as above)
- Surgery. Beware cutaneous nerve branches. Can be difficult to dissect from radial artery. Trace deeply to origin from edge of joint and excise all of root if possible.

Carpometacarpal boss

Pathology
Swelling over the second–third carpometacarpal joint. Osteophyte and sometimes bursa. Perhaps due to instability of the 2nd CMJ (usually a very stable joint with very little movement).

Symptoms and signs

Bone-hard swelling, distal and radial to the usual site of a dorsal ganglion. Sometimes tender, sometimes pain on stressing the joint.

Investigation

True lateral X-ray centred on the swelling.

Treatment

- Leave if asymptomatic
- Surgery. Transverse skin crease incision. ECRL and ECRB elevated subperiosteally and retracted sideways.. Osteophyte excised to either side of joint. Periosteum closed dissolvable suture. Subcuticular dissolvable skin closure. May recur; if so, and if painful, consider CMC fusion using K-wires or circular plate and graft from Lister's tubercle.

Articular synovitis

Radioscaphoid arthritis: soft, diffuse swelling, over the dorsoradial aspect of the wrist, with underlying tenderness and reduced range of movement especially radial tilt and flexion. Pathognomic if radioscaphoid OA. Confirmed by plain X-ray.

Treatment

- Cortisone injection—will help the wrist pain for a while.
- Excision is pointless unless the underlying OA is also addressed.

Tenosynovitis

24 tendons run across the wrist (ECRB, ECRL, ECU, EIP, EDC ×4, EDM, FCU, FDPx4, FDSx4, PL, FCU, FPL, APL, APB, EPL). These, except palmaris longus, run in a synovial sheath and are subject to synovial thickening from whatever cause. The precise tendon involved can be localized clinically; ultrasound can help further.

Soft tissue tumours

Many soft tissue tumours can be found over the wrist, e.g. giant cell tumour (= pigmented villonodular synovitis), xanthoma of tendon etc. Ultraound and biopsy can elucidate further.

Dorsal impingement syndrome

Unusual condition. Similar to occult dorsal wrist ganglion. Thickened synovium impinges between the dorsal lip of the distal radius and the lunate. Pain on forced passive extension (press-ups, pushing doors). Tenderness precisely over dorsum of radius–lunate joint.

Investigation

MRI. Arthroscopy if clinical diagnosis not clear.

Treatment

Cortisone injection can be curative, may need repeating.
Arthroscopic removal of thickened synovium.

Avascular necrosis

The carpal bones rely on an extrinsic vascular supply. The lunate and very rarely the scaphoid may develop ischemia or frank necrosis if the blood supply fails.

Kienbock's

Described by Robert Kienbock (1910).

Aetiology

Unknown. Various theories
- *Vascular:* ?failed arterial inflow (only single nutrient vessel in 20%). ?Obstructed venous outflow.
- *Mechanical:* about 70% of patients have a negative ulnar variance, i.e. the radius is long relative to the ulna. This may alter the load carried by the lunate.

Clinical features

- *Symptoms:* commonest age of presentation 20–40. May be asymptomatic. Central wrist pain, not always related to activity. Fluctuates over time.
- *Signs:* tender over mid-carpus. Initially range of movement preserved, but if the carpus collapses then reduced range of movement and reduced grip strength.

Radiology

Plain X-ray

In earliest stage, the lunate on plain X-rays is normal. Plain X-rays may show a relatively long radius or vague increased density of the lunate. In established disease, plain X-rays show degree of lunate collapse and associated mid-carpal collapse and secondary osteoarthritis.

Intercarpal ratio: As the lunate collapses, the scaphoid tends to flex. The relative height of the lunate:capitate diminishes, carpal ratio falls below normal of 0.54.

MRI scan

A gadolinium-enhanced MRI scan will demonstrate the condition even if plain X-rays are normal. Reduced marrow fat on T1-weighted sequence. Low signal on T2-weighted sequence. Signal changes isolated to ulnar corner of lunate more likely ulnocarpal abutment especially if positive ulnar variance (cf. Kienbock's diffuse lunate changes, negative ulnar variance)

CT scan

Limited extra information over plain X-rays. Shows lunate collapse and intracarpal arthritis.

Classification

Table 15.2 Classification of Kienbock's disease (Lichtman)

Stage	X-ray, MRI	Treatment
1	Normal X-ray, changes on MRI	Cast 3 months Vascularized bone graft
2	Lunate sclerosis on plain X-ray, fracture lines sometimes present	Vascularized bone graft If negative ulnar variance: radial shortening If positive ulnar variance: radial dome osteotomy
3a	Fragmentation of lunate, height preserved	Proximal row carpectomy
3b	Collapse of lunate, proximal migration of capitate, fixed scaphoid rotation	Scaphocapitate fusion STT fusion PRC
4	Mid-carpal or radiocarpal arthritis	PRC Total wrist fusion Wrist replacement

Treatment

Non-operative

Not all patients progress symptomatically (even with quite advanced or progressive radiological signs). Therefore observation and simple treatment are justified. Rest (in a cast for exacerbations); NSAIDs; splint.

There are many surgical operations and comparative outcome studies are rare; surgery to be tailored for each individual patient's radiological stage, symptomatology and expected outcome.

Joint-preserving surgery

- Joint neurectomy: used as an adjunct to other procedures
- External fixator: temporary unloading of lunate with external fixator across carpus. May be an adjunct to revascularization.
- Vascularization: for grade 0 or 1 Kienbock's with symptoms but well preserved lunate. 2nd intermetacarpal vascular bundle can be implanted or a block of distal radius bone based on the 3–4 or 4–5 extensor compartment retinacular artery.
- Radial shortening osteotomy: for negative ulnar variance. Anterior approach, 2–3mm excised with cooled saw. Rigid compression fixation.
- Ulnar lengthening osteotomy (alternative to radial shortening if negative ulnar variance. More complex than radial shortening).
- Radius tilting osteotomy (alters load on lunate, radius tilted radialwards).
- Limited intercarpal fusion: to unload the lunate and restore a normal lunate–capitate ratio. The lunate may be excised at the same time. STT fusion or scaphocapitate fusion are both reasonable options; the latter probably gives a lesser range of movement.

- Lunate replacement: silastic or metal implants do not restore normal kinematics so not routinely used.
- Proximal row carpectomy: if the capitate–lunate and radius–lunate joints are preserved (check arthroscopically).
- Total wrist fusion: for symptomatic grade IIIb and IV.
- Wrist replacement: in lower-demand patients requiring some preservation of wrist movement.

Preiser's disease

Aetiology
Very rare condition. Usually older than 40. Associated with steroid use.

Clinical features
Radial-sided wrist pain and tenderness. Reduced range of movement and grip in later stages. MRI may detect early changes. Plain X-ray shows sclerosis and, later, fragmentation and collapse.

Treatment
Simple non-operative methods.
Surgery: sparse guidance in literature. Ischaemia without collapse—revascularization. Scaphoid collapse with intrusive symptoms—scaphoid excision with either proximal row carpectomy or four-corner fusion. Wrist replacement.

Wrist operations

Wrist arthroscopy

Indications

- Diagnosis (of conditions that may not always be diagnosed by non-invasive tests, e.g. small TFCC perforations, some interosseous ligament tears, early osteoarthritis, extrinsic ligament tears).
- Quantification of pathology (e.g. degree of interosseous ligament instability, presence of osteoarthritis in certain parts of wrist, a prelude to limited carpal fusion, assessment of instability of the TFCC).
- Therapeutic arthroscopy: debridement of synovitis, debridement of chondral lesions, removal of loose bodies, debridement of unstable TFCC perforations, arthroscopic repair of TFCC detachment; capsular shrinkage for mid-carpal instability; guidance of reduction and percutaneous pinning of fractures, excision of distal surface of ulnar head; excision of radial styloid; proximal row carpectomy, capsular resection and debridement of intra-articular fibrosis for joint stiffness; debridement of hamate–lunate arthrosis, partial lunate resection (Grade III Kienbock's); partial scaphoid excision.

An arthroscopic finding is only pathological when it fits the history and examination. In cadavers, interosseous ligament tears and TFCC perforations not uncommon.

Operative procedure

General anaesthetic or regional block. Two fingers suspended in expandable mesh supports ('Chinese finger traps'). Distraction through finger traps by a vertical tower or by weight off the edge of operating table (4–5kg). Bone landmarks outlined with pen. Portals identified (📖 see p. 486). Joint distended with saline (7–10ml) using hypodermic needle through 3/4 or 6R portal. Vertical skin incision. Soft tissues gently spread with fine mosquito clip. Capsule perforated with tip of clip. Blunt trochar into 3/4 portal (proximal carpal joint) or mid-carpal portal (mid-carpal joint); replaced by arthroscope; optional DRUJ portal (need very small scope). Systematic assessment.

Remember: some changes are normal variations—e.g. early chondral change, TFCC perforations, laxity or tears of interosseous ligaments, mild synovial thickening. *Arthroscopic findings must correlate with suspected clinical diagnosis to be denoted as pathological.*

Outerbridge classification of cartilage change

I Softening
II Fraying
III Partial cartilage defect
IV Subchondral bone visible

Arthroscopic instruments

Small diameter scope (1.9–2.7mm); small hooked probe; suction punch; scissors; angled punches; straight and curved punches; rongeurs. Small serrated graspers; rotating shaver; bone burrs; radiofrequency probes (for thermal ablation and thermal cutting).

Closure
Thorough washout. Marcain around portals and into joint. Adhesive paper sutures. Light dressing.

Postoperative care
Depends upon procedure performed. Early mobilization usually encouraged. Dressing reduced and paper sutures removed at 10–14 days.

Complications
The complication rate is approximately 3%. Infection. Persistent leakage. Cutaneous nerve damage. Reflex sympathetic dystrophy.

Total wrist fusion

Indications
- Relief of pain from radiocarpal and mid-carpal or pancarpal arthritis that has not been solved by a motion-preserving procedure.
- Stabilization of radiocarpal joint or mid-carpal joint.
- Correction of severe deformity (e.g. cerebral palsy, head injury, post-traumatic deformity).
- Radial nerve palsy

Contraindications
- Skeletally immature
- Active sepsis
- Poor soft-tissue envelope
- Tetraplegia (if tenodesis required)

Procedure
Above-elbow tourniquet. General or regional anaesthesia. Dorsal midline approach. EPL and ECRB retracted radialwards, EDC retracted ulnarwards. Longitudinal capsulotomy. Excision of joint surfaces with osteotome or rongeurs. Bone graft (local source, iliac crest or bone substitute) packed into spaces. The 3rd carpometacarpal joint should be denuded and bone graft applied. If ulnar head too long after joint excision, excise triquetrum. *Do not delete the ulnar head.*

Options for fixation
- *Purpose-designed wrist fusion plate* (larger screws proximally for radius, smaller screws distally for 3rd metacarpal, contour for depression at back of carpus, predefined dorsal angulation of distal edge of plate).
- *Crossed K-wires.*
- *Intramedullary Steinmann pin.* Usually for rheumatoid arthritis with soft, collapsing, spontaneously fusing carpus. Pin passed either through 3rd metacarpal neck (Mannerfelt technique) or through 2nd/3rd metacarpal space. Bone graft not always needed, especially if wrist is spontaneously fusing.
- *Sliding bone graft* (slither of bone from dorsum of radius elevated, passed distally and then secured from dorsal to palmar with screws).

Complications

Non-union. Wound failure. Persisting pain. Dystrophy. Tendon impingement on metalwork. Extrusion of Steinmann pins. Failure of fusion of 3rd carpometacarpal joint. Metalwork failure (usually subsequent to non-union). Ulnocarpal impaction.

Position of fusion

For best grip, wrist fused in approximately 20° extension. If both wrists fused, then non-dominant wrist fused in neutral or perhaps even slight flexion, or consider wrist replacement, to help with personal care. In coronal plane, fuse with middle finger aligned with radius (plate fixation) or very slight ulna deviation (Steinmann pin between 2nd/3rd metacarpal space).

Outcome

Residual pain on activity in most. Relieves rest pain in most. Grip strength about 65% of normal. Functional difficulties persist (personal care, hair combing, securing buttons and zips, gloves). Return to work not predictable, especially if flexion essential (plumbing, decorating etc.). Passive tendodesis effect of wrist is lost, so finger excursion reduced.

Proximal row carpectomy

Principles

Purpose is preservation of functional wrist movement by articulating the head of capitate in the lunate fossa. The lunate fossa joint cartilage is usually preserved in arthritis subsequent to scaphoid non-union (SNAC) or scapholunate ligament failure (SLAC). If doubt about the integrity of the cartilage in lunate fossa or head of capitate, preliminary wrist arthroscopy should be performed.

Indications

- Scaphoid non-union.
- Scaphoid union with subsequent radioscaphoid arthritis (stage II).
- Scapholunate ligament failure with secondary radioscaphoid arthritis (stage II).
- Stage II and III Kienbock's disease with preservation of lunate fossa and capitate head.
- Lunotriquetral ligament failure.

Procedure

Wrist arthroscopy to confirm integrity of capitate and lunate cartilage. If degraded, then alternative salvage procedure required.

Dorsal midline incision. EPL, ECRB and ECRL retracted radialwards, EDC retracted ulnarwards. 1cm of PIN excised. Ligament preserving capsulotomy (see below). Scaphoid, lunate and triquetrum removed with osteotome and rongeurs. If needed, supplementary incision over scaphoid tubercle to remove anterior remnants of scaphoid. Capitate placed into lunate fossa of radius. Check for impingement of capitate on radial styloid by fluoroscopy; remove tip of styloid if impingement. Capsule closed. If any chance of instability or subluxation, then percutaneous K-wire to stabilize lunate-capitate joint. Skin closure. Plaster cast for three to four weeks. Removal of wire then gentle mobilization.

Complications
Infection. Scar pain. Instability. Progressive arthritis (12/16 patients at 10 years.[1]

Outcome
- Many reports. Grip strength 70–90% of normal side. Flexion–extension arc approximately 70–90° of other side.
- Recent studies have shown pain relief and good function for at least 10 years.

Scaphoidectomy with four-corner fusion

Principles
Joint-preserving procedure. Even in late stages of SLAC wrist and SNAC wrist the lunate fossa is preserved. Preferable to proximal row carpectomy if there is secondary arthritis in the lunate–capitate joint (found in later stages of SLAC and SNAC wrist).

Indications
- Radioscaphoid arthritis secondary to scaphoid non-union or scapholunate ligament failure.
- Symptomatic SNAC and SLAC, following failed alternative reconstructive treatment.
- Lunate–capitate arthritis.
- Lunotriquetral ligament instability after failed reconstruction.
- Mid-carpal instability.

Procedure
Dorsal midline incision. ECRB and ECRL retracted radialwards, EDC and EDM retracted ulnarwards. 1cm PIN excised. Ligament-sparing capsulotomy (see below). Scaphoid excised. Lunate reduced to neutral position (usually hyperextended) using K-wire as a 'joystick'. Reduced lunate held against capitate with K-wire. Lunate–triquetrum and triquetrum–hamate–capitate secured with provisional K-wires. Joint between lunate, hamate, capitate and triquetrum denuded (circular bone routers particularly suitable). Space packed with graft (scaphoid, beneath Lister's tubercle, iliac crest, bone substitute). Fusion secured with circular plate, K-wires, staples or cannulated compression screws. Check for impingement of capitate against radial stolid with fluoroscopy. Ecise tip of styloid if needed. Capsule closure. Plaster cast 6 weeks. X-rays to confirm union. Union difficult to confirm as usually persisting lunate–triquetrum gap.

Outcome
Similar to proximal row carpectomy.
Studies vary. Grip strength approximately 75–80% normal; range of movement 55–70% of normal.

Complications
Non-union. Metalwork failure. Loss of extension (due to unreduced lunate or circular plate impingement on dorsal lip of distal radius). Later radiocarpal arthritis is possible.

1. Imbriglia et al. (2000). Hand Clinics.

PRC vs scaphoidectomy with four-corner fusion (SFCF)

No randomized comparisons. Overview of literature and indirect comparative studies suggest no difference in grip, range of movement or function.

PRC

- Lower complication rate
- Technically easier

SFCF

- Intrinsically higher complication rate (metalwork, non-union).
- Technically more demanding.
- Probably slightly better resistance to torsion.

Radioscapholunate fusion

Principles

Motion-preserving procedure. About 50% wrist motion at radiocarpal joint, 50% at mid-carpal joint. For deletion of radiocarpal joint when mid-carpal joint preserved. The distal pole of scaphoid should also be removed to allow better radial tilt and flexion.

Indications

Radius–scaphoid–lunate arthritis, usually from malunited intra-articular distal radius fracture. SLAC wrist, SNAC wrist (but PRC or 4CF better options). Radiocarpal instability.

Procedure

Dorsal midline incision. EPL, ECRB and ECRL retracted radialwards, EDC retracted ulnarwards. 1cm PIN excised. Ligament-sparing capsulotomy. Lunate and scaphoid reduced to radius with provisional K-wires. Radiocarpal joint surface denuded with rongeurs or osteotome. Distal pole of scaphoid excised (scaphoid unable to flex and crosses mid-carpal joint; excision increases mid-carpal movement from 60° to 120°). Space packed with graft from scaphoid, beneath Lister's tubercle, iliac crest or bone substitute. Secured with K-wires, cannulated compression screws, staples or locking plates. Capsular closure. Wound closure. Plaster of Paris. X-ray at six weeks. Hand therapy.

Outcome

Few reports. Grip strength about 50–70%. About 50° flexion–extension arc.

Complications

High non-union rate. About one-third develop painful mid-carpal arthritis within a few years.

Scapho–trapezio–trapezioid fusion

Indications

- STT arthritis (📖 see p. 258).
- Kienbock's disease (allows power transfer across the wrist bypassing lunate
- Scaphoid instability (prevents anterior rotation of the scaphoid) e.g. ligamentous laxity, SLIL injury.

Procedure

Transverse dorsoradial approach. STT identified behind ECRL. Capsule reflected. Joint surfaces denuded. Maintain original dimensions of STT joint with a spacer. Set scaphoid angle at 55–60° relative to long axis of radius. Hold with K-wires. Pack cancellous graft from distal radius. Excise radial styloid, preserving origin of volar ligaments. Plaster cast 6 weeks.

Outcome

Reports vary. 60% range of motion; 75% grip strength.
Longer-term arthritis in other joints theoretical but rarely reported.

Complications

Up to 50% in some series. Non-union, radial styloid impingement, metal-work problems, stiffness, persisting pain.

Other limited carpal fusions

Various combinations have been described.
- Scaphocapitate fusion (for lengthening mid-carpus and decompressing lunate in Kienbock's).
- Lunotriquetral fusion (for lunotriquetral ligament failure, low union rate).
- Lunocapitate fusion (isolated mid-carpal arthritis. Low union rate. No kinematic advantage over SFCF).
- Scapholunate fusion (for scapholunate ligament failure. Difficult to secure union. Considerable loss of wrist movement due to obstructed scaphoid flexion and extension. Likely secondary arthritis. Proximal row carpectomy or SFCF better option if scapholunate reconstruction fails).

Radiolunate (Chamay) fusion

Principles

Lunate fused to radius. Good wrist movement preserved as the lunotriquetral ligament and scapholunate ligament still function.

Indications

Rheumatoid arthritis with impending ulnar slide of carpus. Isolated radiolunate arthritis. Radioscapholunate ligament failure with marked dorsal tilt of lunate.

Procedure

Dorsal midline incision. EPL/ECRL/ECRB retracted radialwards, EDC retracted ulnarwards. Ligament-sparing capsulotomy. Lunate reduced and held to radius with provisional K-wire. Joint surface denuded and packed with bone graft from distal radius, iliac crest or substitute. Fixation with K-wires, cannulated compression screws, staples or low-profile locking plate.

Outcomes

Variable reports. About 70% of normal flexion–extension.

Complications

Metalwork failure (especially soft rheumatoid bone). Infection. Progressive instability. Persisting pain.

Capsular exposure of the wrist

To preserve optimum movement after exposure of the wrist joint, the capsule can be divided along the line of the fibres of the dorsal intercarpal ligament and dorsal radiocarpal ligament.

Denervation

Principles

Regardless of pathology, afferent pain can be reduced by denervation. Many salvage procedures on the wrist cause unacceptable loss of movement and grip strength. Denervation can preserve movement and grip strength without primarily addressing the original pathology.

Procedure

Full denervation described by Wilhelm (1966)—multiple incisions to divide all nerve fibres crossing the wrist (superficial radial, anterior interosseous, posterior interosseous, medial, ulnar, dorsal branch of ulnar, lateral cutaneous nerve of forearm, medial cutaneous nerve of forearm, palmar branch of median nerve.. Some authors only divide the PIN and, if located via the interosseous membrane through same dorsal incision, the AIN.

Some precede denervation by trial of lidocaine around the posterior interosseous nerve and other nerves. However, this is a non-specific test. Small dorsal transverse incision. Posterior interosseous nerve divided beneath EDC tendons. Small window made in interosseous membrane, anterior interosseous nerve retrieved with small hook and divided. Further denervation can be achieved around the antero-radial border of the wrist (small nerves alongside radial artery, division of plane between subcutaneous tissues and wrist capsule/tendon sheaths on radial side of wrist). Ulna-sided neurectomy performed through a small anterior and also dorsal incision, again sweeping subcutaneous plane away from the capsular/tendon sheath plane.

Outcome

Results in literature difficult to interpret—small series, short follow-up, different techniques, synchronous procedures, vague outcome measures.

Probably worth trying as a chance of a good persisting result with wrist architecture preserved, minimal complication rate and further salvage procedures not compromised.

Complications

Charcot joint not reported. Wound infection and dystrophy possible but very rare.

Total wrist replacement

Indications

When wrist motion is to be preserved but an alternative procedure (proximal row carpectomy, radio–scapho–lunate fusion, four-corner fusion) is not suitable. Because longevity and resilience of implants not established, reserve for lower-demand individuals especially if hand function diminished by pathology elsewhere (i.e. rheumatoid).

Contraindications
- Previous infection
- Resorption of carpus from rheumatoid, previous silicone implant;
- Severe osteopaenia
- Lack of bone stock.
- Use of walking stick
- Ligamentous laxity
- Sporting or heavy labouring ambitions

Implant design
- *Silastic:* flexible hinge. Implant fracture, silicone synovitis
- *Previous designs:* ball-and-socket, hinge: problems with imbalance, breakage, subsidence, loosening (usually distal component).
- *Modern design:* metal stems attached to carpus (rather than metacarpals) by screw or impaction. Intercarpal fusion. Broad, ellipsoidal semi-constrained plastic contoured liner allowing movement in 3 planes. Metal radius component, press fit, minimal bone resection. Option to presserve ulnar head. Cemented or uncemented options. Cutting guides.

Procedure
The manual for the implant should be consulted. Observation and cadaver/model bone practice recommended.

Complications
- *Early:* dislocation, infection, dystrophy
- *Late:* loosening, dislocation, component failure, infection, erosion.

Outcome
- *Previous implants:* range of movement approx 30° flexion to 30° extension, 5° radial and ulnar deviation. High failure rates, although improving with newer designs.
- *Biaxial wrist:* 80% survival at 5 years, usually metacarpal loosening.
- *Recent implants:* (universal 2): About 35° flexion, 35° extension. Consistently good pain relief. Early results show good maintenance of position.

Direct comparison of wrist fusion and contralateral wrist replacement in the same patient shows patient preference for the arthroplasty. Generally good patient satisfaction.

Radial styloidectomy

Indications
Radial styloid arthritis (SLAC, SNAC, malunited Chauffeur's styloid fracture, spontaneous arthrosis). Impingement after STT fusion, PRC or SFCF.

Anatomy
Dorsal ligamentous attachments: RLT. Palmar ligamentous attachments: RSL, RSC, LRL. Act as a sling around scaphoid.

Technique
Open: incision over front or radial side of styloid, respect SRN and radial artery. Excise no more than 4mm to preserve ligamentous attachments.
Arthroscopic: preferred. 3/4 portal (scope) 1/2 portal (burr).

Results
Pain relief usually good; movement rarely improves.

STT fusion
📖 See p. 258.

Tuberculosis

Clinical features

Very rare. In wrist, usually presents as an established arthritis. May be associated features of TB in hand (tenosynovitis) or systemically. Can resemble rheumatoid (but rheumatoid usually bilateral, TB almost always unilateral).

Gradual onset of pain, stiffness and weakness.

Wrist swollen and warm, painful to move. Flexor tendon compartment may be involved—large fluctuant swelling either side of transverse carpal ligament (compound palmar ganglion).

Investigation

General: chest X-ray. ESR, CRP.

X-rays: localized osteopaenia and irregularity of radiocarpal and intercarpal joints; sometimes bone erosion.

Biopsy: important to secure diagnosis.

- Zeihl–Neelsen staining (positive = acid-fast bacilli).
- Histology—granulomata with central caseation.
- Culture on Lowenstein–Jensen medium for 6 weeks at 37° for *MycobacteriumTuberculosis*.

Treatment

Antituberculous drugs and wrist splint. If abscess forms, drainage. If carpus destroyed and painful, systemic treatment continued until the disease quiescent then wrist arthrodesis.

Children

General considerations

Congenital upper limb anomalies

- Congenital hand anomalies are common (1 in 500 live births).
- Children's hands are still growing. This must always be kept in mind, and makes their treatment different from adult practice.
- These cases should be treated in specialist centres.

Aetiology

- Spontaneous genetic mutation
- Inherited conditions
- Intrauterine damage
- Drugs
- Infection
- Ionizing radiation

Initial consultation

- The parents and child are likely to be anxious, and may previously have been given conflicting information.
- There may be issues of maternal guilt, parental anger and resentment.
- Families may have unrealistic expectations about the outcome and possibilities of surgery.
- It is important to gain the confidence of the family at the initial consultation, and remember that they are likely to be long-term patients.
- It is important to give a *diagnosis, prognosis, reassurance about the future* and *a long-term plan*, including a *schedule of surgery*, which may be in several stages.
- Many children manage well into adulthood with untreated congenital anomalies, and the requirement for surgery is not always clear.
- Be wary of operating on adults with untreated congenital hand anomalies:
  - They will have adapted to the condition, with established patterns of use.
  - There may be complex psychological reasons for seeking surgery.

Syndromic conditions

- Many congenital hand anomalies are part of a syndrome.
- The surgeon must ensure that the child has been investigated appropriately, and if necessary refer to other specialists.
- Genetic counselling should be made available for inherited or unusual conditions, and may be helpful in reaching a diagnosis.

Examination

- The clinic should be held in a child-friendly setting.
- Toys should be available to allow children to play in an unrestrained manner, which permits close observation of hand function.
- The absence of skin creases suggests congenitally abnormal or absent joints which do not move.
- It is often easier to examine a child sat on its parent's lap.

Reasons to operate

Function

- E.g., pollicization of the index finger to reconstruct an absent or hypoplastic thumb

Progression of deformity

- E.g., division of syndactyly of unequal length (e.g. ring and little fingers) to prevent progressive deviation of the fingers with growth.

Appearance

- The hand is second only to the face in self-consciousness of appearance.
  - If it looks normal, a child is more likely to use it normally.
  - If it looks abnormal, the child will hide it away.
  - This concept is known as 'dynamic cosmesis'.

Pain

- This is a less common indication.
- An example is a tender fingertip in constriction ring syndrome when there is poor soft tissue cover over the bone.

Dressings

- Small children wriggle out of dressings easily.
  - This is distressing to the family
  - It may result in disastrous complications, and compromise your careful surgery (it is always best to get it right the first time).
- In general, use above-elbow dressings or casts, secured to the skin with adhesive tape.
- Dressings can be left on for several weeks until wounds and grafts are healed.
- Dressing changes should be performed under GA or sedation:
  - Reduces the psychological impact of aversive hospital experiences.
  - Allows fitting of splints (if required) by hand therapists at the same time.

Embryology

- Hand and upper limb development occurs in weeks 4 to 6.
- Initiation of upper limb bud is dependent on fibroblast growth factors (FGF) acting on predetermined cells (mesoderm), governed by *HOX* genes.

Timing

Day 27

- The arm bud appears as an ectodermal-covered mesenchymal proliferation at the level of the 8–12 somite.

Weeks 4–5

- The limb bud differentiates proximal-to-distal.

Week 6

- Hand initially develops as a paddle.
- Fingers start to separate by dorsal grooving.

Week 8

- Fingers separate fully.

Weeks 7–12

- Formation of bone, cartilage, neurovascular and other structures.
- Mesenchyme differentiates into cartilage, which then forms primary ossification centres.

Limb bud development

- The limb bud develops along three axes. These 'tell' cells how they are orientated, by producing 'morphogen' diffusible protein factors.

Proximal to distal axis

Humerus or finger

- The key organizer is the **apical ectodermal ridge** (AER), a thickening of the ectoderm running around the rim of the limb bud, in an anterior to posterior direction.
- Undifferentiated mesenchymal cells lie beneath the AER at the apex of the limb bud, in an area known as the **progress zone** (PZ).
- The AER produces FGF-4 (under the influence of the *HOX* gene), and this controls proximal to distal differentiation of the undifferentiated mesenchyme in the PZ.
  - Short time in PZ produces proximal structure.
  - Long time in PZ produces distal structure.
- Removal of the AER causes limb truncation.

Anterior to posterior axis

Radial or ulnar

- This axis is controlled by an area of mesenchyme on the posterior part of the limb known as **the zone of polarizing activity** (ZPA).
- The ZPA expresses a factor which controls differentiation into anterior and posterior structures.
- The cells of the ZPA express the sonic hedgehog gene, and produce the sonic hedgehog protein, which may influence the morphogen factor.

Dorsal to ventral axis
Flexor or extensor

- This axis is controlled by the **dorsal ectoderm**, which produces a morphogen factor controlled by the *wnt7a* gene.
- High concentration produces ventral structures.
- Low concentration produces dorsal structures.

Ossification

Clavicle

- The first bone to ossify
- Appears in membrane before there is any cartilage in the embryo
- **Week 5:** two centres ossify, and fuse rapidly
- Elongation oocurs at the sternal end in secondary cartilage
- Epiphysis at sternal end appears during late teens and fuses during twenties

Scapula

- **Week 6:** whole scapula becomes cartilaginous
- **Week 8:** bony centre appears in lateral angle
- **Birth:** blade and spine ossified
- **10 years:** coracoid process ossifies, and fuses soon after puberty
- **Puberty:** secondary centres appear in acromion, medial border, inferior angle, lower margin glenoid cavity
- **25 years:** all secondary centres fused

Humerus

- **Week 6:** whole humerus becomes cartilaginous
- **Week 8:** primary centre in mid-shaft
- **Birth:** upper and lower ends cartilagenous

Secondary centres (upper end)

- **Year 1:** head of humerus
- **Year 3:** greater tuberosity
- **Year 5:** lesser tuberosity
- **Year 7:** all fuse to single epiphysis
- **Year 20:** single epiphysis fuses

Secondary centres (lower end)

- **Year 2:** capitellum and lateral ridge of trochlea
- **Year 5:** medial epicondyle (stays separate)
- **Year 12:** rest of trochlea
- **Year 13:** lateral epicondyle
- **Years 13–18:** all except medial epicondyle fuse
- **Year 18:** union of all centres with shaft

Radius

- **Week 6:** whole humerus becomes cartilaginous
- **Week 8:** primary centre in mid-shaft
- **Birth:** upper and lower ends cartilagenous
- **Year 1:** secondary centre for lower end
  - The epiphyseal line of the lower end is extracapsular
- **Year 4:** secondary centre for upper end
- **Year 12:** upper end fuses
- **Year 20:** lower end fuses

Ulna

- **Week 6:** whole humerus becomes cartilaginous
- **Week 8:** primary centre in mid-shaft
- **Year 6:** distal ulna (growing end) ossifies
- **Year 10:** epiphysis appears at upper end
- **Year 18:** upper end fuses
- **Year 20:** distal ulna fuses with shaft

Carpus

- **Birth:** whole carpus cartilaginous
- **Year 1:** capitate ossifies
- **Year 2:** hamate ossifies
- **Year 3:** triquetral ossifies
- **Year 4:** lunate ossifies
- **Year 5:** trapezium ossifies
- **Year 6:** scaphoid ossifies
- **Year 7:** trapezoid ossifies
- **Year 10:** pisiform ossifies

Metacarpals and phalanges

- **In-utero:** shafts ossify
- **Birth:** cartilagenous epiphysis at head of 2nd to 5th MCs
- **Birth:** cartilagenous epiphysis at base of 1st MC
- **Birth:** cartilagenous epiphysis at base of phalanges
- **Years 2–3:** cartilagenous epiphyses ossify
- **Year 20:** fusion of all epiphyses

Functional hand development

- 0–3 months: ulnar-sided grasp
- 3–6 months: palmar grasp
- 6–9 months: wrist extension
- 9–12 months: palmar pinch

IFSSH classification of congenital limb malformation

- *Swanson* has classified '*congenital limb malformation*' into seven major categories on behalf of the International Federation of Societies for Surgery of the Hand (IFSSH).
- Some conditions do not fit easily into one category, or may fit into several
  - E.g. thumb hypoplasia in '*Failure of formation*' or '*Undergrowth*'.
- Many conditions have their own classification, e.g.:
  - *Wassell* classification of thumb duplication
  - *Blauth* classification of thumb hypoplasia

I. Failure of formation
Transverse arrest
Longitudinal arrest
Radial ray (pre-axial)
- Radial dysplasia

Ulnar ray (post-axial)
- Ulnar dysplasia

Central ray (cleft hand)
- Cleft hand (typical cleft hand)
- Symbrachydactyly (atypical cleft hand)

Intersegmental/intercalated (phocomelia)

II. Failure of differentiation
Soft tissue
Arthrogryposis
Poland's syndrome
Syndactyly
Camptodactyly
Thumb-in-palm
Trigger digit
Skeletal
Elbow synostosis
Symphalangism
Clinodactyly

Tumerous
Vascular
- Haemangioma.
- Vascular malformation.

Neurological
Skeletal

III. Duplication
Polydactyly

IV. Overgrowth
Macrodactyly

V. Undergrowth
Brachymetacarpia
Brachysyndactyly
Brachydactyly

VI. Constriction ring syndrome
VII. Generalized conditions

Radial dysplasia (radial club hand)

Definition

- Longitudinal radial ray deficiency
- Affects all soft tissues, as well as skeletal structures
- Forearm—wrist—hand most commonly affected
- Radial dysplasia usually associated with thumb hypoplasia
  - EXCEPTION: thrombocytopenia—absent radius (TAR) syndrome where thumbs are normal

Incidence

- 1 in 30 000 to 1 in 100 000 live births
- Male > female
- Right > left
- Half bilateral
- An anomaly of the radius is present in 50% of patients with thumb hypoplasia

Aetiology

- Sporadic
- Syndromal
- Teratogens:
  - Thalidomide
  - Valproic acid
  - Radiation

Associated disorders

- These are common, and are syndromic and non-syndromic.

Haematological disorders
Fanconi anaemia

- Autosomal recessive
- Anaemia, thrombocytopenia, leucopenia
- Cardiac, renal, gut anomalies
- Mental retardation in 20%
- Small/absent thumb in 80%
- Radial dysplasia in 20%

Thrombocytopenia—absent radius (TAR) syndrome

- Autosomal recessive
- Thrombocytopenia and leukocytosis
- Bilateral radial aplasia, **but thumbs present**
- Cardiac, gut, and skeletal anomalies
- Normal intelligence in 90%

Heart disorders
Holt–Oram syndrome

- Autosomal dominant
- ASD in one third
- Triphalangeal thumb
- Radial dysplasia
- Radioulnar synostosis

Craniofacial disorders
- Cleft lip in 7% radial aplasia

Nager syndrome

Hemifacial microsomia

Vertebral disorders

VACTERL (VATER)
- **V**ertebral anomalies
- **A**nal atresia
- **C**ardiovascular anomalies
- **T**racheo-esophalgeal fistula
- **R**enal anomalies
- **L**imb defects

Non-syndromic disorders
Cutaneous
- Syndactyly

Skeletal
- Tri-phalangeal thumb
- Radioulnar synostosis
- Sprengel's deformity
- Scoliosis
- Congenital dislocation of the hip
- Club foot

Neurological
- Hydrocephalus
- Deafness

Pulmonary
Cardiac
- Patent ductus arteriosus
- Ventriculo-septal defect

Gastrointestinal
- Tracheo-oesophalgeal fistula
- Anal atresia

Genitourinary

Classification

Bayne and Klug classification of radial dysplasia

Type 1	Radius shorter than ulna
Type 2	Hypoplastic distal radius
Type 3	Partial absence of radius
Type 4	Complete absence of radius

Incidence
- Type 4 (66%)
- Type 1
- Type 3
- Type 2

Clinical features
- Wrist flexed, with supination and radial deviation of hand.

Skeletal
- Radial deficiency from mildly hypoplastic to absent depending on grade.
- Fibrous '*anlage*' is a band of fibrotic tissue, representing a mesenchymal remnant of the distal radius, which can tether the wrist to the proximal forearm, causing a progressive deformity.
- Forearm short, with ulna only 60% of normal length.
- Bowing of ulna in Types 3 and 4.
- Humerus may be short with distal defects, contributing to reduced elbow ROM.
- No radiocarpal joint. Abnormal articulation of ulna with carpus, and absent TFCC.
- Hypoplastic carpus, with absence or hypoplasia of trapezium and scaphoid.
- Thumb hypoplasia or absence.
- Stiff abnormal fingers, improving from radial to ulnar.

Muscle
- Muscle anomalies related to degree of radial deficiency
- Absent or hypoplastic muscles:
  - Forearm—PT, brachioradialis
  - Extrinsic flexors—FCR, FPL,
  - Extrinsic extensors—ECRL and ECRB, EDM, EI
  - Thumb extrinsics—APL, EPL, EPB,
  - Thenar muscles—APB, FPB, AP
- FDS often fused to FDP
- FDP to index may be absent
- FCU usually present
- Ulnar nerve-innervated intrinsics usually present

Nerve
- Ulnar nerve usually normal
- Musculoskeletal nerve usually absent, with median nerve innervation of anterior compartment of arm.
- Radial nerve usually stops at elbow (SBRN absent)
- Median nerve usually supplies sensibility to radial side of hand and forearm.

Vascular
- Brachial artery usually divides high.
- Ulnar artery usually present.
- Radial artery usually absent.

Management
Manage the patient
- Assess for associated conditions (paediatricians)

Manage the deformity
- There are three treatment options, depending on the patient and the deformity

No treatment
- See list of contraindications for surgery below.
- Most Type 1 patients improve with stretching and splinting.

Educate parents about stretching and splinting
- Types 1 and 2
- Treatment should start as a neonate

Surgery
- Correction of the wrist in severe Type 2, and Types 3 and 4.
- Distraction lengthening of forearm in some Type 2, and Types 3 and 4.
- Ulnar osteotomy when required in Types 3 and 4.

Contraindications for surgery
- Mild anomaly
- Severe associated systemic conditions, with poor prognosis
- Untreated adult (who has grown up and adjusted to deformity)
- Lack of elbow flexion:
  - Straightened hand will not reach mouth or perineum
  - In bilateral cases with stiff elbows, only correct one hand
- Severe soft tissue contracture, where correction is tethered by nerve or vessels

Surgical principles
- Correct the deformity
- Reduce radial and palmar carpal dislocation
- Stabilize wrist
- Realign hand on ulna whilst maintaining wrist movement

Increase the length of the forearm
- Avoid further damage to (already reduced) growth potential

Improve hand function
- Improve prehension, grip and pinch
- Pollicization when required, **after** correction of the wrist

Appearance
- Although improvement in appearance is important, it should not override functional considerations, especially in untreated adults.

Splintage
- All procedures require support using splints postoperatively.

Timing of surgery

Early

Before 6–9 months
- Correct wrist in types 3 and 4:
  - Pre-surgical distraction
  - Centralization/radialization

9–18 months
- Pollicization, or other thumb reconstruction

Late
- Revision of wrist correction as required
- Distraction lengthening of ulna
- Ulnar osteotomy
- Opposition transfer

Operative options

Pre-surgical distraction
- Can achieve correction where stretching and splinting have failed.
- May need to release anlage at time of frame application.
- Allows tension-free wrist correction.
- Additional lengthening reduces pressure on ulnar epiphysis (and less compromise of growth) in severe types.
- Reduces requirement to excise carpal bones to achieve wrist correction.

Centralization
- Resection of central carpal bones to create a slot for the ulna.
- Shaving of distal ulnar cartilage, preserving the epiphyseal plate.
- Insert ulna into slot and pin fixation.
- Rebalancing of ECU and FCU tendons.
- Compromises carpal growth.

Radialization
- Need full passive wrist correction pre-operatively
  - Pre-surgical distraction may be required
- No resection of carpal bones
- 2nd metacarpal aligned with axis of ulna, placing carpus radially, by pin fixation
- Rebalancing of tendons as necessary
- Can maintain limb length and wrist ROM
  - Less damage to carpus and ulnar physis

Distraction lengthening of ulna
- May be used to correct length of ulna, and alignment of wrist

Ulnar osteotomy
- May be performed at same time as wrist correction, or later
- Distraction lengthening technique may also be used to correct radial bowing of ulna

Ulnocarpal arthrodesis
- For wrists at or near skeletal maturity
- For untreated patients
- For recurrence of deformity after previous treatments

Complications
Early
- Pin infection/extrusion
- Broken pin

Late
- Recurrent radial deviation of wrist
- Reduced growth of wrist and forearm
- Stiff wrist

Ulnar dysplasia (ulnar club hand)

Definition
- Longitudinal ulnar ray deficiency

Incidence
- 1 in 100 000 live births
- Unilateral > bilateral (4:1)
- Males > females (3:2)
- Left > right

Aetiology
- Sporadic
- Not related to thalidomide
- Injury to zone of polarizing activity

Associated disorders
- Not associated with systemic anomalies (**unlike** radial dysplasia)
- Mainly skeletal; 50% associated with other musculoskeletal anomalies
- Contralateral limb anomalies in 45% of unilateral cases:
  - Phocomelia, transverse arrest, digital absence, radial deficiency
- Lower limb deficiency in 44%:
  - proximal femoral focal deficiency
  - fibular ray deficiency

Classifications

Forearm and elbow anomalies in ulnar dysplasia (Bayne)

Type 1: hypoplastic ulna
- Distal and proximal ulnar epiphyses present
- Digital absence/hypoplasia common

Type 2: partial aplasia of ulna
- Distal ulna absent
- Proximal ulna present
- Fibrous anlage tethers radius, causing bowing of ulna
- May get radial head dislocation
- Digital absence (usually little finger)

Type 3: total absence of ulna
- Forearm straight as no anlage
- Elbow unstable with posterior dislocation
- Elbow flexion deformities
- Carpal and digital deficiencies

Type 4: radiohumeral synostosis
- Elbow stable and extended
- Ulna absent
- Anlage causes radial bowing, with ulnar deviation of hand
- Hand anomalies always present
- Pronation of forearm and internal rotation of humerus

Hand anomalies in ulnar dysplasia (Manske)

Type A: normal 1st webspace and thumb

Type B: mild 1st webspace and thumb deficiency

Type C: moderate to severe 1st webspace deficiency
- Loss of opposition
- Malrotation of thumb into plane of other digits
- Thumb—index syndactyly
- Absent extrinsic tendon function

Type D: absent thumb

Clinical features
- Hypoplasia of whole limb, with absence/hypoplasia of humerus and shoulder girdle
- Elbow malformed and unstable:
  - radial head dislocation
  - radiohumeral synostosis
- Carpal hypoplasia
- Ulna hypoplastic or absent
- Radius bowed
- Hypoplastic or absent digits:
  - usually ulnar digits, but radial digital absence/hypoplasia, thumb duplication and syndactylies present in 50%
- Syndactyly in 30%
- Thumb or 1st web anomaly in 70%

Management
Manage the patient
- Assess for associated conditions (paediatricians)

Manage the deformity.
Educate parents about stretching and splinting
- Treatment should start as a neonate

Indications for surgery
- Syndactyly
- Thumb hypoplasia
- Tight 1st webspace
- Progressive curvature of radius
- Pronation deformity of forearm
- Internal rotation of forearm

Surgical principles and options
- The limb is more useful than one would expect from the abnormal anatomy.
- The majority of procedures are done in the hand.

Hand
- Separate syndactyly
- Widen and deepen 1st webspace
- Rotational osteotomy to enable opposition of digital tips
- Thumb reconstruction

Wrist
- Splint for the first few years to improve alignment
- The wrist is usually stable—stabilize if necessary
- Excise anlage to correct deformity

Forearm and elbow
- Elbow function usually good despite radial head dislocation:
  - Radial head excision (+/- formation of one-bone forearm) for loss of rotation or elbow instability
- Radial osteotomy for pronation deformity (+/- wedge osteotomy for bowing)

- Tendon transfers to rebalance forces
- Radius or ulnar distraction lengthening when short
- Rotational osteotomy of humerus for internal rotation deformity

Timing of surgery
Early

Before 6–9 months
- Excision of anlage
- ? separation of syndactyly

9–18 months
- Other hand procedures

Late
- Radial osteotomy
- Excision of radial head
- Humeral osteotomy

Complications
- Non-union of one-bone forearm in 30%

Cleft hand

Definition
- Longitudinal central ray deficiency
- Known as '*Typical*' or '*True cleft hand*'.
- Should distinguish it from the central deficiency form of **symbrachydactyly**, which was previously called *Atypical cleft hand*' (□ see p. 544).

Incidence
- 1 in 10 000 to 1 in 90 000 live births
- 50% bilateral

Aetiology
- Sporadic, or autosomal dominant, with variable penetrance in families
- Split hand/split foot gene (*SHFD1*) on chromosome 7

Associated disorders
- May have clefting of one or both feet.
- EEC syndrome most common association:
  - Ectrodactyly
  - Ectodermal dysplasia
  - Cleft lip and palate.
- Associated with many other syndromes, including cardiac, visceral, ocular, auditory, and skeletal abnormalities.

Classification
- *Manske* has classified the thumb webspace, which is useful (and more important than the cleft itself) to plan the treatment

Manske classification of thumb webspace in cleft hand

Type	Webspace	Treatment
I	Normal web	Close cleft
		Excise transverse MC
IIa	Mildly narrowed	Close cleft
		Z-plasties 1st webspace
IIb	Severely narrowed	Close cleft
		Flap to 1st webspace
III	Syndactylized	Close cleft
		Release syndactyly + flap
IV	Missing index finger	No cleft to close
		1st webspace merged into cleft
V	Absent web	Reconstruct thumb

Clinical features

- V-shaped cleft in the centre of the hand.
- Varies from a minor cleft with normal digits (microform) to severe forms.
- Metacarpal abnormalities:
  - Absent metacarpals
  - Transverse metacarpals, which widen cleft with growth
  - Bifid metacarpal supporting two digits
  - Two metacarpals for one digit.
- May be absence of one or more digits.
  - If only a single digit remains, this is the little finger.
- 1st webspace often abnormal and tight
- May be syndactylies of the digits bordering cleft.
- May be angulation and rotation of digits, with delta phalanx.
- Flexion contracture of PIPJs with stiffness.

Management

- Cleft hand has been described by *Flatt* as 'a functional triumph, but a social disaster'.
- Treat to improve function, but consider aesthetics.
- Some families with several affected generations will prefer to leave hands untreated, as function is so good.

Surgical principles and options

Prevent progressive deformity

Transverse bones

- Remove bone, with preservation of the MCPJ capsule, +/− collateral ligament reconstruction.

Unequal (deforming) syndactyly

- Divide to prevent progressive deviation.
- Cleft skin may be used for FTSG if no flap for 1st webspace

1st webspace and closure of the cleft

- This requires one or more of the following procedures:

Release of thumb-index syndactyly, including release of intrinsics

Rotational osteotomy of index

- If index finger is in the plane of the thumb

Transposition of 2nd metacarpal to 3rd metacarpal remnant

- Check rotation, especially in flexion, before fixation

Creation of an intercarpal ligament

- Suture flaps from the adjacent A2 pulleys

Close the cleft skin, and use it as a flap for the 1st webspace

- The following four techniques are combined with 2nd to 3rd metacarpal transposition
- Snow–Littler procedure:
  - Palmar flap transposed from cleft to 1st webspace
  - *Technically complex, with risk of flap necrosis*
- Miura–Komada technique:
  - Ulnar translocation of index ray, using dorsal incisions to close cleft.

- *Ueba* technique:
  - Palmar flap to dorsum, and dorsal flap to palmar surfaces.
- Bilobed flap:
  - Can be used if there is vestigial middle finger in the cleft.

Formation of a new webspace commisure between the index and ring fingers
- Include a small diamond-shaped flap to make a neat commisure on the ulnar side of the transposed digit, and avoid formation of a tight web.

Management of the absent thumb
- Separate syndactylized radial ray and create webspace using flap
- Pollicization of ulnar digit
- Toe transfer

Treat clinodactyly (p. 558) and camptodactyly (see p. 552)
The feet
- As a congenital hand surgeon, you may be involved with the management of the feet.
- Ensure that parts which could be used for hand reconstruction are not discarded.

Timing of surgery
- Removal of transverse bones or separation of unequal syndactyly should be performed early to prevent progression of deformity.
- Other intervention can be performed at the same time, or later.

Symbrachydactyly

Definition
- Translated as 'short fingers with stiff joints'
- Occurs in a teratogenic sequence, from short middle phalanges, through central ray absence causing a U-shaped defect, to absence of the whole hand
- Finger nubbins, with nail remnants, are characteristic
- Difficult to distinguish from true transverse absence

Aetiology
- Thought to be mesodermal.
  - This explains the ectodermal remnants in the form of finger nubbins.
- Usually sporadic, and unilateral.

Associated disorders
- Poland's syndrome

Classification

Yamauchi classification of symbrachydactyly
Type 1: triphalangeal
- No missing bones; all fingers have three phalanges
- Middle phalanx may be short
Type 2: diphalangeal
- One phalanx (usually middle) is missing in one or more digits
Type 3: monophalangeal
- Finger or fingers with only one phalanx
Type 4: aphalangeal
- All three phalanges missing in a digit or digits
Type 5: ametacarpia
- Absence of a metacarpal plus three phalanges in a digit or digits
Type 6: acarpia
- Absence of all the digits and partial or complete absence of the carpus
Type 7: forearm amputation
- Absence of the distal portion of the forearm
- May be rudimentary digits on the stump

Management
Short finger types (Types 1, 2 and 3)
- Function good
- Syndactyly release if indicated
- No other surgery required

Missing and absent fingers (Types 4 to 7)
- The number, position and function of the digits determines treatment.
- Reconstruction of absence proximal to the CMCJs is not possible.

Surgical principles

- The detailed planning of reconstruction is described in *Green's Operative Hand Surgery*.[1]
- The hand is explored for proximal '*enabling structures*' (tendons and nerves), as well as recipient vessels, **prior** to harvest of toe transfers, which should not proceed if these are absent.

Operative options

Deepening of webspace
Transposition of existing rays
Augmentation of an existing digit

- Non-vascularized toe phalangeal transfer
  - Use 3rd toes, and reconstruct with bone graft to prevent floppy toes at donor site
  - Preserve 2nd toes for microsurgical transfers
- Distraction lengthening
- Microsurgical on-top-plasty toe transfer

Microsurgical free toe transfers

Timing of surgery

- Non-vascularized toe phalangeal transfer must be done early for growth to occur.

1. Green DP, Hotchkiss RN, Pederson WC *et al.* (2005). *Green's Operative Hand Surgery*, 5th edn, Elseiver.

Arthrogryposis multiplex congenita (AMC)

Definition
- A syndrome of joint contractures which is present at birth, due to lack of movement during fetal life (from a variety of causes).
- *Arthrogryposis* means curved joints.

Incidence
- 1 in 3000 live births.

Aetiology.
- Unknown.

Associated disorders
- There are many disorders which have features of arthrogryposis:
  - Freeman–Sheldon (whistling face) syndrome (autosomal dominant)
  - Beal's syndrome
  - Wind-blown hand

Classification of AMC	
Group 1	Isolated features of Group 2
Group 2	Classic features (described below)
Group 3	Associated with syndromes or complex anomalies

Clinical features
- Wasted shoulders, held in internal rotation
- Elbows stiff in extension
- Wrists flexed
- Fingers flexed at MCPJs with ulnar deviation.
- Thumbs held in the palm (in flexion and adduction)
- Intellectually normal
- Lower limbs similarly affected by adducted and internally rotated hips, flexed knees and club feet
- Muscle wasting
- Lack of subcutaneous tissue

Management
- The goal is to achieve independent function.
- Passive stretching and splinting in first instance.
- Increase in passive range improves function, and increases possibilities of surgical reconstruction.
- Surgery performed at a later age must take into account established patterns of prehension.

Surgical principles and options
Humerus
- Rotational osteotomy
- Beware of muscle release to correct internal rotation:
  - These children use the humerus to grasp against the chest
  - Transfers for elbow flexion may be compromised.

Elbow

- Posterior capsular release and triceps lengthening to restore passive ROM
- Restore active flexion:
  - Microsurgical functional gracilis transfer
  - Pectoralis major (Clarke's) transfer
  - Steindler flexorplasty
  - (Triceps transfer)—useful to keep for elbow extension especially for wheelchair users.

Wrist

- Correct position by osteotomy, carpectomy, or distraction.
- FCU to ECRL tendon transfer

Fingers

- Release skin, retinacular fibres, and abnormal tendons as for windblown hand +/− camptodactyly correction.
- Tendon transfers

Thumb

- Release adductor contracture
- Correction of 1st webspace
- Further splinting
- Immediate, or delayed (after splinting) tendon transfer(s) for extension and abduction:
  - EI often absent

Poland syndrome

Definition
- Congenital chest and upper limb girdle defect, associated with hand anomalies. Described by *Alfred Poland* in 1841, whilst a medical student at Guy's Hospital.

Incidence
- 1 in 20000 to 30000
- Male = female
- Right > left (2:1)

Aetiology
- Mostly sporadic
- Vascular hypothesis, from hypoplasia and kinking of subclavian artery

Associated disorders
- 1 in 500 000 have *Poland* and *Moebius* (bilateral VI and VII cranial nerve palsy) syndromes.

Clinical features
Hand
- Always hypoplastic
- May be small thumb with tight 1st webspace.
- Single or multiple syndactyly
- Hypoplasia of middle phalanges with symphalangism (ulnar-sided)
- Symbrachydactyly

Upper limb
- Usually hypoplastic forearm, and sometimes hypoplastic upper arm
- Absent sternal (and sometimes clavicular) head of pectoralis major
- Hypoplastic/absent pectoralis minor, serratus anterior, latissimus dorsi and shoulder muscles

Ipsilateral chest
- Hypoplastic/absent ribs, costal cartilage, breast and nipple.

Management
Hand
- Treat anomalies, usually separate syndactyly and 1st webspace.

Chest
- Reconstruct as required (unusual).

Axillary fold
- Reconstruct for appearance (not function), using ilpsilateral (pedicled) or contralateral (microsurgical) latissimus dorsi transfer.

Breast
- Refer to plastic surgeons for reconstruction around time of puberty.

Syndactyly

Definition

- Conjoined digits, usually congenital, but can be caused by scarring following injury, or flap reconstruction

Incidence

- Second most common congenital hand anomaly, after polydactyly.
- 1 in 2000 live births
- Male > female (2:1)
- Bilateral in 50%
- Highest incidence in 2nd post-axial web (3rd webspace on hand)
  - 50% 3rd webspace
  - 30% 4th webspace
  - 15% 2nd webspace
  - 5% 1st webspace

Aetiology

- Familial in 10–40%
- AD inheritance with incomplete penetration and variable expression

Associated disorders

- May be isolated, part of a complex anomaly, or syndromic (Apert's)

Classification

- **Complete** (whole digit) or **incomplete**
- **Simple** (soft tissue only) or **complex** (soft tissue and bone)
- **Acrosyndactyly** tips fused with proximal separation
- **Single** or **multiple**

Management

- Assess nail complex, skin and bony involvement to plan surgery.
- X-ray hand, to detect bony involvement, or hidden polydactyly.

Surgical principles

Surgical problems

- Skin—there is always a skin shortage
  - The circumference of two conjoined digits *is less than* two separate digits (*Flatt*).
- Fascial sheets span the conjoined digits.
- Neurovascular bundles:
  - Distal divisions beyond webspace
  - Neural loops
- Joints:
  - Shared joints
  - Symphalangism
- Bone:
  - Conjoined +/− abnormal bones

Surgical principles

- Create a good webspace:
  - Free, U-shaped, transverse edge
  - Hour glass shape
  - No scar contracture
  - Slopes from dorsal to palmar at 45°
- Minimal scarring on dorsum of digit
- Avoid longitudinal scars on digits
- Avoid hair-bearing skin for use as graft
- Avoid separation of syndactylies on both sides of a digit to avoid vascular compromise

Timing of surgery

- Early separation for complex syndactyly, and digits of unequal length (e.g. ring and little fingers) to prevent differential growth

Operative options

Web reconstruction

- Design carefully to create good webspace, and avoid 'web creep'.
- Dorsal, proximally based, rectangular flap used most commonly.
- 'Gull-wing' design avoids the use of skin grafts by redistributing dorsal skin.
- Many other designs, including triangular dorsal and palmar flaps.

Digital separation

- Use interdigitating, zig-zag flaps.
- Ensure you have drawn correctly (so they interdigitate) when planning!
  - Draw the dorsal flaps on the drapes.
  - Draw the palmar flaps—the orientation is the same.
- Do not suture under excessive tension to achieve closure—better to leave small gaps.
- Some incomplete syndactylies can be treated by other local flaps ('Jumping-man' 5-flap Z-plasty, X-to-M-plasty)

Nailfolds

- Reconstruct the nailfold in complete syndactyly:
  - Buck–Gramco pulp flaps

Skin grafts

- Usually required to cover defect left by webspace flap.
- Harvest laterally in the groin, to avoid pubic hair-bearing skin.

Complications

- Injury to, or inability to separate digital neurovascular bundles.
- Loss of skin graft/delayed healing, leading to scar contracture.
- Web creep.
- Deformity of digit:
  - Differential growth from length inequality before separation
  - Scar contracture.
- Hyperpigmentation of skin graft (common in groin skin).
- Hairy grafts.

Camptodactyly

Definition
- Flexion deformity of the PIPJ in a dorsal–palmar plane of one (usually little finger), or more, digits.

Incidence
- Common, affects 1% of population, mostly affecting the little finger.
- Bilateral in 2/3.
- Many cases are mild, and asymptomatic.
- Two peaks of presentation; in childhood, and early adolescence.

Aetiology
- Imbalance between flexors and extensors.
- Most commonly abnormal lumbrical and abnormal FDS.
  - Many other anatomical anomalies can cause camptodactyly.
- Secondary joint changes and skin shortage.

Differential diagnosis
- Congenital trigger digit
- Absence of extensor mechanism
- Distal arthrogryposis
- Collagen disorders

Associated disorders
- More than 70 associated craniofacial (and other) disorders.

Classification of camptodactyly		
Type 1	Infants	Male = female
		Usually little finger
Type 2	Adolescence	Mainly females
		Usually little finger
		Does not improve spontaneously
		May progress to severe flexion deformity
Type 3	Syndromic	Affects multiple digits of both hands

Clinical features
- The MCPJ may be hyperextended, especially when PIPJ flexion is severe.
- Check whether PIPJ can be passively extended.
  - Yes with MCPJ in flexion, no in extension, probably due to abnormal lumbrical insertion.
- Examine with all other fingers extended, and then allow flexion of ring finger (to see whether connection between FDS IV and FDS V)
- Lateral X-ray shows characteristic appearance:
  - Grooving of the base of the middle phalanx.
  - Chisel-shaped, flexed head of the proximal phalanx.

Management
- Splinting (day and night) for all in the first instance.
- Educate parents, and encourage them to achieve compliance in infants (gradually increase splinting time).

- PIPJ flexion under 40° does not interfere with activity, and should be treated conservatively.

Indications for surgery
- Severe (progressive) deformity that has failed conservative treatment.
- Warn parents and children that results of surgery are inconsistent, and success is not guaranteed.

Surgical principles and options
- Have a surgical scheme which can be tailored to your anatomical findings.
- Explore through palmar zig-zag or mid-lateral *extensible* approach.
- Anticipate and plan for skin shortage (may need local flap or FTSG).
- Release abnormal structures (always explore lumbrical and FDS).
- Consider FDS lasso (Zancolli) to produce MCPJ flexion.
- Consider tendon transfer of FDS or EI through lumbrical canal to extensor mechanism to augment PIPJ extension.
- Total anterior teno-arthrolysis for severe cases/salvage procedure

Complications
- Recurrent camptodactyly
- Skin loss
- Tendon adhesions
- Loss of flexion, and stiffness

Congenital clasped thumb (CCT)

Definition
- Child holds thumbs in an adducted and flexed position, under flexed fingers, beyond 3 months old.
- This is not the same as the spastic thumb-in-palm deformity seen in cerebral palsy (where the diagnosis is clear).

Aetiology
- Familial in up to one-third of cases.
- Commonly part of complex disorder.

Associated disorders
- Wind-blown hand
- 'Whistling face' *Freeman–Sheldon* syndrome (craniocarpotarsal dysplasia)
- Club foot
- Congenital dislocation of the hip
- Camptodactyly

Classifications

Weckesser classification of congenital clasped thumb
Group 1
- Extensors weak or absent
- No other abnormalities
- Passively correctable, so splinting may be successful

Group 2
- Extensors weak or absent
- Flexion contractures of thumb and other digits
- Represents mild arthrogryposis

Group 3
- Thumb hypoplasia

Group 4
- All other cases

McCarroll classification of congenital clasped thumb
Group 1
- Simple CCT with full passive ROM

Group 2
- Complex CCT (all others), not passively correctable

Clinical features

- Often bilateral
- Male > female (2:1)
- Flexion of the MCPJ and adduction of the 1st metacarpal so that the thumb lies across the palm

Management

- It is normal for babies to hold the thumb in the palm for the first 3 months, so the diagnosis should not be made before then.
- It must be distinguished from congenital trigger thumb.
- Conservative treatment by splinting and stretching for passively correctable groups.
- Surgery if splinting unsuccessful.

Surgical principles

Soft tissue release

- May convert complex CCT to simple CCT, which then responds to splinting.
- May require use of local flap from radial border of index finger.

Tendon transfers

- To restore thumb extension, abduction and opposition.
  - EI can be absent

Trigger digit

Definition
- A trigger digit is fixed (usually in flexion) due to a nodule on the tendon, which catches on the edge of an annular pulley.
- As the sensation of triggering is unpleasant, most children hold the digit (usually the thumb) in a fixed (flexion or extension) position.

Incidence
- Trigger thumb commoner than other digits (single or multiple)
- Can be bilateral

Aetiology
- Unknown

Clinical features
- The child usually presents with loss of extension (or flexion) of the thumb IPJ, or finger PIPJ.
- There is often a palpable (Notta's) nodule on the flexor tendon.
- Most present in the first year, but can present later.

Management
- Observe during first year of life, as some resolve spontaneously.
- Can splint, but not tolerated well in very young children.
- Surgery to release A1 pulley in those that do not resolve.

Surgical principles
- GA and tourniquet, and loupe magnification.
- Make a transverse incision across MCPJ flexion crease.
- Expose A1 pulley, using skin hooks to retract skin, and longitudinal blunt dissection, protecting digital nerves.
- Divide A1 pulley on radial side, to avoid injury to oblique pulley.
- Confirm pulley is fully divided, and check full excursion of tendon.

Complications
- Injury to digital nerves
- Hypertrophic scar
- Bowstringing if oblique pulley damaged

Radioulnar synostosis

Definition
- Congenital fusion of the radius and ulna, fixed in pronation.

Incidence
- Rare, bilateral in 60%, male = female

Aetiology
- Autosomal dominant in some

Associated disorders
- **One third** associated with other syndromes (Apert's syndrome, arthrogryposis, fetal alcohol syndrome, Kleinfelter's) and anomalies (thumb hypoplasia, symphalangism, club foot).

Classification

Cleary and Omer classification of radioulnar synostosis
- Fibrous synostosis
- Bony synostosis
- Bony synostosis with posterior dislocation of radial head
- Bony synostosis with anterior dislocation of radial head

Clinical features
- Present between 2 and 6 years with painless absence of forearm rotation, and slight elbow flexion contracture.
- Child holds objects backhanded or in hyperpronated position, and has difficulty catching a ball or other activities requiring supination.
- The synostosis is usually proximal.
- Synostosis initially cartilaginous, which ossifies later.
- The radial head may also be dislocated.

Indications for surgery
- Extreme pronation (> 60°) which interferes with function.
  - Supination required to hold bowl in rice-eating cultures.

Operative options
- Rotational osteotomy, proximal (or distal) through synostosis.
- Excision of synostosis, with interposition of vascularized fascia.
- Surgery to restore forearm rotation is unsuccessful.

Complications
- Vascular compromise and compartment syndrome, especially after rotation >85°.
- Posterior interosseous nerve injury.
- Non-union.

Clinodactyly

Definition
- Deviation of digit in the radioulnar plane, usually at level of PIPJ (or IPJ in the thumb).
- Clinodactyly is usually congenital, but may be acquired following injury to growth plates (e.g. frostbite).

Incidence
- Common, and often familial (autosomal dominant)
- Most commonly radial deviation of little finger at PIPJ, often bilateral.
- Can also affect thumbs

Aetiology
- Deformity may be due to;
  - Minor abnormality of P2
  - Abnormal middle phalanx (delta phalanx), with C-shaped, longitudinally bracketed, epiphysis
  - Short middle phalanx (brachymesophalangia).

Associated disorders
- Clinodactyly is associated with many syndromes, chromosome abnormalities, and complex hand anomalies.
  - Down's syndrome (high incidence)
  - Kleinfelter syndrome
  - Holt–Oram syndrome
  - Treacher–Collins syndrome
  - Apert's syndrome

Management
- Splinting is not successful:
  - doesn't change the shape of the abnormal middle phalanx.
- Reassure anxious parents that there are few functional problems.

Indications for surgery
- Significant angulation (>50–70°)
- Scissoring of fingers
- Progressive deformity from delta phalanx

Surgical principles
- Skin release
- Correct skeletal defect
- Reconstruct skin defect (may need Z-plasty, local flaps or skin graft)

Operative options
- Epiphysiolysis (bracket resection) +/– fat graft—prevents progression
- Closing wedge osteotomy (shortens)
- Opening wedge osteotomy (lengthens)
- Reversed wedge osteotomy (lengthens)

Thumb duplication (radial or pre-axial polydactyly)

Definition
- Thumb duplication (radial, or pre-axial polydactyly)

Incidence
- 0.08/1000 live births (6.6% of all congenital hand anomalies)
- Type 4 commonest, followed by Type 2, and then Type 3.
- Male > female
- Right > left

Associated disorders
- Most occur sporadically
- Radial polydactyly can be associated with syndromes:
  - Holt–Oram syndrome
  - Fanconi anaemia
  - VACTERL
  - Trisomy 21

Classification

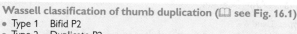

Wassell classification of thumb duplication (📖 see Fig. 16.1)
- Type 1 Bifid P2
- Type 2 Duplicate P2
- Type 3 Bifid P1, duplicate P2
- Type 4 Duplicate P1, duplicate P2 (📖 see Fig. 16.2)
- Type 5 Bifid metacarpal, duplicate P1 and P2
- Type 6 Duplicate metacarpal, P1 and P2
- Type 7 Triphalangeal thumb component

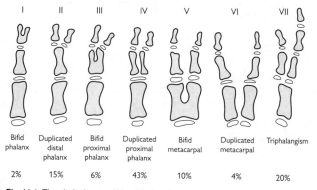

I	II	III	IV	V	VI	VII
Bifid phalanx	Duplicated distal phalanx	Bifid proximal phalanx	Duplicated proximal phalanx	Bifid metacarpal	Duplicated metacarpal	Triphalangism
2%	15%	6%	43%	10%	4%	20%

Fig. 16.1 Thumb duplication. Wassell's classification showed seven types of duplication: Type 4 was the most common.

Clinical features

- Varies according to the level of duplication.
- There may be Z-deformities, and/or unstable joints

Management and surgical principles

- Flatt states that *'It is wise to explain to the parents that they should look on the two thumbs as the result of splitting of one [normal] thumb.'*
- The treatment is more than simple excision of the duplicate thumb.
- Decide which thumb to keep—remove the smaller (usually radial) digit.
- If thumbs are equal size, try to keep ulnar thumb, to preserve ulnar collateral ligament.

Type 1 and 2

- When unequal sizes, remove smaller component.
- When equal size and small, can use *Bilhaut–Cloquet* sharing procedure

Types 3 and 4

- Separation better than sharing.
- Explore for abnormal connection between flexor and extensor tendons (pollex abductus).
- Detach insertion of APB and RCL from base of radial digit and reattach to ulnar digit (☐ see Fig. 16.2).
- Closing wedge osteotomies to the P1 and metacarpal prevent a secondary Z-deformity.

Types 5 and 6

- Similar to Types 3 and 4, with rebalancing of intrinsic muscles.
- 1st webspace may be tight and require Z-plasties or a local flap.

Complications

- Small thumb with stiff joints
- Secondary Z-deformity:
  - Untreated bone or joint deviation
  - Untreated pollex abductus or other tendon anomalies
- Unstable joints

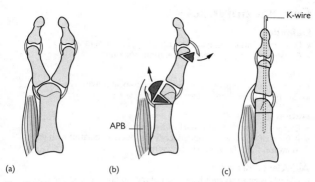

Fig. 16.2 Type 4–dual osteotomy. (a) When the articular surfaces of both joints are not at 90° to the long line of the thumb, a dual osteotomy may be needed. (b) Closing wedge osteotomies are used, and the portion of the metacarpal head corresponding with the discarded thumb is removed. (c) The abductor pollicis brevis (APB) and the collateral ligament are reattached after the K-wire has been passed.

Central polydactyly

Definition
- Extra digit within the hand and not along its borders.
- Commonest in ring, then middle, then index fingers.

Incidence
- Uncommon compared with pre- or post-axial polydactyly
- Can be bilateral, with autosomal dominant trait.

Aetiology
- Occurs in isolation or as part of a syndrome.
- A form of ring finger synpoydactyly has been associated with gene mutation (*HOXD13*) on chromosome 2.

Associated disorders
- Closely related to cleft hand (sometimes in contralateral hand).

Classification

Tada modification of Stelling classification of central polydactyly	
Type I	Soft tissue mass not adherent to existing skeleton
Type II	Duplication of digit (whole or part)
• Type IIA	Not adherent to adjacent digits
• Type IIB	Adherent to adjacent digits (central synpolydactyly)
Type III	Complete duplication of digit and metacarpal

Clinical features
- Extra digit may be hidden within syndactyly (synpolydactyly).

Management
- Separate (Type I, Type IIA and Type III digits) can be excised, including the metacarpal ray if appropriate.
- It may be difficult to decide whether to separate abnormal digits, which may result in unsightly, thin, angulated fingers.
- These may be better left conjoined, or sometimes amputated.
  - better than unsatisfactory, multi-staged attempts at reconstruction.

Ulnar (post-axial) polydactyly

Definition
- Extra little finger

Incidence
- Commonest congenital hand anomaly
- Eight times more common than polydactyly of other digits
- Commoner in African and Asian populations

Aetiology
- Autosomal dominant inheritance, with variable penetration.

Associated disorders
- May be associated with syndrome, chromosomal abnormality, or other anomaly (e.g. cleft lip) in Caucasians

Classification

Stelling classification of ulnar polydactyly	
Type A	Well-formed digit
	Articulation against metacarpal
Type B	Small poorly formed digit
	Narrow soft tissue pedicle to hand

Management
Type A
- Similar to thumb polydactyly.
- Usually excise ulnar digit.
- Detach and reconstruct ADM and UCL.

Type B
- Preferable to excise rather than tie off with cotton by midwives—this can leave painful nodule with underlying neuroma.
- Can do under LA when young (under 3–4 months):
  - Bring baby in starved, and put first on list.
  - Get mum to feed just before procedure; baby will usually then go to sleep.
- Ensure neurovascular bundle dissected out, diathermied, and cut back under tension so nerve end is not in wound.

Macrodactyly

Definition
- Congenital enlargement of a digit in the hand or foot.

Incidence
- Uncommon (0.9% of all congenital hand anomalies), mostly sporadic.

Aetiology
- Primary, of unknown cause.
- Associated with enlargement and fatty infiltration of peripheral nerve.

Associated disorders
- Secondary causes:
  - Neurofibromatosis
  - Gigantism
  - Vascular malformation syndromes (Mafucci, Klippel–Trenauney)
  - Ollier's disease
  - Proteus syndrome
- Syndactyly in 10%

Classification

> **Flatt's classification of macrodactyly**
>
> Type I: lipofibromatosis (most common form)
> - Associated with fatty infiltration of peripheral (often median) nerve
>
> Type II: neurofibromatosis
> - Often seen in plexiform NF. Frequently bilateral.
>
> Type III: hyperostotic form
> Type IV: hemihypertrophy of all digits, sometimes whole limb
> - Proteus syndrome

Clinical features
- Often seen at birth or within first 3 years
- Can be *static* (maintains relationship to the rest of the hand with growth) or *progressive* (disproportionate growth) types.
- Often unilateral.
- Most commonly seen in a single digit, or in the territory of a single nerve.
- Frequently affects more than one digit, which become divergent.
- Index (and middle) most commonly affected.
- Digits stiffen with growth.

Management
- Examine affected digits and limb. Compare with normal side.
- Look for swelling over affected nerve (and signs of nerve compression) and triggering.
- Look for stigmata of secondary causes.
- Compare size with hand of same sex parent.
- X-ray:
  - OA, trapezoidal bones, hyperostotic form.

Indications for surgery
- Functional (digits are stiff, and get in the way).
- Aesthetic (stigmatizing, teasing by peers).
- The family should be informed that this condition is difficult to treat, and surgery is unlikely to produce a normal digit.

Surgical principles and options
Surgery to limit growth

Epiphysiodesis
- When the digit reaches size of same-sex parent's normal digit
- Can include wedge osteotomy to correct deviation

Digital nerve stripping, debulking, or excision

Correction of deviation

Wedge osteotomy

Surgery to reduce size
- Debulking
- Usually one half at a time

Ray amputation
- May be better than multiple procedures resulting in a stiff, functionless digit.
- Avoid in thumb.

Thumb hypoplasia

Definition
- Congenital hypoplasia or aplasia of the thumb.

Incidence
- 4.6% of all congenital hand anomalies.

Aetiology
- Isolated, or as part of many other conditions or syndromes.

Associated disorders
- Radial or ulnar dysplasia (as part of it)
- Thumb duplication (one or both thumbs small)
- Symbrachydactyly and transverse absence
- Constriction ring syndrome

Classification

Blauth classification of thumb hypoplasia

Type III modified by Manske and McCarroll.

Type I	Mild hypoplasia, with normal function
Type II	Tight 1st webspace, with adduction contracture
	Lax UCL
	Hypoplasia of thenar muscles
Type IIIA	Extrinsic and intrinsic musculotendinous deficiencies
	Intact 1st CMCJ
Type IIIB	Extrinsic and intrinsic musculotendinous deficiencies
	Absent 1st CMCJ
Type IV	Soft tissue pedicle; no skeletal attachment (*Pouce flottant*)
Type V	Absent thumb

Clinical features
- These are described in the classification above.

Pollex abductus
- This is an abnormal connection between the FPL and EPL:
  - Also seen in thumb duplication
- Movement is poor at the IPJ with poorly defined skin creases.
- Attempted flexion at the IPJ produces abduction of the thumb.

Management
- Assess thumb deformity
- Look for other anomalies
- X-ray hand and forearm

Indications for surgery

Type I
- Usually not required

Type II and IIIA
- Triple procedure:
  - Augment 1st webspace, UCL reconstruction, opposition transfer.

Type IIIB
- Most prefer pollicization of index (or other digit).
- Can reconstruct, using vascularized free MTPJ transfer.

Type IV and V
- Pollicization of index (or other digit).

Operative options

Augment 1st webspace
- Z-plasty techniques:
  - Standard, 4-flap, 5-flap (Jumping man)
- Dorsoradial flap from index (usually closes directly)
- Dorsal flap from thumb (usually requires FTSG)
- FTSG
- Regional, distant or free flaps:
  - A free groin flap gives the least conspicuous donor site in children.

UCL reconstruction
- Free tendon graft (PL, plantaris, 2nd toe extensor)
- Can use slips of FDS when combined with opposition transfer

Opposition transfer
- ADM (Huber–Nicholayson)—also provides some thenar bulk
- FDS III or IV

Pollicization
- Must have a good-quality index finger (this can also be hypoplastic).
  - If not, it will not be used by the child after pollicization, so consider other digit.

Brachydactyly

Definition
- Short fingers (usually middle phalanx), or metacarpals, where all the bones are present, but one or more are small.

Incidence
- Rare as an isolated condition feature (autosomal dominant)

Aetiology
- Isolated, sporadic, part of syndrome, following trauma (e.g. frostbite) or metabolic disease (e.g. pseudohypoparathyroidism).
- Some types now mapped to chromosomes 2 and 9.

Associated disorders
- Associated with many syndromes.

Classification

Modified Bell classification of brachydactyly

Type A: all have short middle phalanges (P2) (the last to ossify):
- A1 (Farabee): short P2, sometimes fused to P3
- A2 (Mohr–Wriedt): short delta phalanx P2 index finger/2nd toe
- A3 (Bauer): short delta phalanx P2 middle finger
- A4 (Temtamy): short P2 index and little fingers
- A5 (Bass): absent P2, hypoplastic P3 and nails

Type B: Mackinder:
- Hypoplastic P3 with absent nails

Type C: Drinkwater:
- Short P2 index/middle. Delta phalanx little finger
- Hyperphalangism (extra bone) index and middle fingers
- Short metacarpals

Type D: Breitenbecker:
- Short P2 thumb

Type E: Bell:
- Short metacarpals with normal length phalanges
- Short stature

Other
- *Pitt–Williams:* short P3 ulnar digits, short MCs, normal stature
- *Sugarman:* short P1 with symphalangism
- *Smorgasbord:* combination of Types A2 and D

Clinical features
- Degree of shortening is variable.
- There may be syndactyly, clinodactyly, and symphalangism.

Indications for surgery

- Minimal functional impairment, apart from short central rays, especially metacarpals, when grip may be reduced if the metacarpal head is in the proximal palm.
- Treat associated conditions, such as sydnactyly and clinodactyly.
- Results for digital lengthening are disappointing, and this should be discouraged.
- Metacarpal distraction lengthening can improve function and appearance (restores normal digital cascade).

Operative options

- One-stage lengthening +/– bone graft:
  - Can combine with wedge osteotomy for correction of angulation
- Distraction lengthening +/– bone graft

Complications

- Digital lengthening can produce stiff, scarred fingers, with downgraded function.

Constriction ring (amniotic band) syndrome

Definition

- Congenital disorder, with constriction rings, acrosyndactyly, and distal amputations. The proximal limb is usually normal.

Incidence

- 1 in 5000 to 1 in 15 000 live births.

Aetiology

- Still not completely understood.
- Exogenous, due to constriction by amniotic band, perhaps from perforation of amniotic sac.
- Endogenous, due to band-like apoptosis.

Associated disorders

- None
- Can be confused with symbrachydactyly p. 544, which has nail remnants.

Classification

Patterson's classification of ring constriction syndrome	
Group 1	Simple ring constriction
Group 2	Ring constriction with distal deformity +/– lymphoedema
Group 3	Ring constriction with distal fusion (acrosyndactyly)
Group 4	Intrautetrine amputation

Clinical features

- Dried-up amniotic bands seen attached to ring constrictions in neonate.
- Constriction rings can affect limbs, trunk and head and neck.
- Acrosyndactyly.
- Tapering amputation stumps, usually without nails.
- Amputation, nerve and lymphatic obstruction.

Management

Group 1: simple ring constriction

- Excise constriction ring, including groove (safe to excise whole ring in one go).
- Suture with multiple Z-plasties.

Group 2: ring constriction with distal deformity +/– lymphoedema

- May require urgent surgery for limb or digital salvage.
- Excision and Z-plasties as above
- Usually requires excision of ring of deep fascia if tight.
- May require decompression of peripheral nerves if symptomatic.
- Can also use multiple Y- to V-plasties for skin closure (less skin distortion)

Group 3: ring constriction with distal fusion (acrosyndactyly)
- Digits are short, oedematous, and distally amputated, with a fenestration at the proximal end of the web.
- Separate (where appropriate) using zig-zag flaps and FTSG (may be available from discarded parts).

Group 4: intrautetrine amputation
Stump revision
- Fingertips usually have poor soft tissue cover, and are painful
- Revision by minor shortening, or use of advancement flaps where appropriate improve function and apprearance significantly

On-top plasty
- Usually to augment thumb with remnant of index finger when this is also missing.

Toe transfers
- Whole or partial (usually 2nd toe) transfers can be used to reconstruct the thumb and other digits.
- The feet may be incomplete if also affected.

Spare part surgery
- In the event of amputation of unsalvageable toes or a leg, the spare parts (skin and toes) should be used to reconstruct the hand.

Trauma

- The principles of the treatment of trauma are covered in Chapter 5, 6, and 7.
- These can all be applied to the treatment of children. There are a few extra considerations.

Surgery

- Use loupe magnification.
- Use absorbable, fine, skin sutures.

Donor sites

- Try to avoid disfiguring donor sites for flap or skin grafts.
- Consider the donor site carefully when choosing flap reconstructions:
  - Good—e.g. free groin flap
  - Bad—e.g. radial forearm flap, scapular flap.

Growth

- Damage to the physis, by the injury, or by surgery, will affect growth.
- Reconstruction must allow, or sometimes import, the ability to grow.
- SSG is tight, and restrains growth.
- Flaps grow with the child, without contractures.
- Scar contracture limiting movement of joints can lead to remoulding of joint surfaces, and established capsular contracture, with loss of range of movement.
- Vascularized joint, or epiphyseal transfers import the potential for bony growth.
- It is safe to place a K-wire across a growing joint for several weeks.

Compliance

- Young children will not comply with postoperative instructions, or complex rehabilitation.
- Dressings have to be foolproof, and may need to be changed under anaesthetic or sedation.
- Tendon repairs should be wrapped up in a boxing glove-type dressing, allowing a limited range of movement, but protecting the repairs, for 4–6 weeks, depending on the age of the child, and the nature of the injury.
- It is difficult to use distant flaps, such as the pedicled groin flap, or techniques such as tissue expansion, in young children.
- Children cannot work with therapists following 2-stage tendon reconstruction much before the age of 7 or 8.

Tumours

Types of tumour

Benign

Bone and cartilage
- Osteoid osteoma
- Osteoblastoma
- Chondroma (enchondroma, periosteal chondroma = ecchondroma)
- Osteochondroma (exostosis)
- Chondromyxoid fibroma
- Fibrous tumours of bone (fibrous cortical defect, non-ossifying fibroma, fibrous dysplasia)
- Unicameral (solitary) bone cyst
- Aneurysmal bone cyst
- Epidermoid cyst
- Giant cell tumour of bone

Soft tissue
- Epidermal inclusion cysts (dermoid cysts)
- Fat tumours (lipoma and lipofibroma)
- Connective tissue tumours (fibroma, dermatofibroma, desmoplastic fibroma)
- Synovial tumours
- Giant cell tumour of tendon sheath (PVNS)
- Vascular tumours (haemangioma, lymphangioma, glomus tumour)
- Nerve tumours (neurilemmoma = Schwannoma, neurofibroma)

Tumour-like lesions
- Ganglia and mucous cysts
- Foreign body responses (granuloma)
- Fibromatoses

Malignant

Bone and cartilage
- Osteogenic sarcoma (= osteosarcoma)
- Chondrosarcoma

Soft tissue
- Liposarcoma
- Fibrohistiocytic tumours (Malignant fibrous histiocytoma (MFH), fibrosarcoma, dermatofibrosarcoma protuberans)
- Rhabdomyosarcoma
- Synovial sarcoma
- Malignant vascular tumours (angiosarcoma, haemangiopericytoma, Kaposi's sarcoma)
- Epitheloid sarcoma
- Clear-cell sarcoma

Benign tumours of bone and cartilage

Benign tumours are generally discovered coincidentally. For example, an X-ray taken following an injury may show a lesion. Benign tumours are well-delineated lesions that do not usually exhibit rapid progression, bone and soft tissue destruction. Clinically, the symptoms are mild. Pain is not a common feature. Benign lesions are staged as follows:

Staging

- **Stage 1:** asymptomatic lesions. They may be latent (non-proliferative) and if so do not require treatment.
- **Stage 2:** active lesions, frequently require surgery. Recurrence is possible.
- **Stage3:** aggressive lesions demonstrating destruction. Treatment requires wide excision.

Enchondroma

Common cartilage-producing tumour. The hand is commonly involved (50% of all enchondromata seen in hand bones). Diagnosis is commonly coincidental after a pathological fracture. Unlike their counterparts in large bones, solitary enchondromata of the hand almost never convert to a chondrosarcoma.

X-rays show a well-delineated osteolytic lesion with thinning of the cortices.

Treatment for asymptomatic enchondroma is therefore not indicated. If the patient presents with a pathological fracture, the fracture is allowed to heal first. The enchondroma is then curetted and grafted.

Ollier's disease

Multiple enchondromatsis. Non-familial.

Mafucci syndrome

Multiple haemanigiomata are seen in addition to enchondromata. Patients with multiple enchondromata should be followed up carefully for possible conversion into chondrosarcoma.

Osteochondroma (exostosis)

Second most common benign bone tumour (after non-ossifying fibroma). The lesion grows from the metaphseal area away from the adjacent joint. The cartilage cap has histologic characteristics similar to a growth plate and stops growing at the same time as the bone itself.

Hereditary multiple exostosis (HME)

Autosomal dominant condition. The conversion rate to chondrosarcoma is 1%. Treatment is by excision.

Epidermoid cyst

Seen almost exclusively in the distal phalanx or skull. The pathogenesis is the same as epidermoid (or dermoid) cysts seen in soft tissue—a compound (crush) injury which thrusts epidermal cells of the nail bed into the distal phalanx. Presents with is with a swollen fingertip. The cyst can be transilluminated. X-rays demonstrate a clearly defined lesion which replaces bone usually on one side of the phalanx. Treatment is by excision (curettage) and bone grafting if required.

Osteoid osteoma

Osteoid-producing neoplasm. Peak incidence is in the second decade. Although the hand and wrist are generally not typical locations, the most common location in the hand is the proximal phalanx. It has also been reported in the carpal bones.

The clinical presentation includes pain which is worse at night and is relieved by aspirin. Less than 10% of osteoid osteomata (OO) are pain-free. The characteristics of pain may change depending on location. The pain is dull and hard to localize if the lesion is in the carpus, in case of phalangeal lesions it is sharp and easily localized. Reactive joint swelling may be seen with juxta-articular lesions and swelling is more obvious with digital lesions (a cause of *dactylitis,* 📖 see p. 383).

Investigation

- **X-ray** shows characteristic osteolytic nidus surrounded by reactive sclerosis. This appearance has many variations, depending on the amount of the two components, i.e. osteolysis and reactive sclerosis.
- **Technetium** 99 three-phase bone scan is nearly 100% sensitive.
- **CT scan** is highly specific.
- **MRI scan** can differentiate hypervascular OO and other hypovascular lesions.

Treatment

- **NSAIDs** for pain relief. Remission may be obtained over a prolonged period (2–20 years!).
- **Surgery:** curettage, or en bloc resection of the area. Precise intra-operative localization is crucial as incomplete excision of nidus is the most important determinant for recurrence. Newer, percutaneous techniques have been described to reduce morbidity. These include drilling, trochar ablation, radio frequency ablation (RFA) and laser. Recurrence rates 5–25% .

Giant cell tumour of bone

Locally aggressive tumour. Variants common in childhood include aneurysmal bone cyst (ABC), chondroblastoma, osteoid osteoma and osteoblastoma. The giant cell reparative granuloma is also similar, however it exhibits spindle rather than giant cells. More common in females. The distal radius is the second common location (after the proximal tibia). Metastasize to the lung in about 2%.

Clinical presentation

Joint effusion and pain. Pathological fracture is also possible although the lesion does not normally break through the articular cartilage into the adjacent joint.

Investigation

- X-rays: lytic lesion at the epiphyseal–metaphyseal junction.
- Chest X-ray to exclude metastasis.

Treatment

Curettage, burring of the tumour walls and adjuvant chemoablation using phenol, hydrogen peroxide or liquid nitrogen. The cavity is then packed with bone cement. The recurrence rate is 10–25%. Therefore more aggressive resection of the tumour and surrounding soft tissue extension is recommended. In the distal radius allograft or free fibular reconstruction should be considered. Radiotherapy is contraindicated as it is likely to increase this recurrence rate.

Chondromyxoid fibroma

Rare tumour. Predominantly seen in males in their second and third decade. Presents with mild pain and slowly growing mass. Radiographs show a similar appearance to a bone cyst with loculations. Histologically, the features may be mistaken for a chondroblastoma or chondrosarcoma. Excision of the lesion with or without bone grafting is recommended.

Aneurysmal bone cyst

Rarely seen in the hand, however phalanges, metacarpals and carpal bones may be affected. X-ray findings are expansion of the bone with formation of septae, and destruction of the cortex which can give the impression of a malignant tumour. Differential diagnosis should also include giant cell tumour (GCT) of bone. Treatment should commence with a biopsy to avoid undue extensive surgery, as these lesions may be left alone to involute forming a layer of reactive bone at the periphery. Healing may be expedited by curettage and bone grafting.

Intraosseous ganglia

These are rare and may present as a coincidental X-ray finding. Symptoms may include weakness and a dull ache. Diagnosis is possible on plain X-rays, however for accurate delineation, use CT or MRI. Treatment may not be required if findings are coincidental and the patient is symptom-free. Curettage of the lesion and bone grafting, usually under X-ray control, is the treatment of choice in symptomatic cases.

Ganglia

Aetiology

Ganglia represent the majority (50–70%) of soft tissue swellings in the hand and wrist. They are seen throughout life. Developmentally, there are two variants.

The first type is seen in young people, typically between second and fourth decades of life. These do not have associated osteoarthritis, however they may be associated with underlying joint laxity.

The second type occurs from the fifth decade onwards, and is generally associated with underlying joint arthritis.

Ganglia may appear suddenly but usually grow gradually. They are attached to an underlying joint, or tendon sheath. Just occasionally there is a convincing temporal relationship with a violent event (e.g. forced flexion of the wrist) to suggest a traumatic aetiology.

Pathology

Ganglion cysts may be uni- or mutilocular with the wall comprising collagen. They do not have an epithelial or synovial lining. The stalk is filled with serial clefts which represent a tortuous duct from the underlying join to the ganglion. Histopathologically, no inflammatory reaction is present. The cyst contains highly viscous jelly-like mucin consisting of glucosamine, proteins, and hyaluronic acid. The pathogenesis is unclear, however it appears that there is a 'microscopic herniation' of mucin forming cells through the fibres of the joint capsule, ultimately forming the ducts and lakes of mucin seen on histologic sections of the stalk. These coalesce to form the visible subcutaneous cyst.

Wrist ganglia

Dorsal

Most common location for ganglia. (Two-thirds of all wrist ganglia.) Typically arise from the confluence of capsule over the scapholunate ligament and capitate ligament.

Occult ganglia

These are very small and may be impalpable or only palpable with wrist hyperflexed. Patients complain of localized pain especially on forced extension under load; on examination they have a localized point of tenderness over the scaphoid–lunate–capitate confluence. The differential diagnosis is dorsal synovial impingement which has the same symptoms and signs.

Dorsal synovitis

Patients with radioscaphoid arthritis, typically males aged 60 onwards, may have a diffuse dorsoradial swelling. This is not a ganglion, but synovial thickening associated with arthritis. Supporting physical signs include painful loss of radial tilt and palmar flexion. X-rays are diagnostic.

Tenosynovitis

Synovitis around the ECRB/ECRL or EDC tendons may mimic a ganglion. Careful examination will distinguish.

Extensor tendon ganglion
Attached to the extensor tendon, small and hard, moves with

Volar
One-third of wrist ganglia are volar; may arise from radiocarpal or STT joint, occasionally pisotriquetral joint. The ganglion may be in close contact with the branches of radial artery and its accompanying veins, or the FCR sheath, making surgical dissection difficult.

Diagnosis
Clinical
This is usually straightforward by inspection and palpation of the cyst. Transillumination (shining of a pen light into the lesion in a dark room) helps if in doubt. A solid lesion will not allow light through whereas ganglion gel will.

Imaging
- *Ultrasound:* specific for differentiating solid from liquid lesions.
- *MRI* is very sensitive. Asymptomatic small ganglia are often seen; as usual with MRI, findings must correlate with the clinical picture.

Rare differential diagnosis of wrist ganglia
- Inflammation (rheumatoid nodules, gout tophi)
- Infection (bacteria, fungi)
- Neoplasms (soft tissue and bone)
- Vascular malformations (aneurysms, A-V malformations)
- Anomalous muscle

Treatment of wrist ganglia
No treatment is required for the majority, unless there is a clear justification to treat. Many ganglia will spontaneously resolve in time.
The following treatments have been tried with varying success.

Aspiration with a large bore needle
This occasionally succeeds. The aspirated material usually re-forms within a matter of days. However, the demonstration of the collapse of the lesion is therapeutic for some, allaying fears of cancer.

Aspiration + injection
Various substances including steroids, hyaluronidase and sclerosing agents have been used with moderate success. Recurrence is usual and infection is a rare but severe complication.

Surgery
This is the only reliable treatment method. It may be done as an open or arthroscopic procedure for dorsal ganglia. It is important to follow the stalk of the ganglion into the joint and excise a cuff of joint capsule around the stalk.

Operative technique for dorsal ganglia

The ganglion is exposed through a transverse skin crease incision. The extensor retinaculum is incised and tendons retracted. The ganglion is bluntly dissected free from the surrounding tissues and its stalk is followed to the wrist capsule. Excision must include a cuff of dorsal wrist capsule around the stalk to minimize recurrence. The capsule is left open. It is important to direct the blade away from the plane of the scapho-lunate ligament (i.e. to hold tangentially to it) to ensure its integrity is not breached. Satellite ganglia are excised if present.

Other types of ganglia

Flexor tendon sheath ganglion (seed ganglion)

Third most common ganglion in the hand and wrist. Arises from weak-spot between A1 or A2 pulley. Paniful on grip.

Diagnosis: palpation of firm and tender mass which does not move with finger flexion/extension.

Treatment: needle aspiration helps 50–60%. Surgery for recurrence.

Operative technique for seed ganglion

A1 pulley is approached through an oblique or Bruner-type palmar incision. Neurovascular bundles retracted. Ganglion removed including healthy cuff of surrounding tissue (pulley). Integrity of A2 pulley must be preserved

Mucous cyst (nail-bed cyst) (DIP joint)

Older age group. Early clinical signs include grooving of the nail plate due to pressure on germinal matrix. Later, the cyst weakens the overlying skin and may rupture and drain—renders cyst vulnerable to infection, which may track into the DIP joint. Heberden's nodes are often present. Treatment is surgical excision if required.

Operative technique for mucous cyst

Cyst is exposed through Y-shaped incision over back of DIP joint if it is relatively proximal. If it under the nail fold, then a longitudinal incision is made over the cyst, reflecting the nail fold sideways . The cyst is traced to its root usually a small osteophyte in the dorsal corner of the DIPJ. The sharp osteophyte and the capsule of the cyst is excised to lessen the chance of recurrence. A transposition flap may be required if the condition of overlying skin is poor.

CMC joints (carpal boss) associated ganglion

Ganglia may be seen growing where a juxta-articular osteochondroma of the CMC joints (most commonly the 3rd CMC joint) is present. This should be excised together with the underlying osteochondroma (exostosis) if it comes to surgery.

PIP joint/extensor tendon

- Ganglia may appear on the extensor tendon similar to the DIPJ. Treatment by aspiration or by surgical excision including cuff of dorsal PIP joint capsule.

First dorsal compartment

Ganglia may occur on the surface of the first dorsal compartment, usually in patients with De Quervain's disease. Diagnosis by palpation of the firm, tender, immobile cyst. Intracompartmental steroid injection can be curative for De Quervain's disease and ganglion. In persistent cases, surgical release of the first dorsal compartment with excision of the ganglion is required.

Ulnar (Guyon's) canal

Ganglia arise from the pisotriquetral joint or triquetro-hamate joint.

The presentation may be with low ulnar nerve palsy (see p. 324). Diagnosis confirmed by USS or MRI. Treatment: surgical exploration of Guyon's canal and excision of the ganglion

Benign tumours of soft tissue

Giant cell tumour of tendon sheath

Second most common soft tissue tumour of the hand. Otherwise kown as pigmented villonodular synovitis (PVNS). Histology: multinucleate cells, haemosiderin deposits, histiocytes. Arises close to tendons sheaths and joints. Several aetiologic factors proposed, e.g. genetic, inflammatory, traumatic, immunological and metabolic. Benign tumour but high rate of local recurrence following surgical treatment, especially if associated with DIPJ. Malignant change has never been reported.

Clinical findings

Slowly growing painless lump, usually in finger. X-rays may show erosion into bone. At surgery, orange-brown, lobulated, and pedunculated appearance of the lesion. Lesion may be fixed to bone or joints or entwined around neurovascular structures. Satellite lesions may be present.

Treatment

Thorough excision preferably en bloc to avoid tumour seeding. Recurrence between 10–30%.

Epidermal inclusion cysts (dermoid cysts)

Third most common soft tissue swelling of the hand. These are aberrant skin islands under the skin probably caused by traumatic implantation of skin elements. Present with firm, sometimes fluctuant (in case of sebum formation) swelling. Excision is straightforward as the lump has a well-defined capsule and is not adherent.

Pyogenic granuloma

Beinign lesion usually post-traumatic. Most common on fingertip. Grows rapidly into peduculated friable red lump. Treatment by silver nitrate if small, surgical excision if larger or recurrent.

Haemangioma

Paediatric haemangioma usually on back of hand. Grows rapidly in the first 2 years of life. Majority resolve spontaeously by age 7 (📖 see p. 606).

Glomus tumours

Arise from the glomus bodies located in the dermis (A-V shunts to regulate temperature). Most common location in the fingertips, particularly nailbed. These lesions can cause intense pain.

Diagnosis

A purple discolouration may be seen through the nail plate. Very localized exquisite tenderness may be elicted by applying pressure with tip of a pen (Love sign). Tenderness diminishes if a tourniquet is applied. Plain X-rays may show scalloping of bone. MR is diagnostic.

Treatment

Careful pre-operative marking. Meticulous surgical excision to prevent recurrence.

Fat tumours (lipomata and lipofibromata)

Fifth most frequent benign tumours. May arise from within muscle (intra-muscular), between muscle planes (intermuscular), from within the tendon sheath. Neural fibrolipoma occurs around nerves and can be found in carpal tunnel (therefore good practice to palpate the carpal tunnel for any possible space occupying lesions at every routine carpal tunnel decompression).

Fibromatoses

Keloid

Scar hypertrophy is an unwelcome complication after an injury or operation. More common in 2nd and 3rd decade as well as in dark-skinned and black individuals. Sloppy surgical technique may contribute to hypertrophy of the scar but keloid is seen only in susceptible individuals. Treatment options include elastic pressure garments, intradermal steroid injection and surgical excision. Radiation has been used in the past but best avoided due to danger of secondary skin tumour development.

Fibroma

- Well-encapsulated lesion arising adjacent to a tendon sheath or nail.
- Treatment: Excision.

Dermatofibroma

Dermatofibromata are locally invasive and recurrent lesions. They include the following:
- Subdermal fibromatosis of infancy
- Infantile dermatofibromatosis
- Infantile digital fibroma
- Juvenile aponeurotic fibroma
- Palmar fibromatosis (Dupuytren's)

These conditions have a strong genetic predilection. The infantile and juvenile forms are either present at birth or appear during the first decade of life. Aggressive local behaviour—recurrent enlargement and extension. Biopsy may be required for differential diagnosis from malignant fibrous histiocytoma and fibrosarcoma. Treatment is mainly expectant for juvenile and infantile lesions unless the lesions interfere with function of the limb (hand/foot) when functional surgery may be required. High local recurrence rate.

Desmoplastic fibroma

This is a very rare and aggressive form of fibromatosis. It is clinically and histopathologically similar to fibrosarcoma. It is locally aggressive but non-metastatic. Treatment is by excision or amputation.

Nerve tumours

See Chapter 11.

Malignant tumours

Malignant tumours in the hand are rare and therefore can be missed. Treatment requires expertise which can only be accumulated if these cases are referred to dedicated musculoskeletal tumour centres for management. The treatment and prognosis are related to factors such as location, size, histological grade and expansion (tissue invasion) of the lesion.

Staging

• **MSTS system** (Musculoskeletal Tumor Society) or Enneking system. Grades lesions according to expansion, i.e. whether intra- or extra-compartmental, histological grades (low or high grade) and whether or not distant metastasis exists. The concept of a compartment is important in Enneking's classification. A compartment may be the bone itself in case of bone and cartilage tumours. It could be a fascial compartment in soft tissue tumours. However, compartments are not so easy to define in the hand. Anatomical spaces (compartments) may extend far beyond their boundaries, i.e. into the wrist and forearm, e.g. extrinsic tendons. For clarity, a lesion in the hand and wrist may only be considered intra-compartmental if:
  • It is superficial to deep fascia i.e. it is subcutaneous
  • It is confined to a single digital ray;

Table 17.1 MSTS (Enneking) staging

Stage	Grade	Site
IA	Low	Intra-compartmental
IB	Low	Extra-compartmental
IIA	High	Intra-compartmental
IIB	High	Extra-compartmental
III	Any	Metastasis

Table 17.2 AJCC staging

Stage	Grade	Size	Depth
IA	Low	<5cm	Sup/deep
IB	Low	>5cm	Sup
IIA	Low	>5cm	Deep
IIB	High	<5cm	Sup/deep
IIC	High	>5cm	Sup
III	High	>5cm	Deep
IV	Any lymph node or distant metastasis		

Sup, superficial to fascia; Deep, deep to fascia.

• **American Joint Committee on Cancer (AJCC) system.** AJCC staging relies on size, histological grade, depth and presence of metastasis.

Malignant tumours of bone and cartilage

Management of malignant bone and cartilage tumours requires a multi-disciplinary approach. These tumours are uncommon, and they are rare in the wrist and hand. Therefore it is essential that cases are referred to centres where expertise has been accumulated.

Ostogenic sarcoma (osteosarcoma)

Most frequent primary malignant bone tumour. Annual incidence is 2–3 per million, peaks at adolescence. About 15% arise in the upper extremity, mainly the proximal humerus., with the hand constituting less than 0.1%. Many subtypes have been described, such as periosteal and parosteal lesions. The tumour arises from the metaphyseal–epiphysial junction. Diagnosis is by recognizing the slowly but relentlessly growing mass, or as a result of a pathological fracture. Early metastasis is common, however only about 20% of patients are diagnosed as having metastasis at first diagnosis.

Investigation

- *X-ray*: radiolucent area surrounded by new bone formation, periosteal elevation with bone formation (Codman triangle) and ossification of soft tissues in a radial 'sunburst' pattern.
- *MRI*: defines the extent of invasion thus providing information to plan surgery.

Treatment

- Radical excision of the tumour, including amputation.
- Adjuvant chemotherapy is routinely used.

Chondrosarcoma

Most common primary malignant bone tumour of the hand, yet only 1% of all chondrosarcomata grow in the hand. Metacarpals and proximal phalanges are the preferred location. Seen in the 5th decade of life or later. Originates from cartilage cells in and around joints. Associated with enchondromatosis but malignant transformation of a solitary enchondroma has not been reported. The male to female ratio is 2:1. Chondrosarcoma presents as a slow-growing mass. The tumour is locally invasive, but metastasis is only seen in about 10% of patients. The lungs are the most common sites of metastasis.

Investigation

- *X-ray*: areas of calcification within cartilage matrix.

Treatment

- Surgical excision.
- Chemotherapy and radiation therapy are not effective.

Soft tissue sarcoma (STS)

- The term sarcoma is derived from the Greek word for *flesh*.
- These are malignant tumours of the soft tissues, of mesodermal and neuroectodermal origin.
- STS represent 1% of all malignant tumours.
- 50% of STS affect the limbs (upper and lower, especially the thigh). Only 5% in the hand and wrist.
- There is a tendency to misdiagnose because of the rarity and diversity of the presentation.
- There is no age or sex predominance.
- They are classified according to their tissue of origin, and each has a different pattern of behaviour.
- They are aggressive tumours, which should only be treated in specialist centres.

Types of soft tissue sarcoma
- Fibrous tissue:
  - Fibrosarcoma
  - Malignant fibrous histiosarcoma
- Fat:
  - Liposarcoma
- Smooth muscle:
  - Leiomyosarcoma
- Skeletal muscle:
  - Rhabdomyosarcoma
- Blood and lymphatic vessels:
  - Epitheliod haemangioendothelioma
  - Angiosarcoma
  - Lymphangiosarcoma
  - Karposi's sarcoma
- Synovial tissue:
  - Synovial sarcoma
- Peripheral nerves:
  - Malignant peripheral nerve sheath tumour

Aetiology
- Usually unknown
- Inherited:
  - Neurofibromatosis
- Acquired:
  - Irradiation
- Chemical:
  - Arsenic
- Lymphoedema

Cardinal features of STS
- Lesion >5cm
- Rapidly expanding
- Deep to the deep fascia

- Recurs despite 'apparently' benign pathology

Diagnosis
- History
- Clinical examination
- Imaging
- Biopsy:
  - Refer without a biopsy if you are suspicious of a soft tissue sarcoma.
  - Biopsy should be performed by the surgeons or the interventional radiologists at the specialist centre.
  - Fine-needle aspiration first line.
  - Ultrasound-guided core biopsy and open (incisional) biopsy must be after detailed imaging within specialist centre within proposed field of excision.
  - Avoid contamination of uninvolved compartments.
  - Use tourniquet, but no exsanguination or compression of tumour.
  - Do not infiltrate biopsy site with LA.
  - Histology should be reviewed by a specialist sarcoma pathologist.

Investigations
- Plain X-ray
- USS
- Angiography
- MRI scan of tumour
- Staging CT, or PET/CT scan

Treatment of soft tissue sarcoma
Excision
- Wide excision, including adjacent uninvolved anatomical plane if close.
- The biopsy tract must be included in the resection specimen.
- There is no place for enucleation of the tumour in sarcoma surgery.
- Preservation of limb function wherever possible rather than compartmentectomy or amputation.

Limb-sparing reconstruction
- Reconstruction of soft tissue envelope using microvascular free tissue transfer for better function, cosmesis, and tolerance of postoperative radiotherapy.
  - Regional flaps extend radiotherapy field.
- Immediate reconstruction of bone (vascularized free fibula), joints (prosthesis), vessels.
- Reconstruct nerves after radiotherapy.

Radiotherapy
- Either by brachytherapy or external beam radiotherapy.
- For higher-grade tumours, marginal excision, large tumours.

Neoadjuvant chemotherapy
- For high-volume tumours to allow surgical resection.
- Causes higher surgical complication rates.

Prognosis for local recurrence

Grading of tumour
- Histopathological type most important
- Vascularity/necrosis
- Histopathological grade

Staging
- Dimensions
- Site

Treatment
- Margin of excision
- Adjuvant treatment

Table 17.3 Soft tissue sarcoma types and incidences in the hand and wrist. The results of the French Sarcoma Database 1980–2000.

Sarcoma type	Incidence (%)
Synovial sarcoma	10 (27.8)
Epitheloid sarcoma	7 (19.5)
Rhabdomyosarcoma	5 (13.9)
Clear cell sarcoma	4 (11.1)
Malignant fibrous histiocytoma	3 (8.3)
Spindle cell sarcoma	2 (5.5)
Kaposi's sarcoma	2 (5.5)
Leiomyosarcoma	1 (2.8)
Malignant Schwannoma	1 (2.8)
Extraskeletal chondrosarcoma	1 (2.8)
Total	**36 (100)**

Epithelioid sarcoma

Presents as a hard subcutaneous growth in the hand, wrist or forearm in a young adult. May also present as ulceration on the palmar aspect of the hand if the tumour undergoes central necrosis. Microscopically, the tumour shows positivity for epithelial markers. It can readily metastasize to regional lymph nodes. Metastasis to lungs, bone and scalp have also been reported. Tumours larger than 5cm have worse prognosis.

Treatment
Wide local excision or amputation followed by radiotherapy is the most effective treatment. The survival rate at 10 years is between 50–74%.

Synovial sarcoma

It is the most common soft tissue sarcoma of the hand constituting 20–30%. The incidence is highest in the third decade of life. Arises around a joint, tendon, or bursa and usually presents as a painful mass, often in the carpus. Highly malignant. Metastasis is present in 25% of patients (via lymphatics).

Treatment
- Wide local excision or amputation.
- Adjuvant radiation therapy and chemotherapy
- Progosis poor; median survival 36 months.

Rhabdomyosarcoma

Rare in the hand but rhabdomyosarcoma is the most common soft tissue sarcoma in children. It is painful and causes local nerve compression. A history of trauma is commonly present. Rapid lymphatic and blood-borne metastasis is common (to lymph nodes, bone, lungs, pancreas, liver, heart and kidneys).

Treatment
- Surgery, chemo- and radiotherapy.
- Prognosis is extremely poor; 5 year survival rates < 10%.

Clear cell sarcoma

Originates from tendons, tendon sheaths and aponeurotic tissue. Immuno-histochemical and karyotypic similarities to melanoma (has been called a 'soft tissue melanoma'.) Slow growing. Affects patients in their 2nd to 4th decade of life. The distal parts of the upper and lower limb are the most common locations. Metastasis is to regional lymph nodes, lungs and bone has been reported, even as long as 10 years after initial diagnosis.

Treatment
- Wide excision.
- Prognosis is guarded with 5-year survival being 50–60%.

Malignant nerve tumours
See p. 344.

Metastatic tumours

In the musculoskeletal system, metastatic tumours are far more frequent compared with primary tumours. However, involvement of the areas distal to the knee and elbow are uncommon. Involvement of the hand is rare with neoplasms of lung and kidney origin representing the majority of such involvement. If a metastatic lesion is discovered in the hand and wrist, the emphasis is usually on local control rather than systemic, as other metastases would have occurred. Metastatic lesions are usually seen in the phalanges, most notably in the proximal and distal phalanx. For distal phalangeal lesions the preferred treatment is amputation. Ray amputation rather than metacarpophalangeal disarticulation is preferred for the proximal phalanx due to the better cosmetic and functional result. Thumb reconstruction may be required after amputation, but the general health and requirements of the patient should be put into context when the indication is considered. In practice, most elderly patients would not benefit from such treatment.

Vascular

Vascular anatomy

Subclavian artery

- This is divided into three parts by the **scalenus anterior** muscle (this lies over the 2nd part).
- It has 5 branches.

The 1st part of the subclavian artery

- This has 3 branches;
  - 1st branch—the vertebral artery
  - 2nd branch—the thyrocervical trunk
  - This divides into **transverse cervical** and **suprascapular arteries,** continuing as **the ascending cervical artery.**
  - 3rd branch—the inferior thyroid artery

The 2nd part of the subclavian artery

- Lies behind the scalenus anterior.
  - 4th branch—the costocervical trunk
  - This divides into the **superior intercostal artery** and **the deep cervical artery**.

The 3rd part of the subclavian artery

- This lies behind the prevertebral fascia (with the trunks of the brachial plexus), which plasters them onto the floor of the posterior triangle.
- The **prevertebral fascia** continues into the axilla as the **axillary sheath**, surrounding the axillary artery.
- The **subclavian** and **axillary veins** are not surrounded by the axillary sheath, allowing them to distend with increased blood flow.
  - 5th branch—the dorsal scapular artery
  - sometimes from the 2nd part
  - runs laterally in front of scalenius medius, through the brachial plexus, and disappears deep to levator scapulae to join the scapular anastomosis.

Axillary artery

- The **axillary artery** is the continuation of the **3rd part of the subclavian artery.**
- Enters the axilla by passing over the first slip of serratus anterior, at the outer border of the 1st rib, behind the midpoint of the clavicle.
- It is invested in fascia, the axillary sheath, which is a continuation of the prevertebral fascia.
- The axillary vein is on the medial side of the artery.
- Becomes the **brachial artery** at the lower border of the teres major.
- Divided into 3 parts by the pectoralis minor.
- The **cords of the brachial plexus** are related to the 2nd part of the axillary artery.
- The medial and lateral heads of the **median nerve** clasp the 3rd part of the brachial artery.

1st part of the axillary artery

Superior thoracic artery

- This runs forward to supply both pectoral muscles.

2nd part of the axillary artery
Thoracoacromial artery
- Pierces clavipectoral fascia
- Divides into 4 branches:
  - Clavicular
  - Deltoid
  - Acromial
  - Pectoral

Lateral thoracic artery
- Follows lower border of pectoralis minor.
- Supplies pectoralis major and minor, and the breast.

3rd part of the axillary artery
Subscapular artery
- Gives off **circumflex scapular artery** posteriorly:
  - Passes between subscapularis and teres major, medial to the long head of triceps
- Continues as the **thoracodorsal artery**:
  - Supplies latissimus dorsi and serratus anterior muscles
  - Thoracodorsal nerve runs with it.

Anterior circumflex humeral artery
- Runs deep to coracobrachialis and both heads of biceps.
- It gives an ascending branch which runs up the intertubercular groove to the long tendon of biceps and the capsule of the shoulder joint.
- It passes around the neck of the humerus to anastomose with the posterior circumflex humeral artery (CHA).

Posterior circumflex humeral artery
- Larger than the anterior CHA
- Passes through quadrilateral space
  - Upper border—subscapularis anteriorly, teres minor posteriorly
  - Lower border—teres major
  - Lateral border—humerus
  - Medial border—long head of triceps
- Runs with axillary nerve to supply deltoid
- Anastomoses with **profunda brachii artery**

Brachial artery
- This is the continuation of the **axillary artery**.
- The **median nerve** is lateral to the brachial artery in its upper part, and crosses obliquely in front of the artery to lie on its medial side below.
- Venae comitans around the brachial artery at the elbow converge to form the **basilic vein**, which perforates the deep fascia opposite the deltoid insertion.
- The ulnar nerve is posterior to the brachial artery, and diverges away from it in the lower part, to pass through the medial intermuscular septum.
- It lies deep to the deep fascia, in the groove between biceps and triceps.
- It passes into the cubital fossa, where it divides into the radial and ulnar arteries.

Branches of the brachial artery

Profunda brachii

- Leaves through the lower triangular space (below teres major, between humerus and long head of triceps) to run in the radial groove with the radial nerve.
- It supplies triceps muscle.
- The descending branch of the profunda brachii provides the blood supply for the lateral arm flap. (📖 See p. 212.)
- It divides into anterior and posterior branches to join the cubital anstomosis.

Superior ulnar collateral artery

- Accompanies ulnar nerve

Inferior ulnar collateral artery

- Divides into anterior and posterior branches
- Contributes to cubital anastomosis

Radial artery

- The radial artery appears as a longitudinal continuation of the brachial artery, with the ulnar artery coming off perpendicularly.
- It runs medial to the biceps tendon, deep to brachiradialis, and gives off the radial recurrent artery.
- It runs across supinator, over the tendon of pronator teres, the radial origin of FDS, the origin of FPL, the insertion of pronator quadratus and the lower end of the radius.
- In the forearm it lies beneath brachioradialis, between it and FCR, where it runs alongside the superficial branch of the radial nerve.
- It gives off a number of small perforator arteries which anastomose with the ulnar, anterior and posterior interosseous arteries.
- It gives off a superficial palmar branch, which contributes to the **superficial palmar arch** (formed by the ulnar artery).
- It then disappears below the tendons of APL and EPB to cross the anatomical snuffbox.
- It passes deep to the tendon of EPL, and then between the 2 heads of the 1st dorsal interosseous muscle, to emerge in the palm between the oblique and transverse heads of the adductor pollicis to form the **deep palmar arch**.
- In a study of 120 patients:
  - Radial artery provides dominant flow in 57%.
  - Ulnar artery and superficial arch provides dominant flow in 21.5%.
  - Radial and ulnar arteries supply equal flow in 21.5%.

Ulnar artery

- The **ulnar artery** gives off **anterior** and then **posterior ulnar recurrent arteries**.
- The **anterior ulnar recurrent artery** lies between brachialis and PT, and anastomoses with the inferior ulnar collateral artery in front of the medial epicondyle.
- It passes deep to PT, where it gives off the common interosseous artery.
- It runs medially where it lies deep to FCU and on top of FDP.
- It continues distally deep to the deep fascia, between FCU and FDS.

- It crosses into the palm in Guyon's canal, lateral to the pisiform and above the superficial carpal ligament, and forms part of the **superficial palmar arch**.

Common interosseous artery
- This is a short trunk which passes backwards to the interosseous membrane, where it divides into the anterior and posterior interosseous arteries.

Anterior interosseous artery
- Descends with the anterior interosseous nerve in front of the interosseous membrane, beneath FPL and FDP.
- It gives off the median artery which accompanies the median nerve.
- It gives off osseous and muscular branches, a branch to the palmar carpal arch, and then penetrates the interosseous membrane to anastomose with the dorsal carpal arch.

Posterior interosseous artery
- This passes backwards over the free edge of the interosseous membrane, between the supinator and APL.
- It gives off the interosseous recurrent branch, which ascends to the elbow under ECU to run on the deep surface of anconeus.
- The main posterior interosseous artery (PIA) descends between the superficial and deep extensor muscles with the deep branch if the radial nerve.
- It gives off a large branch to the radius between supinator and APL.
- It descends between ECU and EDC, giving muscular and fasciocutaneous perforators.
  - These provide the blood supply for the posterior interosseous artery flap.
- It anastomoses distally with the anterior interosseous artery and dorsal carpal network, by a connecting vessel under EIP at the level of the distal ulna.

Becker flap perforator
- A cutaneous perforator arises 3–5cm proximal to the pisiform. This is the basis of the *Becker* ulnar artery perforator flap.

Carpal arches
Dorsal carpal arch
- This is formed mainly by the radial artery, deep to the thumb extensors.
- The skin over the extensor retinaculum is supplied by the rete carpi dorsale, with contributions from the radial, anterior and posterior interosseous, and the dorsal carpal branch of the ulnar artery.

Palmar carpal arch
- The flexor aspect of the wrist is supplied by branches of the radial and ulnar arteries, with contributions from the median artery if present.

Dorsal metacarpal arteries
- The dorsal carpal arch lies deep to the extensor tendons across the distal carpal row.
- The dorsal matacarpal arteries usually arise from the dorsal carpal arch.

- Each artery gives off a skin perforator approximately 1cm proximal to the webspace, on which small skin flaps can be designed.

Superficial palmar arch

- The superficial palmar arch is formed maily by the ulnar artery and completed by the superficial palmar branch of the radial artery.
- It lies deep to the palmar fascia at the level of the 1st web of the extended thumb.
- It lies superficial to the branches of the median nerve.
- It gives off the ulnar digital artery (UDA) to the little finger and 3 common digital arteries:
  - Radial digital artery (RDA) little/UDA ring finger
  - RDA ring/UDA middle finger
  - RDA middle/UDA index finger
- The RDA to the index arises from the deep palmar arch:
  - the radialis indicis
- Near the metacarpal heads, they receive communicating branches from the deep palmar arch.
- As they pass distally on the lumbricals, they lie dorsal to the digital nerves.

Deep palmar arch

- This is formed mainly by the **radial artery**, and completed by the **deep palmar branch of the ulnar artery**.
- The radial artery emerges between the 2 heads of adductor pollicis in the palm and gives off the **princeps pollicis artery** (to the thumb) and the **radialis indicis artery** (to the index finger), and passes medially, deep to adductor pollicis.
- The deep arch gives off 3 palmar metacarpal arteries to the palmar interossei.
- The deep arch then gives off a branch to the hypothenar muscles.

Digital arteries

- These are the main blood supply to the digits.
- Each common digital artery divides into an ulnar and a radial digital artery to adjacent digits.
- The UDA of the little finger is formed by the superfical palmar arch.
- The RDA of the index is a branch of the deep palmar arch, the radialis indicis.
- Short dorsal branches to the dorsal web skin are given off in the webspaces.
- The digital arteries run deep (dorsal) to the digital nerves.
- In the thumb, the digital arteries and nerves converge towards the midline over the proximal part of the proximal phalanx.
  - Because of the pronated position of the thumb, they appear to lie towards the **ulnar** side of the thumb when looking at the hand with the palm upwards.
- Digital artery diameter:
  - 1mm in the proximal finger
  - 0.5mm at the DIPJ
- The diameter of the UDA is bigger than the RDA in the thumb, index and middle fingers.

- The diameter of the RDA is bigger than the UDA in the ring and little fingers.
- Each digital artery gives off 3 dorsal branches.
- The distal palmar digital arteries continue and converge in an H-shaped or cruciate anastomosis.

Venous system

Venous drainage of the hand

- There are small veins, mainly distal, on the palmar side of the digits.
- The veins are mainly on the dorsum of the digits, joining up with the superficial dorsal venous arch of the hand.
- The loose dorsal skin allows dilatation of the dorsal veins, which are not compressed during gripping actions.
- The veins of the thumb and index fingers join the radial side of the dorsal venous arch, which continues proximally as the cephalic vein.
- The ulnar digits drain to the ulnar side of the arch, which becomes the basilic vein.

Venous drainage of the forearm

- The forearm is drained by 3 major veins:
  - Cephalic vein: runs on the radial border of the forearm, continues on lateral border of biceps, then enters the deltopectoral groove.
  - Basilic vein: runs along the ulnar border of the forearm, and receives the median vein of the forearm and median cubital vein just below the elbow.
  - Median vein of the forearm.
- They lie on the anterior (flexor) aspect of the forearm.

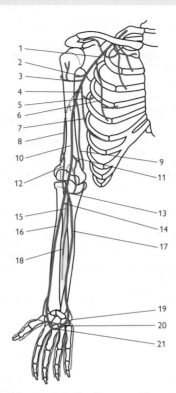

Fig. 18.1 Arteries of the upper limb: (1) axillary artery; (2) posterior circumflex humeral artery; (3) anterior circumflex humeral artery; (4) subscapular artery; (5) circumflex scapular artery; (6) laeral thoracic artery; (7) subscapular artery; (8) arteria profunda brachi; (9) ulnar collateral artery; (10) brachial artery; (11) inferior ulnar collateral artery; (12) anterior branch of arteria profunda brachi; (13) ulnar recurrent artery; (14) interosseous artery; (15) dorsal interosseous artery; (16) radial artery; (17) ulnar artery; (18) volar interosseous artery; (19) deep ulnar artery; (20) deep palmar arch; (21) superficial palmar arch.

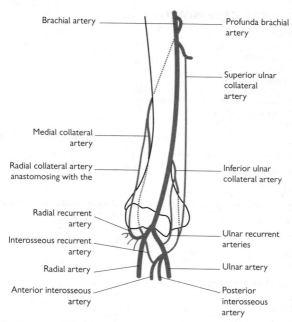

Fig. 18.2 Arrangement of collateral arteries participating in the anastomosis around the elbow joint. Branches given off by the arteries to supply muscles and skin have been omitted.

Vascular assessment

History

- Duration of symptoms:
  - Congenital
  - Recent onset
- ? related to injury:
  - penetrating or blunt
  - Repetitive injury, e.g. industrial
- Presence of swelling
- Timing of symptoms
- Precipitating factors
- Pain
- Family history of blood disorders

Past medical history

- Diabetes
- Reynaud's disease or previous cold injur;y
  - Unilateral Raynaud's is suggestive of vascular occlusion or thrombosis

Social history

- Occupation
- Smoker
- Drugs
- IV drug abuse

Clinical examination

Appearance

- Colour:
  - Pale and ischaemic
  - Red
  - Blue, with venous stasis or congestion
  - Nicotine stains
- Pulsatility
- Sweating
- Swelling:
  - Discrete
  - Generalized
- Oedema, with loss of dorsal skin creases
- Loss of fingertip pulp volume
- Nail changes
- Calcinosis

Capillary refill

- Time taken for colour to return to nail bed or skin after squeezing.
- 'Normal' less than 2 seconds, but compare with other digits, especially opposite hand.

Pulse

Radial artery

- Palpable in radial wrist groove.
- Can also be felt in anatomical snuffbox.

Ulnar artery
- Palpable on radial side of pisiform in distal wrist.

Digital arteries
- Common digital arteries can be palpated in the webspaces, and the digital arteries can be felt in slim fingers more distally.

Allen's test
- This is usually performed at the wrist on the radial and ulnar arteries.
- It can be used on the finger, a **digital** Allen's test.
- The examiner places the index and middle fingertips of each hand over the patient's radial and ulnar arteries in the wrist, with the thumbs resting on the dorsum of the patient's wrist.
- The patient is asked to raise and clench the fist to squeeze the blood out of the hand, and the examiner occludes the radial and ulnar arteries. The hand should be white.
  - It takes 11 or more pounds of pressure to occlude the vessels, and this causes discomfort in most patients.
- The examiner releases the radial artery, and notes the time taken for the colour to return.
- Revascularization times:
  - Rapid fill—less than 6 seconds
  - Delayed fill—6–15 seconds
  - Absent fill—no refill after 15 seconds.
- The test is repeated for the ulnar artery.

Investigations
Plain radiograph
- Previous fractures, vascular lesions and bony erosions may be visible on plain X-ray.
- Skeletal overgrowth may be associated with some vascular malformations.

Doppler ultrasound
Hand-held Doppler probe
- The hand-held Doppler may be used in the clinic or operating theatre to detect the presence of pulsatile flow in a vessel.
- This is useful for pre-operative mapping of specific perforating vessels when designing flaps.
- It may also be used to monitor flow across an anastomosis, pre- or postoperatively.

Duplex colour Doppler
- This is a more sophisticated, non-invasive method of mapping flow in small vessels, which combines ultrasound imaging techniques and colour-coded Doppler.
- It is non-invasive and reproducible, and has reduced the need for more invasive arteriography.
- The machine is large and not easy to move, so this is usually only available in the radiology department.

Digital plethysmography (pulse volume recordings)

- This technique quantitates flow by the analysis of limb of digit volume change, usually by the use of an air-filled cuff connected to a pressure transducer.
- The normal triphasic wave patern is altered in occlusive disease or stenosis.
- It is non-invasive, reproducible and cheap.

MRI

- Can be used to image vascular lesions.

Magnetic resonance angiography (MRA)

- High resolution MRA images arterial and venous structures.
- Gadolinium cntrast is necessary to see small vessels.
- This technique is less invasive than conventional angiography, but the resolution is not as good.

Angiography

- This is still the 'gold standard' modality for static upper extremity vascular imaging.
- Computer digital imaging combined with subtraction techniques means less contrast material is required.
- Surgeons should communicate directly with the radiologists to ensure the correct information is obtained from the study.

Complications of angiography

- Arterial injury at injecton site
- Displacement of emboli
- Catheter-induced vasospasm
- Failure to see distal arterial reconstruction because of vasospasm.
- Allergic reaction to contract agents.

Hand–arm vibration syndrome (Vibration white finger)

Pathophysiology

Prolonged exposure to significant vibration affects the nerves, small vessels and muscles. The risk is proportional to the magnitude of vibration, and the duration of exposure.

Symptoms

- **Blanching** of fingers in cold weather, initially just at the tips of one or more fingers, followed by **cyanosis** and then painful **redness** (vibration white finger—VWF)
- Loss of dexterity
- Reduced sensitivity to touch and temperature
- Carpal tunnel syndrome (over and above peripheral neuropathy)
- Pain and stiffness in the hands and wrists (the cause is not so clear)
- Permanent circulation failure (dusky discolouration) and even gangrene (very rare)

The condition worsens over time with continued exposure to vibration. Initially there is just cold intolerance. The symptoms do not necessarily occur during vibration—they occur whenever exposed to cold.

Classification

- The Taylor–Pelmear classification has now been superseded by the Stockholm Classification.

Table 18.1 Stockholm classification of hand–arm vibration syndrome (HAVS)

Vascular		
Stage	**Grade**	**Description**
0		No attacks
1	Mild	Occasional attacks affecting only tips of 1 or more fingers
2	Moderate	Occasional attacks affecting distal and middle phalanges of one or more fingers
3	Severe	Frequent attacks affecting all phalanges of most fingers
4	Very severe	As stage 3 + trophic finger tip changes
Sensorineural		
Stage		
0SN	—	Exposed to vibration but no symptoms
1SN	—	Intermittent numbness, no tingling
2SN	—	Intermittent or persistent numbness, reduced sensation
3SN	—	Intermittent or persistent numbness, reduced tactile discrimination and or dexterity

History
Exposure
It is difficult to measure the duration of vibration exposure accurately. Tools can be measured for vibration magnitude with special equipment

Exclude other causes
- Primary Raynaud's disease
- Raynaud's phenomenon
- Idiopathic peripheral nerve compression (e.g. carpal tunnel, cubital tunnel)
- Peripheral neuropathy (e.g. diabetes, alcohol, drugs)
- Cervical spondylosis

Objective tests
Vascular component
- Cold-provocation to induce attacks and thus prove reported symptoms.
- Blood flow measurements (ultrasound, plethysmography)

Neurological component
- Two-point discrimination
- Vibration thresholds
- Temperature threshold measurement
- Nerve conduction studies (to distinguish carpal tunnel syndrome, itself caused sometimes by vibration but usually sporadic), from the peripheral neuropathic changes of HAVS.

Prevention
- Hazardous jobs and tools should be identified
- Reduction of vibration exposure with job rotation, new tools, new techniques, new processeses
- Tool design (damping)
- Protective gloves
- Surveillance
- Training of employees and employers

Treatment
- Prevention is the key.
- If symptoms occur, then vibration must be eliminated or reduced as far as possible.
- Avoidance of cold weather, use of gloves in cold weather.
- Avoidance of smoking (peripheral vasoconstrictor).
- Carpal tunnel release will usually relieve the proportion of symptoms due to median nerve compression, but the background small nerve neuropathy will persist.

Outcome
- Avoidance of vibration will possibly allow vascular symptoms to improve a little.
- Neurological symptoms tend not to improve even after cessation of exposure.

Vascular anomalies

- The terminology used to describe vascular lesions (strawberry naevus, port wine stain, cystic hygroma) is confusing and contradictory.
- The term 'haemangioma' has (inaccurately) become synonymous with any vascular anomaly in children.
- Congenital vascular anomalies can be separated into two groups, defined by the biology of their endothelial cells.
- **Haemangioma.**
- **Vascular malformation**
- This difference between haemangioma and vascular malformation was described in a classification defined by endothelial characteristics, published by Mulliken and Glowacki in 1982.

Haemangioma

Growth characteristics of haemangioma

- Haemangioma appears in the first few months after birth.
- Proliferative phase:
  - There is rapid growth over a period of approximately 12 months.
  - This is due to endothelial cell proliferation.
- Involutional phase:
  - The haemangioma shrinks spontaneously to an end point, usually leaving a fibro-fatty remnant.
  - 70% resolution by 7 years.
  - Rate of regression is unrelated to sex, age, site or size.

Clinical features of haemangioma

- A red area seen at birth develops into a red, raised, strawberry-like lesion.
- Lesions on the fingertips and nail may become infected following sucking.
- Haemangioma of the axilla or webspaces may ulcerate.
- Compression of underlying nerves or musculotendinous units does not occur.
- The start of involution is marked by grey spots of ischaemic necrosis ('herald spots') on the surface of the haemangioma.
- Haemangioma is commonest in the head and neck.
- Haemangiomas of the upper limb can involve the chest, abdomen and lower limb.
- More than half of vascular anomalies seen in the upper limbs of children are haemangiomas.

Investigation of haemangioma

- Recognition by clinical features
- USS
- MRI

Management of haemangioma

- Most haemangiomas can be managed conservatively by allowing them to involute spontaneously.
- Parental reassurance is necessary, and it may be difficult for a family to understand that the best result will be obtained by allowing the haemangioma to proliferate, and then involute naturally.

- Although haemangiomas of the upper limb do not usually need urgent treatment, hand surgeons should be aware that extensive haemangiomas involving the airway, or around the orbit, must be treated immediately in specialist centres.
  - Urgent treatment is by intralesional injection of steroid or α-2a interferon, or surgery.
- Following involution, excision of the fibro-fatty remnant may be indicated for improvement of contour and appearance, especially on the dorsum of the hand and forearm.

Vascular malformations

- Vascular malformations are biologically quiet lesions in which there is no endothelial cell turnover.
- Many are not present at birth, but appear within the first 2–5 years of life, and grow proportionally with the child.
- Vascular malformations do not involute (unlike haemangiomas).

Classification of vascular malformations
Predominant cell type

- They are classified according to their predominant cell types, into capillary, venous, lymphatic, arteriovenous, and combined (☐ see Table 18.2).
- Combined malformations can involve any combination of vascular cells.
  - They are often complex, and may be associated with skeletal overgrowth.
  - They are known by various eponyms (☐ see Table 18.2) .

Flow

- **Fast flow**. These have the worst prognosis, and are the most difficult to treat.
- **Slow flow**.
  - These do not progress into fast flow lesions.
  - They are diffuse, and often difficult to resect.

Table 18.2 Types of vascular malformations, and associated syndromes

CM	Capillary malformation
VM	Venous malformation
LM	Lymphatic malformation
AVM	Arteriovenous malformation
AVF	Arteriovenous fistula
CLM	Capillary-lymphatic malformation
CVM	Capillary-venous malformation
CVLM	Capillary-venous-lymphatic malformation
Klippel–Trenaunay syndrome	CVLM, with skeletal overgrowth
Parkes–Weber syndrome	CVLM, with AVF
Proteus syndrome	CM, VM, macrodactyly, hemihypertrophy, lipoma, pigmented linear naevi, scoliosis
Mafucci syndrome	LVM and multiple enchondromas
Ollier's syndrome	Multiple enchondromas and no vascular anomalies

Venous malformations (VM)
- These are the most common vascular malformations.
- They are slow flow and may involve any tissues.
- Usually more extensive than they appear from the outside.
- Become engorged when held in a dependent position.
- Symptoms are due to enlargement, the mass effect and pain, especially when located along neurovascular structures.
- Ulceration is uncommon.
- They are subject to hormonal influence in women, during adolescence and pregnancy. The enlargement from pregnancy is permanent.

Investigation
- Plain radiograph shows bony changes.
- MRI is the gold standard to determine size and extent of lesions. T1-and T2-weighting, and gadolinium contrast can help to distinguish low-flow from high-flow lesions, and to discern venous and lymphatic channels.
- Angiography is reserved for pre-operative planning prior to major resections.

Treatment
- Initially conservative with pressure garments.
- Surgery should be reserved for specific goals, e.g. nerve compression, painful varices.
- Excision and debulking must be planned carefully to achieve a clean excision with preservation of tendons, joints and neurovascular structures, and may need to be done in several stages, avoiding further surgery to scarred areas.
- Sclerotherapy has limited success although necrosis may result.

Capillary malformations (CM)
- Cutaneous port wine stains, which may involve single digit or whole upper limb.
- Commonly unilateral.
- Bright red colour in young ('naevus flammeus') which becomes purple and pedunculated with age.
- May be associated with deeper vascular anomalies, and skeletal overgrowth.

Treatment of capillary malformations
- Usually conservative.
- Investigate for possible associated problems.
- Dye laser can be effective.

Lymphatic malformations (LM)
- May present as localized lymphoedema or circumscribed lesions.
- All tissues of the upper limb may be affected, but most are in the skin and subcutaneous tissue, displacing muscle and NVBs.
- Those affecting the axilla, infiltrating into the chest, neck and mediastinum were known as cystic hygromas.
- The skin over a LM may be covered with vesicles containing clear or blood-stained fluid.
- Secondary infection with β-haemolytic *Streptococcus* is common.

- Symptoms are related to the size and position of the lesion, and pain is unusual.
- Leakage of lymphatic fluid stains clothing, macerates the skin, and smells unpleasant.
- Compression neuropathies are uncommon.
- There is no hormonal effect.

Investigation of LMs
- This is similar to VMs.
- MRI can distinguish LMs, and categorize them into macro- and micro- cystic lesions.

Treatment of LMs
- Mostly conservative using pressure garments and compression pumps.
- Compression garments are difficult to tolerate, and compression pumps may displace the fluid from one area to another.
- Surgery is indicated for size, weight, and skin changes.
- Complete removal of all involved tissue is essential, and this often requires reconstruction.
- Staged surgical excision is difficult, as wound healing is complicated by leakage and infection.
- Massive diffuse lesions in functionless limbs are best treated by amputation.

Combined capillary–venous–lymphatic (CVLM) and lymphatic–venous malformations (LVM)
- These may contain any vascular component.
- They are characterized by:
  - Skeletal overgrowth and deformation
  - Capillary port wine stains (CM)
  - Massive size
- These are associated with many syndromes. Klippel–Trenaunay and Parkes–Weber are the most common, and have 3 dominant features;
  - Cutaneous capillary malformation
  - Venous component with large varicosities
  - Limb hypertrophy
- Klippel–Trenaunay syndrome mainly venous with a good prognosis.
- Parkes–Weber syndrome contains high-flow with a poor prognosis.
- Mafucci syndrome consists of CVLM and multiple enchondroma

Investigation of CVL and LV malformations
- The cutaneous component is not indicative of the extent of the underlying lesion.
- MRI demonstrates the three-dimensional nature of these leions, which are like icebergs.
- Angiograms and venograms visualize the large saccular components, and not the smaller channels.

Treatment of combined CVL and LV malformations
- This follows similar principles to VMs and LMs.

Arteriovenous malformations (AVM)
- The least common of all vascular anomalies.
- Bimodal presentation:
  - 40% present at birth
  - 60% not clinically apparent until later childhood/adolescence.
- Type A fast-flow lesions.
  - Static vascular anomalies, with either single or multiple arteriovenous fistulae
  - Aneurysms of large- and medium-sized vessels
  - Ectasia of the arterial circulation
  - May involve more than one major artery
- Type B fast-flow lesions.
  - Micro- or macro-fistulas of a single axial artery of the limb
  - Progressive
  - May be associated with distal steal and ischaemia.
- Type C fast-flow lesions.
  - Diffuse arteriovenous lesions with connections to all tissues.
  - Progressive, and symptomatic because of distal steal.
  - Massive lesions result in high-output cardiac failure.
  - Progressive type C lesions may lead to amputation.
- Warmth, soft tissue enlargement, palpable thrills and bruits, hyperhidrosis, and pain after exercise are seen in all groups.
- Type C lesions usually progress to a steal phenomenon with distal ischaemia.
- Growth is affected if a significant proportion of the cardiac output is shunted to the malformaton.
- May present as compartment syndrome.
- May develop compression neuropathies.
- May present with ulceration of fingertips or at the site of previous surgery.
- Hormonally influenced in women.

Investigation of AVM
- Clinical examination
- Baseline angiography for later comparison.
- Doppler scanning provides haemodynamic information.
- MRI can determine the true extent of the lesion.
- Direct puncture angiography should be undertaken before surgery for planning.

Treatment of AVM
- Arterial embolization is used pre- and intra-operatively as an adjunct to surgery.
- Multiple procedures are often necessary.
- Type A and B lesions can often be treated by embolization.
- Soft tissue loss requires reconstruction.
- Ischaemia may result in amputation, especially in Type C AVMs.

Acute vascular injury

Causes of acute vascular injury

Open
- Sharp injury
- Crush injury
- Iatrogenic (i.e. cannulation, producing an arteriovenous fistula)

Closed
- Blunt trauma, including crush injury
- Fracture
- Dislocation

Clinical features and pathophysiology
- Innocuous entry wounds may disguise vascular compromise.
- Symptoms depend on the presence or absence of collateral circulation, post-traumatic sympathetic tone, and vasomotor control mechanisms.
- Complete arterial transection with adequate collateral circulation may be asymptomatic.
- Disruption of the brachial artery, or both the radial and ulnar arteries presents as a critically ischaemic limb (cold, pale, pulseless).
- **Critical ischaemia** is defined as vascular insufficiency which will produce necrosis without vascular reconstruction.
- Arterial reconstruction is recommended in closed brachial artery injury associated with supracondylar fractures in children.
- Crush injuries may present with **delayed** symptoms as swelling, hypotension, and intimal injury combine to cause late thrombosis and vascular insufficiency, often leading to compartment syndrome.

Investigations
- Creatine kinase should be checked in all devascularizing injuries, especially where there has been crush, when this is likely to be very high.
- Plain X-ray to exclude fractures.
- Angiogram (if necessary on table to avoid delay) to assess extent of vascular injury.

Treatment of acute vascular injury

Critical arterial reconstruction
- Usually requires reversed interposition vein grafts, especially for brachial artery.
- Adequate wound excision, stable fracture fixation and good soft tissue cover (using reconstructive flaps is required) are all equally important to obtain a good result.
- Consider fasciotomy and excision of necrotic muscle before revascuarization if there has been a delay of several hours from injury.

Non-critical arterial reconstruction
- Reconstruction is suggested to:
  - Restore physiological flow (especially in case of future injury).
  - Prevent cold intolerance.
  - Enhance nerve recovery.
  - Improve healing.

- There may be a thrombosis rate of 10–20% by experienced surgeons under ideal conditions. This is likely to be higher by inexperienced surgeons in suboptimal conditions.
- Factors causing thrombosis are multifactorial:
  - Surgical technique
  - Tension across anastomosis (avoid by using vein grafts)
  - Mechanism of injury
  - Timing of repair
  - Vessel injured

Occlusion

Causes

Localized arterial occlusion

- Thrombosis:
  - Hypothenar hammer syndrome
- Aneurysm:
  - True
  - False
- Embolism
- Tumour

Systemic arterial disorders

These conditions may affect all the limbs and end circulations.

- Degenerative disease:
  - Atherosclerosis
  - Diabetes mellitus
- Vasospasm:
  - Raynaud's disease
- Tobacco smoking.

Hypothenar hammer syndrome

- This term is used to describe thrombosis of the ulnar artery in Guyon's canal.
- It occurs when the ulnar border of the hand is used as a blunt instrument.
- It is usually associated with cold intolerance, pain and sometimes ulceration of the ring finger.
- Resection of the thrombosed section of the ulnar artery in Guyon's canal with reconstruction with an interposition reversed vein graft cures the condition, and provides the additional beneficial effects of local sympathectomy.

Aneurysm

Causes of aneurysms

False aneurysm (pseudoaneurysm)
- Penetrating injury:
  - Arterial puncture and cannulation
  - Regional anaesthetic blocks
  - Stab wounds
  - Gunshot wounds
- Non-penetrating injury:
  - Fractures
  - Crush
  - Haemophiliac recurrent bleeding
  - Mycotic infection

True aneurysm
- Arteriosclerotic
- Congenital
- Metabolic
- Osteogenesis imperfecta
- Buerger's disease (thromboangiitis obliterans)
- Haemophiliac

False aneurysm (pseudoaneurysm)
- These occur after penetration of the vessel wall with extravasation of blood into the surrounding tissue planes.
- They are saccular.
- The haematoma becomes organized and fibrosed, and then recanalizes.
- The lumen of the false aneurysm is in continuity with the true vessel.
- The endothelial layer is absent.

True aneurysm
- These occur after injury to the vessel which permits gradual dilatation, usually repetitive blunt trauma.
- They are fusiform.

Presentation
- Pulsating masses may appear spontaneously on the palmar surface of the hand or digits, or volar forearm.
- Progress is usually slow and insidious.
- Most pseudoaneurysms occur after injury or iatrogenic puncture wounds.
- Palmar punctures occur from pencils and pens, glass or small knives
- Forearm puncture wounds occur from glass and metal lacerations, knives, low energy transfer ballistic injury and needle punctures.
- A bruit may be present.
- The digits are cold.
  - Ring finger in ulnar artery aneurysm.
  - Index finger in radial artery aneurysm.
- Ulceration is rare in children

Diagnosis
- This is mainly clinical:
  - History of injury or puncture wound.
  - Slow progression.
  - Painless, pulsatile mass.
  - Pain from soft tissue or nerve compression.
  - Distal signs from embolization.
- Colour duplex Doppler scanning identifies most aneurysms.
- Arteriography allows assessment of collateral circulation, defines the extent of the lesion, and is useful for pre-operative planning.

Management options
- Resection and ligation
- Excision of damaged section and vein patch
- Resection and end-to-end repair
- Resection and reversed interposition vein graft

Embolism
- Presents as a painful, pale, pulseless hand.
- Proximal events cause muscle ischemia, but not distal to musculotendinous junctions of extrinsic muscles.
- Secondary vasospasm may compromise undamaged collateral circulation.
- Digits turn blue, then white, then black.
- Upper limb emboli account for less than 20% of all arterial embolic events.
- Mainly from heart (70%), subclavian artery and superficial palmar arch.

Diagnosis
- Clinical features:
  - Pain
  - Pallor
  - Pulseless
  - Petechiae
  - Cyanosis
- Echocardiogram
- Arteriography

Treatment
- Anticoagulation with systemic heparin infusion
- Local infusion of thrombolytic agents
- Embolectomy
- Reperfusion may cause compartment syndrome.
  - This should be anticipated in limbs which have been ischaemic for several hours.
  - In this case, the compartments should be decompressed, and ischaemic muscle excised **before** revascularization, to prevent reperfusion syndrome (□ see Compartment syndrome, p. 618).
- Embolic events in the hand often require surgical exploration to remove the source and revascularize.

Raynaud's disease

- There are two types:
  - **Primary Raynaud's disease**
  - **Secondary Raynaud's phenomenon**.
- The symptoms are similar, precipitated by cold and characterized in sequence by:
  - Pallor
  - Cyanosis
  - Painful vasodilation

Primary Raynaud's disease

- 10–20% prevalence. Precipitated by cold, sometimes by emotional stress
- Symmetrical blanching
- Toes, nose and ears often affected
- Strong familial association

Raynaud's phenomenon

- Secondary to, or associated with, many conditions:
  - Vibration (📖 see p. 604)
  - Rheumatoid
  - Connective tissue disorders (25% of people with SLE have Raynaud's phenomenon, 80% with scleroderma)
  - Atherosclerosis
  - Thoracic outlet syndrome (📖 see p. 329)
  - Blood dyscrasias (e.g. cryoglobulinaemia)
  - Drugs (ergot, Beta–blockers)
  - Frostbite

Compartment syndrome

Definition
A persistent rise in the pressure within a confined fibroosseous compartment that leads to partial, or complete infarction, and fibrosis of the vital components of that compartment.

Aetiology
- Bleeding
- Crush
- Ischaemia and reperfusion
- Electrical burns
- Injection
- Posture
- Iatrogenic

Pathophysiology
- Swelling, or a space-occupying lesion, compresses vasculature.
- Venous outflow of tissue compartment obstructed before arterial inflow, as lower pressure system.
- Arterial inflow continues in presence of reduced venous outflow, and compartment pressure increases.
- Eventually, compartment pressure rises above systolic pressure and compartment becomes ischaemic.

Clinical assessment
- Clinical suspicion is the main indicator.
- Pulses are **NOT** a useful sign—peripheral vascularity does **not** correlate with compartment status.
- The degree of distal ischaemia is **variable** with compartment syndrome.
- Compartment pressure measurement is the only useful investigation.
- Fasciotomy should be performed before pulses are lost.
- Damage varies with pressure differential and time.

Symptoms
- **Pain:**
  - Severe and unremitting
  - Unrelieved by analgesia (look at drug chart showing increasing amounts of painkillers)
  - Progressive
  - Worse on passive stretch of fingers or wrist
  - Unrelieved by immobilization

Signs
- Limb feels tense
- Pain on passive stretch
- Reduced sensibility in distribution of nerves that pass **through** the compartment
- Weakness of muscles in compartment
- Presence of pulse does **not** exclude compartment syndrome.

- Loss of pulse is an end-stage sign by which time muscle necrosis has occurred.

Investigations

Direct compartment pressure measurement is the most useful investigation. There is no place for any other imaging in the management of acute compartment syndrome.

Instruments to measure compartment pressure
- Stryker® dedicated device (Stryker Pressure monitor [ref 295-1] and Quick pressure monitor system [ref 295-2]. Stryker Instruments, 4100E. Milham, Kalamazoo, Michigan, USA 49001. Telephone 2693237700 [USA]. Stryker Instruments, BP 50040-95946 Roissy CDG, France. Telephone 0033148175000 [Europe].).
- Connect saline-filled infusion set with hypodermic needle (19G or 21G) on 3-way tap to pressure transducer from central venous pressure (CVP) monitor.

Measuring compartment pressure
- Calibrate instrument.
- Insert needle or catheter into compartment and take pressure reading.
- Take measurements from different sites in the compartment (compartments are not fluid, so pressure varies within compartment).
- Measurements depend on technique and may vary between operators.
- Look at trend if single measurement equivocal.
- Can compare with contralateral unaffected limb if unsure.

Blood tests
- Creatine kinase (CK)
- Urea and electrolytes (U&E)

A very high CK may indicate muscle necrosis. This may lead to acute renal failure, so monitor U&E and consider early renal dialysis if indicated (discuss with intensive care unit (ITU) and/or renal physicians).

When to perform a fasciotomy
- Clinical suspicion is the main indicator
- Raised compartment pressure
  - 30mmHg for 8 hours or unknown period
  - 20mmHg below diastolic pressure
- Clinical suspicion plus compartment pressure of 30mmHg
- Revascularization of a limb (always)

Fasciotomy of the upper limb
General principles
- General or regional anaesthesia.
- Apply a high tourniquet to the arm for safe initial exposure.
- Remove any rings from the digits.
- Position the patient supine on the operating table with the arm on a hand table.
- Clean the arm to the axilla with surgical disinfectant.
- Drape the arm just below the tourniquet.
- Incisions must be complete and full length.
- Incise the skin (dermotomy) and deep fascia (fasciotomy).

- Design incisions to avoid exposed nerves or tendons.
- Try to minimize cutaneous nerve damage and preserve longitudinal veins.
- Closed, subdermal fasciotomy is **NOT** indicated in trauma.
- Examine the epimysium of individual muscle bellies systematically and incise when tight (epimysiotomy).
- Excise obviously dead muscle with the tourniquet inflated or prior to revascularization to reduce the risk of acute renal failure from myoglobinaemia.
  - If in doubt, do not excise it, and look again after the tourniquet is deflated.
  - Dead muscle does not bleed, is soft and mushy, does not twitch, and is either dark or very pale (not pink).
- Release the tourniquet to assess muscle viability.
- Perform a second look at 24 to 48 hours.

The hand

This is confusing unless you understand the anatomy of the compartments of the hand in cross-section.

Ten compartments:

- Dorsal interossei (4)
- Palmar interossei (3)
- Adductor (often neglected)
- Thenar
- Hypothenar

Dorsal incisions

The dorsal (4) and palmar (3) interosseous and adductor (1) compartments are all decompressed through 2 dorsal incisions between the 2nd and 3rd metacarpals and the 4th and 5th metacarpals. Incise the skin, preserving the dorsal veins where possible.

- Through the 2 dorsal incisions, incise the fascia over each of the four dorsal interosseous compartments, retracting the skin to gain access to the 1st and 3rd dorsal interossei, which are not directly under the incisions. Avoid damage to the superficial branch of the radial nerve when dividing the fascia over the 1st dorsal interosseous muscle.
- The 1st palmar interosseous and adductor compartments are reached through the radial incision by inserting tenotomy scissors perpendicularly along the ulnar border of the 2nd metacarpal, with the blades in the line of the metacarpal, and spreading them widely. You need to feel the dorsal fascia of the palmar interosseous compartment give way as you push the scissors into it.
- The 2nd and 3rd palmar interosseous compartments are reached similarly through the ulnar incision by inserting the scissors along the radial side of the 4th metacarpal (2nd palmar interosseous) and 5th metacarpal (3rd palmar interosseous).

Palmar incision

- The median and ulnar nerves, and the thenar and hypothenar muscles in the palm, are decompressed using one incision.
- Make a lazy-S incision from the distal wrist crease over the carpal tunnel in the midline between thenar and hypothenar eminences to

the proximal palmar crease. This may be continued into the palm in a zig-zag fashion as necessary.

- Deepen the incision through the flexor retinaculum to decompress the contents of the carpal tunnel, taking care to protect the median nerve branches, in particular the thenar motor branch of the median nerve passing radially into the thenar muscles in the distal part of the carpal tunnel.
- Incise the fascia over the thenar muscles to decompress the thenar compartment.
- Deepen the incision in an ulnar direction to decompress the ulnar nerve in Guyon's canal (superficial to the flexor retinaculum of the carpal tunnel, and more superficial than you think).
- Continue into the hypothenar muscles, preserving the deep motor branches of the ulnar nerve, and the ulnar artery as it divides into the superficial palmar arch and deep palmar branch.
- If the digits require decompressing, incise along the mid-axial line (see below) of the digits, on the non-dependent side (the ulnar side of the index, middle and ring fingers and the radial side of the thumb and little fingers).
- The mid-axial line is safe as it is dorsal to the NVBs of the fingers. It is drawn by flexing the fingers into the palm, drawing a dot at the apex of the skin creases of the MCP, PIP and DIP joints, and then joining the dots with the finger in extension. The dissection is continued dorsal to the NVB, volar to the flexor tendon sheath, and then dorsal to the NVB on the opposite side.

The forearm
Three compartments:
- Extensor mobile wad
- Common flexor mass
- Pronator quadratus.

Flexor incision
- Extend the midline incision in the palm ulnarwards along the distal wrist crease.
- Continue for 5cm along the ulnar border of the forearm (providing a flap to cover the ulnar and median nerves) and then radially and proximally towards the radial side of the antecubital fossa.
- Continue ulnarwards across the antecubital fossa in the line of the flexion crease allowing extension into the upper arm as necessary.
- Examine the long flexors of the wrist and digits systematically.
- Examine the pronator quadratus deep to the long flexors.
- Explore the median and ulnar nerves in the wrist and forearm.
- Avoid the palmar cutaneous branch of the median nerve (arises 5cm proximal to the wrist crease on the radial side and passes distally).
- Avoid the dorsal sensory branch of the ulnar nerve (arises 5cm proximal to the pisiform, passing dorsally and ulnarwards).
- Explore the median nerve in the antecubital fossa to release constriction from the lacertus fibrosus next to the biceps aponeurosis, and the proximal edges of the flexor digitorum superficialis and the pronator teres.

Extensor incision
- Make a single longitudinal midline incision on the extensor aspect of the forearm.
- Examine the extensor muscles systematically.

Upper arm

Two compartments:
- Flexor compartment
- Extensor compartment

Flexor and extensor compartments
- Continue the incision proximally over the postero-medial aspect of the biceps brachii to decompress the biceps compartment, brachial artery and branches of the brachial plexus.
- The posterior triceps compartment can be reached through this incision if necessary, avoiding damage to the radial nerve.

Wound closure
- Fasciotomy wounds cannot usually be closed directly. It may be possible to close them partially with sutures, or to close one side of the limb, preferably the flexor surface.
- Healing by secondary intention often produces overgranulating wounds and hypertrophic scars.
- Close open fasciotomy wounds with very thin split skin grafts (which will contract and facilitate later excision). Refer to plastic surgery or use a powered dermatome to minimize skin graft donor site morbidity.
- Splint the limb for 5 days after skin grafting to allow graft take.
- Leave the donor site dressing intact for 14 days.
- Avoid deep tension sutures or other methods of closure relying on tension, such as vascular slings looped between staples. These are slow to heal, and leave ugly, unstable scars.

Postoperative rehabilitation
- Mobilize the limb under supervision of physiotherapists for 6–12 weeks to prevent adhesions and stiffness once wound is closed/skin graft is stable.
- Night splints (full length volar splint in functional position) for 4–6 weeks to prevent development of flexion contractures.

Outpatient follow-up
- See in dressing clinic until wounds healed.
- Review at 6 weeks and 3 months.
- Consider excision of skin grafts or scar revision at 9–12 months.
- Consider tendon transfer or microvascular functional muscle transfer following significant loss of flexor or extensor compartment in upper limb (refer to plastic surgery).

Summary
- Acute compartment syndrome is common and dangerous.
- Adverse consequences can be prevented.
- Vigilance and suspicion are needed.
- Pressure measurement is the only useful investigation.
- Fasciotomy is the only useful treatment.

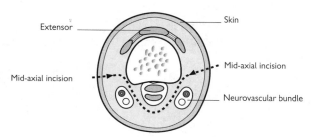

Fig. 18.3 Compartments of the hand and surgical approach.

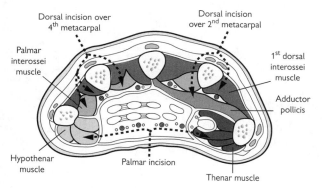

Fig. 18.4 Compartments of the hand.

Index